D0611331

Current Topics in Microbiology
262 and Immunology

Springer
Berlin
Heidelberg
New York
Barcelona
Hong Kong
London
Milan
Paris
Tokyo

Arenaviruses I

The Epidemiology, Molecular and Cell Biology of Arenaviruses

Edited by M.B.A. Oldstone

With 30 Figures and 23 Tables

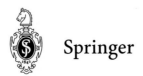

Springer

Professor Dr. MICHAEL B.A. OLDSTONE
Division of Virology
Department of Neuropharmacology
The Scripps Research Institute
10550 North Torrey Pines Road
La Jolla, CA 92037
USA
e-mail: mbaobo@scripps.edu

Cover Illustration: The upper panel depicts the morphology of the arenavirus, lymphocytic choriomeningitis virus (LCMV) by electron microscopy (first three panels from the left courtesy of P. Lampert and M.B.A. Oldstone), while the right panel is a photomicrograph of a cryomicrograph of LCMV (courtesy of M. Buchmeier).

The lower panels show the distribution of some of the Tacaribe-complex of arenaviruses in the New World and of the Old World Lassa fever virus.

ISSN 0070-217X
ISBN 3-540-42244-7 Springer-Verlag Berlin Heidelberg New York

This work is subject to copyright. All rights are reserved, whether the whole or part of the material is concerned, specifically the rights of translation, reprinting, reuse of illustrations, recitation, broadcasting, reproduction on microfilm or in any other way, and storage in data banks. Duplication of this publication or parts thereof is permitted only under the provisions of the German Copyright Law of September 9, 1965, in its current version, and permission for use must always be obtained from Springer-Verlag. Violations are liable for prosecution under the German Copyright Law.

Springer-Verlag Berlin Heidelberg New York
a member of BertelsmannSpringer Science + Business Media GmbH

http://www.springer.de

© Springer-Verlag Berlin Heidelberg 2002
Library of Congress Catalog Card Number 15-12910
Printed in Germany

The use of general descriptive names, registered names, trademarks, etc. in this publication does not imply, even in the absence of a specific statement, that such names are exempt from the relevant protective laws and regulations and therefore free for general use.

Product liability: The publishers cannot guarantee the accuracy of any information about dosage and application contained in this book. In every individual case the user must check such information by consulting other relevant literature.

Cover Design: *design & production GmbH*, Heidelberg
Typesetting: Scientific Publishing Services (P) Ltd, Madras
Production Editor: Angélique Gcouta
Printed on acid-free paper   SPIN: 10763105   27/3020 5 4 3 2 1 0

Preface

Viruses are studied either because they cause significant human, animal or plant disease or because they are useful materials for probing basic phenomena in biology, chemistry, genetics and/or molecular biology. Arenaviruses are unusually interesting in that they occupy both categories. Arenaviruses cause several human diseases known primarily as the hemorrhagic fevers occurring in South and Latin America (Bolivia: Machupo, Argentine, Junin virus, and Brazil: Sabia virus) and in Africa (Lassa fever virus). Because such viruses produce profound disabilities and often kill the persons they infect, they are a source of health concern and economic hardship in the countries where they are prevalent. Further, they provide new problems for healthcare persons owing to the narrowing of the world as visitors from many countries travel increasingly to and from endemic areas and may incubate the infectious agent taking it from an endemic area into an area where the virus is not expected. Such cases are now being recorded with increasing frequency. In addition to these hemorrhagic fever viruses, the arenavirus lymphocytic choriomeningitis virus (LCMV) can infect humans worldwide, although the illness is most often less disabling and severe than those elicited by the other arenaviruses. Yet, LCMV is of greater concern to non-arenavirologists and experimentalists using tissue culture or animals, etc., because normal-appearing cultured cells or tissues from animals used for research may be persistently infected with LCMV without manifesting clinical disease or cytopathology and may transmit that infection to laboratory workers. For example, in 1975 Heinemann et al., recorded 48 cases of LCMV infection among personnel in the Radiotherapy Department and vivarium at the University of Rochester School of Medicine. These persons had contact with Syrian hamsters into which tumors, unknown to be infected with LCMV, were injected. The tumor cells were obtained from an outside, well-known, research supplier who distributed tumor cell lines to numerous laboratories primarily interested in SV40 and polyoma virus research. A subsequent investigation of the 22 tumor lines revealed that 19 yielded infectious LCMV. Thus, both production of SV40 and/or polyoma virus from these cells or the use of hamsters infected with such tumors provided an unanticipated human biohazard. In the Rochester scenario infection was spread from those doing basic research, presumably via air ducts to multiple individuals at the medical school/hospital including healthcare workers and patients undergoing radiologic procedures. Similarly, the Centers for Disease Control (CDC), USA, has recorded multiple cases of LCMV infection in families scattered from the northeast coast of the United States (New York) to the western region (Reno, Nevada) originating from hamsters sold by a single pet store supplier in the southeast (Florida). In addition, several investigators found that their hybridomas making monoclonal antibodies were infected with LCMV. The likely source was infected spleen feeder layers from clinically healthy but persistently infected mice purchased from a well-known commercial source which supplies mice to many universities and institutes in North America. Thus, researchers studying such diverse areas as the molecular biology of SV40, biological effects of *Chlamydia*, immune response of mice, and producing hybridoma cells or ascites fluids have found their preparations contaminated with LCMV. In these cases, the potentially dangerous effects of LCMV were not anticipated because the virus does not cause footprints associated with most acute viruses (i.e., necrosis, inflammatory response). The recognized arenaviruses of man, vectors and laboratory models used for their study are listed in Table 1.

LCMV has proven to be a Rosetta stone for uncovering numerous phenomena in virology and immunology. For example, research on both the acute and persistent infections of mice with LCMV led to the first description of virus-induced immunopathologic disease, of the role of the thymus in the immune response, of T cell-mediated killing and of the MHC restriction phenomenon associated with cytotoxic CD8 cells. In addition, recent studies with LCMV have detailed the kinetics of memory cells generated following an immune response for both CD8 and CD4 T cells and have defined the kinetics of B cell differentiation into plasma cells and the in situ location of such cells challenging previously held concepts. Lastly, LCMV has been instrumental in defining the concept of virus alterations of luxury or differentiated cells effecting differentiated products leading to disturbances in homeostasis and disease in the absence of observed cytolytic destruction of the involved tissues. These events are tabulated in Table 2.

Since the topic of arenaviruses was visited by *Current Topics in Microbiology and Immunology* 14 years ago, enormous ad-

vances have been made in this area. The receptor for several of
the arenaviruses, alpha-dystroglycan has been uncovered, the cell
biology and replication strategy has been decoded and a reverse
genetics system for studying viral gene function and its application to study viral biology is well underway. These findings, in
addition to the molecular phylogeny, discussion of rodent reservoirs and description of clinical diseases found in both new world
and old world arenaviruses, are the topics included in the first
volume. The second volume in this series deals with the biology
and the pathogenesis of arenaviruses primarily through the study
of LCMV. Interestingly and appropriately, the fundamental observation of MHC restriction and CD8 cytotoxic T lymphocyte
killing derived initially from studies with LCMV in the mouse
has been expanded to studies of most human pathogens, viral,
bacterial, parasitic, as well as events in cancer. The scope and
importance of this observation was recognized by awarding
the Nobel Prize in 1996 to Rolf Zinkernagel and Peter Doherty,
long-time workers in the field of LCMV and arenavirus biology.

Over the last 14 years many of the principles for understanding viral pathogenesis and the biology of animal viruses
have been defined, in great part, from the lessons learned by
studying LCMV. Those lessons and their implications are the
subject of this second volume on the arenaviruses. In terms of
virus-induced immune complex disease, the genetic and host
control over such complexes has now been defined and extended
to the injuries caused by immune complexes and the role of such
complexes in persistent RNA and DNA viral infections of
humans. In terms of T cell responses, a most remarkable finding
is that over 60%, and frequently 80%, of a primary T cell
response after viral infection reflect antigen-specific T cell
expansion. A closely related discovery is the mechanisms by
which apoptosis and other means cause such cells to contract
numerically three to four days after the peak T cell response. In
addition, the pool of virus-specific CD8 and CD4 memory T cells
has been quantitated and their kinetics established. The constant
level of antigen-specific CD8 T memory cells over an individual's
lifetime contrasts with the gradual decline of CD4 T memory
cells. This continuous decline of antigen-specific CD4 T memory
cells may have broad implications with respect to the high incidence of cancers and enhanced susceptibility to infectious diseases in the aging human population as well as the potential need
for revaccination of individuals every 10–15 years following
primary immunization.

Recent understanding of persistent viral infection, as opposed to the acute infection that is cleared by antigen-specific

Table 1. Recognized arenavirus diseases of humans

Group	Virus	Locality	Disease	Clinical picture	Hemorrhagic fever syndrome in humans
Old World arenaviruses	Lymphocytic choriomeningitis virus (LCMV)	Probably originated in Europe, now worldwide	Lymphocytic choriomeningitis	Grippe and aseptic meningitis most common; more severe central nervous system disease of meningoencephalomyelitis occasionally occurs. May cause transient hydrocephalus during acute infection or congenital hydrocephalus and chorioretinitis after fetal infection	No
	Lassa fever virus (LFV)	West Africa	Lassa fever	Severe systemic illness with changes in vascular permeability and vasoregulation. Worst cases often associated with bleeding	Yes
New World arenaviruses	Junin virus	Argentine pampas	Argentine hemorrhagic fever (AHF)	Classical viral hemorrhagic fever Similar to Lassa, except thrombocytopenia, florid bleeding, and neurological manifestations much more common	Yes
	Machupo virus	Beni region of Bolivia	Bolivian hemorrhagic fever (BHF)	As in AHF	Yes
	Guanarito virus	Venezuela	Venezuelan hemorrhagic fever	Probably similar to AHF	Yes
	Sabia	Brazil	Not yet named	Likely similar to AHF; extensive hepatic necrosis seen; only 3 cases	Yes

Group	Person to person transmission	Expected mortality	Binding affinity to alpha-dystroglycan receptor	Laboratory model of human infection	Year isolated	Reference(s)
Old World arenaviruses	Never documented	<1%	High	Mouse	1933	ARMSTRONG and LILLIE 1934
	Frequently by blood contamination	15%	High	Monkey, guinea pig strain(s). LCMV WE in guinea pig	1969	FRAME et al. 1970
New World arenaviruses	Occasionally	15–30%	Low	Guinea pig	1958	MOLTENI et al. 1961; PARODI et al. 1958
	Occasionally	25%	Low	Monkey	1963	JOHNSON et al. 1965
	Occasionally	25%	Low		1990	SALAS et al. 1991
	Not known	33%	Low	Not known	1990	CLEGG 1993

Table 2. Contributions to biology and medicine from the study of the LCMV model

Observation	Reference
Immune mediated injury in viral disease: role of the thymus	ROWE (1954)
Definition of T cells in immune response disease	COLE et al. (1972)
T cell killing + MHC restriction	ZINKERNAGEL and DOHERTY (1974, 1996)
Quantitation and kinetics of B and T cell memory regulation of T cell pool (apoptosis, clonal exhaustion)	MOSKOPHIDIS et al. (1993) RAZVI et al. (1995) BUTZ and BEVAN (1998) MURALI-KRISHNA et al. (1998) SLIFKA et al. (1998)
Model of persistent viral infection/ tolerance/negative and positive T cell and positive T cell selection (thymic education)	TRAUB (1936) BURNET and FENNER (1949) HOTCHIN and CINTIS (1958) OLDSTONE and DIXON (1967) VOLKERT AND LARSEN (1965) ZINKERNAGEL et al. (1978)
Etiology and pathogenesis of immune complex disease	OLDSTONE (1975) OLDSTONE and DIXON (1967)
Cytopathology and disturbance of complex homeostasis in the absence of cytocidal injury	OLDSTONE et al. (1977, 1982)
Immunocytotherapy to cure persistent viral infection	OLDSTONE et al. (1986) AHMED et al. (1987) BERGER et al. (2000)

immune responses, has now established the requirements for immunocytotherapy that can clear these persistent pathogens. Thus, the numbers of antigen-specific CD8 cells required to clear virus infection and the numbers of antigen-specific CD4 cells required to maintain those CD8 cells is now known to be 50 CD8 to 1 CD4 T cell. The clinical implication of these findings for adoptive immunotherapy for human diseases like those caused by cytomegalovirus, human immunodeficiency virus and Epstein-Barr virus are clear. Further, these results indicate the number of CD8 and CD4 T cells required following vaccination to prevent or control an acute infection, to cure persistent or latent infections and to shrink tumors.

The concept that virus infects differentiated cells in vitro and in vivo was developed during the study of persistent LCMV infection in the mouse. Such long-term infection disturbs cellular functions thereby altering the cells' homeostasis and causing disease without killing the cell. These well-established observations have now been extended to the understanding of neurologic and hormonal diseases. Related studies in vitro have determined both the host genes and the viral genes involved. Finally, several groups have applied the knowledge of T cell biology and LCMV to construct transgenic mice as experimental models. By cell-specific promoters, i.e., the rat insulin promoter, myelin basic protein promoter, neuron enolase-specific promoter, viral genes or host genes are expressed in specialized cells. For example, viral genes, MHC molecules and cytokines have been expressed in neurons, thymi, beta cells of the islets and oligodendrocytes. The use of such models is presented in this volume. These model systems have provided new information on how autoimmune diabetes and autoimmune CNS diseases occur, have defined the coactivating accessory molecules of the immune system that are required to potentiate or initiate disease and have addressed basic questions about thymic selection and T cell biology.

Other issues in this volume concern selection of viral variants. Those chapters were written by the authorities who initiated or developed the model systems involved.

MICHAEL B.A. OLDSTONE

References

Ahmed R, Jamieson BD, Porter DD (1987) Immune therapy of a persistent and disseminated viral infection. J Virol 61:3920–3929

Armstrong C, Lillie RD (1934) Experimental lymphocytic choriomeningitis of monkeys and mice produced by a virus encountered in studies of the 1933 St. Louis encephalitis epidemic. Public Health Report 49:1019–1027

Berger DP, Homann D, Oldstone MBA (2000) Defining parameters for successful immunocytotherapy of persistent viral infection. Virology 266:257–263

Burnet FM, Fenner F (1949) The production of antibodies. New York, MacMillan

Butz EA, Bevan MJ (1998) Massive expansion of antigen-specific CD8+ T cells during an acute virus infection. Immunity 8:167–175

Clegg JCS (1993) Molecular phylogeny of the arenaviruses and guide to published sequence data. New York, Plenum

Cole G, Nathanson N, Prendergast R (1972) Requirement for theta-bearing cells in lymphocytic choriomeningitis virus-induced central nervous system disease. Nature 238:335–337

Frame JD, Baldwin JM, Gocke DJ, Troup JM (1970) Lassa fever, a new virus disease of man from West Africa. I. Clinical description and pathological findings. Am J Trop Med Hyg 19:670–676

Hinman AR, Fraser DW, Douglas RG Jr, Bowen GS, Kraus AL, Winkler WG, Rhodes WW (1975) Outbreak of lymphatic choriomeningitis virus infections in medical center personnel. Am J Epidemiol 101:103–110

Hotchkin JE, Clintis M (1958) Lymphatic choriomeningitis infection of mice as a model for the study of latent virus infection. Canad J Microbiol 4:149–153

Johnson KM, Wiebenga NH, Mackenzie RB, Kuns ML, Tauraso NM, Shelokov A, Webb PA, Justines GJ, Beye HK (1965) Virus isolations from human cases of hemorrhagic fever in Bolivia. Proc Soc Exp Biol Med 118:113–118

Molteni HD, Guarinos HC, Petrillo CO, Jaschek FRJ (1961) Estudio clinico estadistico sobre 338 pacientes afectados por la fiebre hemorragica epidemica del Noroeste de la Provincia de Buenos Aires. Semana Med 118:838–855

Moskophidis D, Lechner F, Pircher H, Zinkernagel RM (1993) Virus persistence in acutely infected immunocompetent mice by exhaustion of antiviral cytotoxic effector T cells. Nature 362:758–761

Murali-Krishna K, Altman JD, Suresh M, Sourdive DJ, Zajac AJ, Miller JD, Slansky J, Ahmed R (1998) Counting antigen-specific CD8 T cells: a reevaluation of bystander activation during viral infection. Immunity 8:177–187

Oldstone MBA (1975) Virus neutralization and virus-induced immune complex disease: virus-antibody union resulting in immunoprotection or immunologic injury – two sides of the same coin. S. Karger, Basel

Oldstone MBA, Blount P, Southern P (1986) Cytoimmunotherapy for persistent virus infection reveals a unique clearance pattern from the central nervous system. Nature 321:239–243

Oldstone MBA, Dixon FJ (1967) Lymphocytic choriomeningitis: production of anti-LCM antibody by "tolerant" LCM-infected mice. Science 158:1193–1194

Oldstone MBA, Holmstoen J, Welsh R (1977) Alterations of acetylcholine enzymes in neuroblastoma cells persistently infected with lymphocytic choriomeningitis virus. J Cell Physiol 91:459–472

Oldstone MBA, Sinha YN, Blount P, Tishon A, Rodriguez M, von Wedel R, Lampert PW (1982) Virus-induced alterations in homeostasis: alterations in differentiated functions of infected cells in vivo. Science 218:1125–1127

Parodi AS, Greenway DJ, Ruggiero HR, Rivero E, Frigerio MJ, de la Barrera JM, Mettler NE, Garzon F, Boxaca MC, Guerrero LB, Nota NR (1958) Sobre la etiologia del brote epidemico de Junin (nota previa) Dia Med 30:62

Rowe WP (1954) Studies on pathogenesis and immunity in lymphocytic choriomeningitis infection of the mouse. Naval Med Res Inst Resp Rep 12:167–220

Salas R, de Manzione N, Tesh RB, Rico-Hesse R, Shope RE, Betaucourt A, Godoy O, Bruzual R, Pacheco DE, Ramos B, Taibo ME, Tamayo JG, James E, Vasquez C, Araoz F, Querales J (1991) Venezuelan hemorrhagic fever. Lancet 33:1033–1036

Slifka MK, Antia R, Whitmire JK, Ahmed R (1998) Humoral immunity due to long-lived plasma cells. Immunity 8:363–372

Traub E (1936) The epidemiology of lymphocytic choriomeningitis virus in white mice. J Exp Med 64:183–200

Razvi ES, Jiang Z, Woda BA, Welsh RM (1995) Lymphocyte apoptosis during the silencing of the immune response to acute viral infections in normal, lpr, and Bcl-2-transgenic mice. Am J Pathol 147:79–91

Volkert M, Larsen JH (1965) Immunologic tolerance to viruses. Prog. Med. Virol. 7:160

Zinkernagel ES, Callahan GN, Althage A, Cooper S, Klein PA, Klein J (1978) On the thymus in the differentiation of "H-2 self-recognition" by T cells: evidence for dual recognition? J Exp Med 147:882–896

Zinkernagel RM, Doherty P (1974) Restriction of in vitro T cell-mediated cytotoxicity in lymphocytic choriomeningitis within a syngeneic or semiallogeneic system. Nature 248:701–702

Zinkernagel RM, Doherty P (1979) MHC-restricted cytotoxic T cells: studies on the biological role of polymorphic major transplantation antigens determining T-cell restriction-specificity, function and responsiveness. Adv Immunol 27:51–177

Zinkernagel RM, Doherty P (1996) Nobel Prize Lecture

List of Contents

List of Contents
of Companion Volume II

List of Contributors

(Their addresses can be found at the beginning of their respective chapters.)

BORROW, P. 111

BUCHMEIER, M.J. 159

CLEGG, J.C.S. 1

FISHER-HOCH, S.P. 75

KUNZ, S. 111

LEE, K.J. 175

McCORMICK, J.B. 75

MEYER, B.J. 139

OLDSTONE, M.B.A. 111

PETERS, C.J. 65

RUEDAS, L.A. 25

SALAZAR-BRAVO, J. 25

SOUTHERN, P.J. 139

DE LA TORRE, J.C.
  139, 175

YATES, T.L. 25

Molecular Phylogeny of the Arenaviruses

J.C.S. CLEGG

1 Introduction

Molecular approaches to the identification of viruses and the delineation of relationships among them has emerged as an important tool in virology only within the
past 10–15 years. The rapidity and precision with which virus genetic sequences can
now be acquired and the development of sophisticated methods for the phylogenetic analysis of this new universe of data are leading to informative new insights
into the biology, origin and spread of many infectious diseases (see HOLMES 1998
and HUNGNES et al. 2000 for general overviews). To take a single example, current
theories about the origins and timescale of the AIDS pandemic as the result of

Centre for Applied Microbiology and Research, Porton Down, Salisbury, Wiltshire SP4 0JG, UK transmission events from other primary species to humans are based to a large extent on the evidence of sequence-based phylogenetic analyses (ZHU et al. 1998; GAO et al. 1999; KORBER et al. 2000). The absence of material in the fossil record which might illuminate the past history of viruses and viral infections is now to some extent being overcome by this new-found ability to extract quasi-archaeological data from the sequences of present-day viruses.

Molecular phylogenetic analysis can provide information on the relationships between viruses at a number of different levels. In the first place, the relationships between species in a single family can be described. Other sorts of relevant data are generally available, such as serological cross-reactivity, genome size and organization, or protein composition. However, sequence-based phylogenetic comparisons of viruses can provide a much more precise, detailed and quantitative description of their relationships and illuminate the evolutionary pathways which have led to the current situation. At a more practical level, such approaches provide tools for detailed epidemiological investigations, in which the patterns and dynamics of spread of individual virus clades can be followed, and their sequence variation tracked over the course of an epidemic. The precise definition of virus lineages through sequence data also allows investigation of possible correlations with variations in virulence, tissue or cell tropism, host range or other important biological properties. Lastly, on a larger scale, phylogenetic analysis also has the potential to indicate linkage patterns among different families of viruses. In this chapter I will review the application of these avenues of investigation to the arenaviruses.

2 Taxonomy of the *Arenaviridae*

The family *Arenaviridae* contains 19 currently recognized viruses (CLEGG et al. 2000) which are listed in Table 1, together with information on their geographic origin and host species. Recent additions to the family are Sabiá (LISIEUX et al. 1994; GONZALEZ et al. 1996), Oliveros (BOWEN et al. 1996a; MILLS et al. 1996), Whitewater Arroyo (FULHORST et al. 1996) and Pirital (FULHORST et al. 1997) viruses. Almost all the viruses are parasites of rodents, with the apparent exception of Tacaribe virus, which has been only isolated from the fruit-eating bat *Artibeus* sp. A possible further species is Pampa virus, an arenavirus isolated, like Oliveros virus, from *Bolomys obscurus* in Argentina (LOZANO et al. 1997). Full recognition as a separate species would depend on identification of features which sufficiently differentiated the virus from Oliveros virus, its closest known relative.

2.1 Species Demarcation Criteria

Species demarcation criteria have been formulated for the family as part of the development of virus taxonomic practice agreed by the International Committee on

Table 1. Virus species of the Family *Arenaviridae*

Species	Major natural host	Region
Old World arenaviruses		
Ippy virus	*Arvicanthis* sp.	Central African Republic
Lassa virus	*Mastomys* sp.	West Africa
Lymphocytic choriomeningitis virus	*Mus musculus*	Europe, Americas
Mobala virus	*Praomys* sp.	Central African Republic
Mopeia virus	*Mastomys natalensis*	Mozambique, Zimbabwe
New World arenaviruses		
Amapari virus	*Oryzomys capito, Neacomys guianae*	Brazil
Flexal virus	*Oryzomys* spp.	Brazil
Guanarito virus	*Zygodontomys brevicauda*	Venezuela
Junín virus	*Calomys musculinus*	Argentina
Latino virus	*Calomys callosus*	Bolivia
Machupo virus	*Calomys callosus*	Bolivia
Paraná virus	*Oryzomys buccinatus*	Paraguay
Pichinde virus	*Oryzomys albigularis*	Colombia
Pirital virus	*Sigmodon alstoni*	Venezuela
Oliveros virus	*Bolomys obscurus*	Argentina
Sabiá virus	Unknown	Brazil
Tacaribe virus	*Artibeus* spp.	Trinidad
Tamiami virus	*Sigmodon hispidus*	Florida, USA
Whitewater Arroyo virus	*Neotoma albigula*	New Mexico, USA

Taxonomy of Viruses (CLEGG et al. 2000). The criteria proposed for the definition of a species in the family *Arenaviridae* (currently comprising the single genus *Arenavirus*) are:

a. An association with a specific host species or group of species
b. Presence in a defined geographical area
c. Etiological agent (or not) of disease in humans
d. Significant differences in antigenic cross-reactivity, including lack of cross-neutralization activity where applicable
e. Significant amino acid sequence difference from other species in the genus

Applying the concept of a virus species as "a polythetic class of viruses that constitutes a replicating lineage and occupies a particular ecological niche" (VAN REGENMORTEL 1992), viruses differing in any two or more of the above properties would be accepted as belonging to two different species.

  Some examples may help to clarify the application of these criteria and demonstrate their utility in providing transparent rules for classifying new arenavirus isolates. Although both Pirital and Guanarito viruses circulate in the plains of central Venezuela, they are distinguished by their different principal rodent hosts, respectively *Sigmodon alstoni* and *Zygodontomys brevicauda* (FULHORST et al. 1997, 1999b). In addition, in ELISA with hyperimmune mouse ascitic fluids, titers differ by at least 64-fold, and sequence analysis shows less than 55% amino acid identity in partial nucleocapsid protein sequences (FULHORST et al. 1997). In another example, both Lassa virus and Mopeia virus share a common rodent host at the genus level, *Mastomys*. However, they are distinguished by their different geographical range (sub-Saharan west Africa and southeast Africa, respectively), different profiles of reactivity with panels of monoclonal antibodies (Ruo et al. 1991; Howard 1993), and by N protein amino acid sequence divergence of about 26% (Wilson and Clegg 1991). Also, Lassa virus is the cause of hemorrhagic fever in humans and other primates, while Mopeia virus is not associated with human disease and does not cause such disease in experimentally infected primates.

2.2 Classical Approaches to Relationships Among the Arenaviruses

The identity of the family *Arenaviridae* as a distinct grouping was built largely on electron microscopic observations and on extensive investigations of serological cross-reactions between these viruses (reviewed in Howard 1993). Virus neutralization, dependent on epitopes located on the surface glycoproteins, is difficult to demonstrate with many arenaviruses. However, the techniques of complement fixation and immunofluorescence using polyclonal sera demonstrated a variety of nucleocapsid protein-based cross-reactions of differing degrees, and suggested the viruses could be divided into Old World and New World groups. Studies using monoclonal antibodies supported this view, and also identified specific epitopes shared between the Old and New World groups (Weber and Buchmeier 1988). Structural studies of the RNA and protein components of many arenaviruses have confirmed their general similarity and strongly support their grouping into a single virus family.

2.3 Sequence-Based Phylogenetic Approaches

Classification or differentiation of viruses using serological methods relies only on differences between antigenic sites on their constituent proteins. Determination and comparison of nucleotide or amino acid sequences captures information from all parts of the gene or protein, rather than just those regions which are antigenically active. Further, sequence-based methods are more amenable to making quantitative estimates of virus relationships. Quantitative estimates of the robustness of these results can also be made. Nonetheless, there is reason to be cautious in uncritically inferring phylogenetic relationships between viruses from results based on sequences of single genes or gene products, or parts of them.

2.3.1 Genetic Recombination

The evolutionary history of a single gene may not always mirror that of the complete virus. For some viruses there is evidence that their genomes may have evolved through the acquisition of genes or groups of genes from other viruses, or from their hosts. Such recombinational events may have contributed to the evolutionary history of many families of viruses (reviewed in Lai 1995; Strauss and STRAUSS 1997; WOROBEY and HOLMES 1999). Nearly half of the full-length genomic DNA sequences of the recently discovered and widely divergent TT viruses showed evidence of homologous recombination among and between genotypes (WOROBEY 2000). Among the RNA viruses (excluding retroviruses), specific examples include the positive-stranded western equine encephalitis virus (WEAVER et al. 1997), dengue viruses (WOROBEY et al. 1999), Coxsackie A9 virus (SANTTI et al. 2000); the double-stranded RNA-containing rotaviruses (SUZUKI et al. 1998); and the negative-stranded hantaviruses (SIBOLD et al. 1999). It is apparent that recombination has the potential to profoundly affect evolutionary processes in a wide variety of types of RNA viruses. Indeed, it has recently been shown that the nucleocapsid and glycoprotein genes of the arenavirus Whitewater Arroyo have divergent phylogenetic histories (CHARREL et al. 2001). Separate analysis of full-length amino acid sequences using maximum parsimony or neighbor-joining methods show that its nucleocapsid protein has the greatest affinity with those of Pichinde virus and Pirital virus, while its glycoproteins are more closely related to those of Junín, Tacaribe, and Sabiá viruses. This is good evidence that the Whitewater Arroyo virus genomic S segment is the product of genetic recombination between two ancestral arenaviruses. It remains to be determined how important such events have been in shaping the evolutionary history of the arenavirus family as a whole.

2.3.2 Genome Segment Reassortment

In the case of viruses with multipartite genomes, the reassortment of genome segments during co-infection of a single cell can also occur, forming the basis of the well-known "antigenic shift" phenomenon in the influenza A viruses. Reassortment of RNA segments is also well-known among members of the *Bunyaviridae* and has been demonstrated to occur naturally among isolates of Sin Nombre virus (HENDERSON et al. 1995). Intraspecies reassortants resulting from laboratory manipulations have long been known in the case of LCMV (KIRK et al. 1980; RIVIÈRE et al. 1985). Also, LUKASHEVICH (1992) described the generation of an interspecific reassortant virus containing the L RNA segment of Mopeia virus and the S RNA segment of Lassa virus in cells co-infected in vitro with the two parental viruses. Potentially, therefore, there is a role for genetic reassortment in the evolution of the arenaviruses. An instance of wild rodent dual infection by two distinguishable genotypes of Guanarito virus has been noted (WEAVER et al. 2000), providing the opportunity for genomic segment reassortment, but it has neither been sought nor discovered so far.

2.4 Sequence-Based Phylogenetic Analysis of the Arenaviruses

In early studies, direct sequencing of the 3′-termini of arenavirus genomic RNA segments demonstrated a characteristic terminal sequence shared among all arenaviruses analyzed (AUPERIN et al. 1982), providing additional evidence for the existence of the *Arenaviridae* as a family. Building on this, the increasing accessibility and efficiency of techniques for the cloning and sequencing of RNA virus genes made detailed sequence-based phylogenetic analysis of the arenaviruses feasible during the 1980s. These technologies were applied both to the nonpathogenic members of the family and to the agents of viral hemorrhagic fevers, Lassa, Junín and Machupo viruses, facilitating understanding of the relationships of these viruses by reducing the necessity for work at the highest levels of laboratory containment. Much of this earlier work has been brought together and summarized previously (CLEGG 1993). The most comprehensive picture of relationships in the family at that time was provided by alignment and phylogenetic analysis of the complete sequences for the N proteins of nine arenaviruses, of seven different species. This clearly confirmed the separation of these amino acid sequences into Old World and New World groups, indicated the close genetic relationship between Junín virus and Machupo virus (GRIFFITHS et al. 1992), and provided an easy-to-grasp, graphic picture of virus relationships which was highly consistent with available serological and cross-protection data. Trees based on amino acid sequences of the G1 and G2 virus glycoproteins were topologically identical (CLEGG 1993), indicating that intergenic recombination had not been a significant feature in the evolution of the viruses analyzed.

    The ease with which RNA sequences of genomic fragments can be generated by reverse transcription, followed by amplification of cDNA by use of the polymerase chain reaction (RT-PCR), has led to a further increase in the scope and complexity of phylogenetic studies. Analysis of subgenomic sequence fragments reduces the computational challenge in constructing sequence alignments and in tree-building and testing, without necessarily impairing the quality of the results obtained.

2.5 Relationships Among the Arenaviruses: Current Position

The most comprehensive such analyses of the *Arenaviridae* are those of BOWEN et al. (1996b, 1997). In the first of these studies, 613–646nt fragments from the S RNA segment of the 12 then recognized New World arenavirus species were generated by RT-PCR, using primers matching well-conserved regions of the N protein gene. After alignment of these sequences, together with corresponding Old World arenavirus sequences as outgroups, phylogenetic analysis was carried out by the Fitch-Margoliash method, and the robustness of the resulting trees assessed by bootstrap analysis. The results confirmed the distant relationship of two groups of arenaviruses, the Old and New World groups, and indicated a well-supported division of the New World viruses into three lineages. Lineage A contained Tamiami, Pichinde, Paraná and Flexal viruses, and lineage B consisted of Sabiá and Tacaribe viruses, together with the sister species Machupo and Junín viruses, and Amapari and Guanarito viruses. Lineage C consisted of Oliveros and Latino viruses. Phylogenies derived by maximum likelihood or maximum parsimony methods were different only in minor details, except for lack of agreement on the position of lineage C. The former method agreed with Fitch-Margoliash in supporting monophyly of groups B and C, while maximum parsimony favored monophyly of groups A and C.

BOWEN et al. (1997) extended this approach to include at least one strain of every currently recognized arenavirus and applied a broad range of phylogenetic methods to the data set. Maximum parsimony generated the tree shown in Fig. 1. In the Old World group, Mopeia and Mobala viruses were relatively closely related to Lassa virus, while Ippy virus and Lymphocytic choriomeningitis virus (LCMV) were more remote, with LCMV occupying the most ancestral position. These relationships are consistent with previously described serological data (WULFF et al. 1978; RUO et al. 1991; HOWARD 1993) and with the property of cross-protection against Lassa virus challenge by Mopeia virus in experimental primate infections (KILEY et al. 1979; WALKER et al. 1982). The division of the New World viruses into three lineages, with the newly described Whitewater Arroyo virus (FULHORST et al. 1996) from North America included in lineage A, was again well-supported, although the exact placement of lineage C remained unclear. Unweighted maximum parsimony analysis favored monophyly of lineages A and C, but the support was largely from characters in the third codon position, which contains most of the highly variable sites. Successive approximations analysis also strongly supported

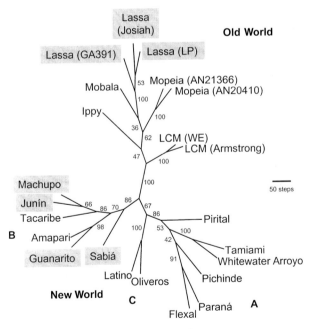

Fig. 1. Phylogenetic relationships among the *Arenaviridae*. Partial N gene nucleotide sequences corresponding to nt 1770–2418 of Tacaribe virus S RNA sequence (GenBank accession no. M20304) were aligned (PILEUP, adjusted manually) and analyzed by maximum parsimony using PAUP. Bootstrap support values for each branch are indicated. Viruses causing hemorrhagic fever in humans are shown in *gray boxes*. (Courtesy of Michael Bowen, C.J. Peters, Stuart Nichol, CDC)

monophyly of lineages A and C, while maximum likelihood analysis did not provide significant support for one topology over the other. The distance-based neighbor-joining method favored monophyly of lineages B and C, whether third base codon positions were included or not. Maximum parsimony methods were also applied to data sets consisting of 11 full-length N genes or 10 full-length GPC genes of representative viruses. The N gene tree supported monophyly of lineages A and C, unless transversion weighting was applied, when lineage B and C monophyly was supported. The GPC gene tree supported the latter topology irrespective of transversion weighting. Resolution of these ambiguities may require the determination of complete gene sequences from all the known arenaviruses.

A view of arenavirus interrelationships somewhat at variance with that described above has been put forward by ALBARIÑO et al. (1998), who suggested that Pichinde virus and Oliveros virus may be more closely related to the Old World group than they are to the other western hemisphere arenaviruses. They discussed a number of hypothetical evolutionary scenarios which might explain this. The closer affinity of these two South American viruses to the Old World group was manifested in maximum parsimony-based analyses of alignments of glycoprotein amino acid sequences. In similar analyses of alignments of the nucleocapsid sequences, the two viruses were placed with the other New World viruses. Similar findings were made using distance-based phylogenetic methods. In the alignments analyzed, sequences of corresponding proteins of Impatiens necrotic spot virus (*Bunyaviridae*; *Tospovirus*) were used as outgroups. In reaching their conclusions, these authors did not take into account the greater interspecies genetic distances among the New World viruses when compared with those among the Old World viruses, nor the effect of the very distantly related outgroup they selected. Both of these factors may have had the effect of distorting the inferred position for the root of the tree (BOWEN et al. 2000). Thus, the evidence for what might be considered an anomalous placement of Pichinde virus and Oliveros virus is not particularly compelling. Moreover, hypotheses about how the different arenaviruses came to occupy their present geographical locations must necessarily take into account the relationships of the viruses with their rodent hosts, a topic which will be discussed below. It is important also to bear in mind the possible impact of genetic recombination, as demonstrated in Whitewater Arroyo virus (CHARREL et al. 2001; see Sect. 2.3.1), on the interpretation of phylogenies based on individual genes or sequence fragments.

There remains an unfortunate lack of sequence information from the L segment of the majority of the arenaviruses, which has prevented the construction of comprehensive phylogenies based on what represents two-thirds of the virus genome, or at least elements from it. However, LUKASHEVICH et al. (1997) calculated maximum parsimony trees, based on the RNA polymerase core amino acid sequences of segmented negative-strand viruses, including sequences from Lassa virus, LCMV, Tacaribe virus, and Pichinde virus. The arenavirus relationships obtained were consistent with those derived from the much more extensive data from the S RNA segment (described above), in that they were clearly separated into Old World and New World groups. It will be necessary to collect further data from other members of the family before the congruence of phylogenies based on S or L RNA segments can be properly assessed.

2.6 Relationship of the *Arenaviridae* to Other Virus Families

RNA viruses have been placed into four main types: those with single-stranded genomes, of either positive or negative polarity, double-stranded RNA viruses, and the retroviruses. The arenaviruses are conventionally placed among the negative-stranded viruses in this scheme, ignoring their exclusive use of ambisense coding strategies on both the S and L genomic RNA segments. Taxonomically, two orders of animal viruses have now been recognized. These are the *Mononegavirales*, comprising the families *Bornaviridae*, *Filoviridae*, *Paramyxoviridae* and *Rhabdoviridae* (PRINGLE 1997), and the *Nidovirales*, which includes the families *Coronaviridae* and *Arteriviridae* (CAVANAGH 1997). Evidence for the assembly of these higher taxa are the similarities in genome structure and organization, gene functions, and in the case of the *Nidovirales*, similarities in morphology. Neither of these orders includes the *Arenaviridae*.

Given the successful use of sequence data in elucidating relationships among viruses at the family level and below, there has been much interest in whether such data might shed further light on higher levels of taxonomic organization. Although there is phylogenetic evidence supporting the relationship of the families comprising the *Mononegavirales* (PRINGLE and EASTON 1997), the sheer diversity of most virus sequences has largely prevented progress. Most effort has gone into schemes based on sequences of the RNA-dependent RNA polymerases necessarily encoded by all RNA viruses. Motifs from these sequences are widely conserved among a wide range of these viruses (POCH et al. 1989). Focusing first on investigations which throw particular light on possible affinities of the arenaviruses with other families, an analysis of 22 negative-stranded RNA viruses by MÜLLER et al. (1994) identified two regions located near the N-terminus of the RNA polymerase which are conserved between two arenaviruses (LCM and Tacaribe viruses) and viruses in four genera of the family *Bunyaviridae*. These were Bunyamwera (genus *Bunyavirus*); Hantaan and Puumala (*Hantavirus*); Rift Valley fever and Uukuniemi (*Phlebovirus*); and tomato spotted wilt (*Tospovirus*) viruses. These two regions apparently conserved between the *Arenaviridae* and the *Bunyaviridae* were supplementary to the more generally conserved motifs described by POCH et al. (1989). These two N-terminal motifs were also present in the L protein of Lassa virus (LUKASHEVICH et al. 1997), but not in the translation product of the L genomic segment of Dugbe virus (*Nairovirus*; *Bunyaviridae*) (MARRIOTT and NUTTALL 1996). As described above, LUKASHEVICH et al. (1997) obtained maximum parsimony trees, based on the polymerase core amino acid sequences of segmented negative-strand viruses, with three major branches. These branches comprised (a) the arenaviruses, the phleboviruses, a nairovirus, and the orthomyxoviruses; (b) bunyaviruses and tospoviruses; and (c) hantaviruses. Similar results for virus sequences from the *Arenaviridae* and the *Bunyaviridae* were obtained when the core polymerase sequences were augmented with the N-terminal conserved sequences described by MÜLLER et al. (1994).

More generally, the existence of three supergroups of positive-stranded viruses have been proposed, from which double-stranded RNA viruses may have arisen on separate occasions (KOONIN 1991; KOONIN and DOLJA 1993; WARD 1993). However, other, phylogenetically incompatible schemes have been proposed (GOLDBACH and DE HAAN 1994; BRUENN 1991), reducing confidence in the validity of RNA polymerase-based approaches. The statistical evaluation by ZANOTTO et al. (1996) further indicated that the lack of sequence similarities among the RNA polymerases of taxonomically distant viruses and the consequent loss of phylogenetic signal produced minimally informative trees which lacked explanatory power when applied to most higher viral taxa, including the *Arenaviridae*.

Protein structural homologies, derived from X-ray crystallographic studies, together with virus architectural considerations have been adduced as evidence of a common evolutionary origin of viruses as disparate as the enteric bacteriophage PRD1 and the adenoviruses. These striking structural parallels are apparent despite the absence of any detectable sequence similarities (BENSON et al. 1999; HENDRIX 1999). It remains to be seen whether such structural, as opposed to sequence-based, approaches will provide a secure basis for a general understanding of relationships among virus families, including the arenaviruses, as knowledge of the three-dimensional structure of viruses and their components expands.

3 Evolution of Human Pathogenic Phenotypes

An important feature, clearly apparent from the tree shown in Fig. 1, is the fact that the property of causing hemorrhagic fever after infection of humans has been acquired on more than one occasion during arenavirus evolution. All the South American viruses causing hemorrhagic disease are monophyletic, all falling into group B, and it is therefore possible that this trait may have evolved only once in this lineage. However, it is clear that in the case of Lassa virus, this phenotypic trait must have evolved independently. It thus appears that this trait has evolved on at least two, and possibly more, occasions during arenavirus evolution. LCMV is capable of eliciting a different type of febrile disease with neurological involvement, which has also evolved independently. It is also important to note that the potential for human pathogenicity has not been exhaustively explored among those arenaviruses not currently recognized as human pathogens. The possibility that other members of the family may have pathogenic propensities is underlined by recent reports that a North American arenavirus, Whitewater Arroyo virus or a close relative, may also be capable of eliciting fatal human disease, with acute respiratory distress syndrome, liver failure, and hemorrhagic manifestations (BYRD et al. 2000). We know nothing of the constellation of virus properties which confer a human pathogenic phenotype or of the molecular mechanisms which underlie it. Despite the similarities in the diseases caused by the agents of hemorrhagic fevers among the arenaviruses, it is by no means clear that easily recognizable common features at the levels of the genome or virus structure exist. Further insights will be required in this area before we can be confident of understanding how the viruses acquired their abilities to cause disease in humans.

4 Phylogeny of α-Dystroglycan Binding Affinity

It has been demonstrated that the cell surface protein α-dystroglycan acts as a receptor for lymphocytic choriomeningitis virus and for Lassa virus (CAO et al. 1998). Soluble α-dystroglycan blocked infection in vitro with these viruses, and cells bearing a null mutation in the gene encoding this protein were resistant to infection. As discussed more fully elsewhere in this volume, the affinity with which different arenaviruses bind to α-dystroglycan varies significantly, with differences in the 300- to 1000-fold range. Those viruses which have been shown to bind with high affinity are the Old World viruses lymphocytic choriomeningitis, Lassa and Mopeia, together with the New World viruses Latino and Oliveros, while the other New World viruses Junín, Sabiá, Machupo, Pichinde and Tacaribe bind with relatively low affinity. The New World high-affinity binders Latino and Oliveros viruses fall into group C (Fig. 1) and are thus phylogenetically distinct both from the Old World high-affinity binders and from New World low-affinity binders, which include members of groups A and B (BOWEN et al. 1997). It seems clear that binding affinity appears to be unrelated to human pathogenicity, since hemorrhagic fever viruses appear in both affinity groups. This may not be particularly surprising, in view of the presence of α-dystroglycan on a wide range of rodent and primate cells (BORROW and OLDSTONE 1992). The propensity of a virus to induce pathophysiological changes leading to hemorrhagic fever in humans presumably depends on the use of alternative receptors, elements of the virus-host interaction downstream of virus binding, or a constellation of such features which remain to be determined.

5 Co-Evolution of Arenaviruses with their Rodent Hosts

The most striking feature of the biology of the arenaviruses is their ability to set up chronic infections in specific rodent hosts, in which infectious virus is present in blood and excreted in body fluids (for detailed review see CHILDS and PETERS 1993). The impact on the host animal can sometimes be significant, but the exquisite balance apparent in many such rodent infections, where virus production takes place over the lifetime of the host with minimal detrimental effects, contrasts dramatically with pathological manifestations which can follow the infection of a human or other primate with some of these viruses. The setting of a chronic infection provides an ideal arena in which competition between members of the viral quasi-species will select for improved adaptation to the host. Indeed, it has long been known from experimental infections with lymphocytic choriomeningitis virus (for example AHMED and OLDSTONE 1988; KING et al. 1990) that viruses better adapted for growth in particular tissues or cells can be readily selected. This precise adaptation to a particular rodent host has led to suggestions that co-evolution of the arenaviruses with them has been a dominant, or at least a major, factor in generating the pattern of virus-host relationships that we see today (JOHNSON et al. 1973; GONZALEZ et al. 1986; BOWEN et al. 1996b, 1997).

Tight linkages between virus and host evolution are well established in other virus families. In the case of the herpesviruses, it has been possible to unambiguously define the divisions of the mammalian and avian viruses into three subfamilies (the *Alpha-*, *Beta-* and *Gammaherpesvirinae*). It has become evident that the branching patterns among the viruses in each of these subfamilies is largely congruent with that of their corresponding host species, arguing strongly for the co-speciation of viruses and hosts. From this can be inferred the antiquity of these virus lineages by reference to the host fossil record, with the last common ancestor of mammalian and avian herpesviruses in existence some 200 million years ago (McGEOCH and COOK 1994; McGEOCH et al. 1995; McGEOCH and DAVISON 1999).

More directly comparable with the arenaviruses, as RNA viruses hosted by mainly rodent species, there is strong evidence of co-evolution of the hantavirus genus of the family *Bunyaviridae* with their natural hosts (reviewed by PLYUSNIN et al. 1996; McCAUGHEY and HART 2000). Genetic relationships of the viruses appear to mirror the affinities of their host species; phylogenies based on the S RNA segment encoding the nucleocapsid protein clearly divide the hantaviruses into three groups, hosted by rodents of the Murinae, the Arvicolinae, and the Sigmodontinae, respectively. An ancient origin for these viruses, around 100 million years ago, has been suggested in this case also. However, detailed analysis of large numbers of hantaviruses from rodents across the USA has demonstrated that, on a background defined by co-evolution, interspecies transmission events have also played a role in shaping the current complex situation (ROWE et al. 1995; MONROE et al. 1999).

With the arenaviruses themselves, the situation remains rather less clear. Paradoxically, this is partly due to the much sparser data available, both in terms of the smaller number of virus species, and the relatively low number of isolates of each species. This makes it more difficult to delineate the large-scale correlations expected of long-term co-evolution and co-speciation. While as we have seen the relationships among the viruses of the family are reasonably well understood, there remain many uncertainties relating to their hosts, which are of two kinds: (a) the identification of the natural host species and (b) the precise phylogenetic relationships among these host species. Until these uncertainties can be clarified, the co-evolution hypothesis cannot be properly tested in respect of the arenaviruses, since in essence it involves mapping the virus phylogeny onto the host phylogeny to examine to what extent they are congruent. There is also some evidence of host-switching, as for the hantaviruses, in which a species acquires and subsequently maintains a virus species which evolved in another species, thus providing another layer of complexity. Our current appreciation of the situation has been comprehensively discussed by BOWEN et al. (1996b, 1997, 2000).

Much of the evidence which is consistent with the co-evolution of arenaviruses with their natural hosts is to be found in the New World group:

- The closely related viruses Junín and Machupo are both hosted by rodents of one genus, *Calomys musculinus* and *Calomys callosus*, respectively.
- Three viruses hosted by rodents of the same genus *Oryzomys* (Flexal, Paraná and Pichinde viruses) were shown to be monophyletic by BOWEN et al. (1997).
- Guanarito virus, a New World group B virus, was found primarily in the rodent species *Zygodontomys brevicauda* (FULHORST et al. 1997, 1999a; WEAVER et al. 2000), while the closely related Amapari virus, also in group B, was associated with *Neacomys guianae* and *Oryzomys capito*. These three rodent genera have been placed in a single tribe, the Oryzomyini, on the basis of DNA hybridization studies (DICKERMAN 1992), morphological cladistic analysis (STEPPAN 1995), and mitochondrial DNA phylogeny (ENGEL et al. 1998):
- Pirital virus, an arenavirus geographically co-located with Guanarito virus in central Venezuela and a member of New World group A, was primarily associated with *Sigmodon alstoni* (FULHORST et al. 1999a), a more distantly related rodent species. Only 1 out of 73 isolates was from *Z. brevicauda*.
- SULLIVAN et al. (1995) demonstrated the close relationship of *Neotoma albigula* and *Sigmodon hispidus* on the basis of mitochondrial DNA sequence data. These species are the respective hosts of the closely related Whitewater Arroyo and Tamiami viruses (FULHORST et al. 1996).

It may also be the case that the longer mean genetic distances among New World arenaviruses observed by BOWEN et al. (2000) are correlated with the exceptionally extensive adaptive radiation of their hosts among the *Sigmodontinae*. As these rodents moved from their origins in North America into the vast new habitat of South America, there occurred one of the greatest radiations of mammals in recent history. Under the co-evolution hypothesis, it would be expected that virus evolution would occur at a similarly unusual rate.

Among the Old World viruses, the monophyly of Lassa, Mobala and Mopeia is reflected in the relationships of their host species of the genera *Mastomys* and *Praomys* within the Murinae. The monophyly of these genera has been suggested on the basis of analysis of chromosomal character states (BRITTON-DAVIDIAN et al. 1995) and DNA hybridization (CHEVRET et al. 1994).

These findings are highly suggestive of a co-evolution scenario for the origin of the present day arenaviruses, but are far from constituting compelling evidence that it is the underlying paradigm. The taxonomy of rodents, particularly that of the taxon Muridae, of which the rodent hosts of the arenaviruses are members, remains in an uncertain and unstable state (NOWAK 1991; MUSSER and CARLETON 1993), but there appears to be little consensus on how to improve the situation. Until the lack of sufficiently reliable phylogenetic studies of the rodent hosts relevant to the arenaviruses is remedied, preferably using molecular methods, no further progress is likely.

In the meantime, there are grounds for believing that co-evolution does not account for all the virus-host relationships observed today. The isolation of Tacaribe virus from *Artibeus* spp. bats (and from mosquitoes) in Trinidad, but not from any rodent species (DOWNS et al. 1963) is clearly inconsistent with any co-evolution scenario, and suggests that interspecies transmission may have also played a part in generating currently observed virus-host relationships. The occurrence of transmission events between rodent species in the past is suggested by the fact that *Calomys* spp. are hosts to viruses of New World lineages B (Junín and Machupo viruses) and C (Latino virus), and that genera of the Oryzomyini tribe (*Oryzomys*, *Neacomys*, and *Zygodontomys*) are hosts to viruses from lineages A (Paraná, Flexal and Pichinde) and B (Amapari and Guanarito) (BOWEN et al. 1997). There is also reason to speculate that interspecies transmission may have occurred recently. Thus, Guanarito virus of genotype 7, localized in a particular locality (Arismendi, Barinas State, Venezuela), has been found not only in its major host *Zygodontomys brevicauda*, but also in *Sigmodon alstoni* (WEAVER et al. 2000). It seems likely that, as with the hantaviruses, the arenavirus-host relationships that we see today are a product of a co-evolutionary base, with an overlay of interhost transmission events.

6 Intraspecies Strain Variation

Recent studies have examined the geographic and temporal basis of genetic diversity within an arenavirus species. Such factors may have important implications for strain-dependent variations in virulence or pathogenicity, in the evolution of epidemics in time and space, and at the practical level, in the tracing of particular routes of transmission. An understanding of the extent of intra-species variation is also essential in the process of developing criteria for the definition of arenavirus species and the recognition of new ones.

6.1 Junín Virus

The endemic area of Argentine hemorrhagic fever has extended over the past three decades from the site of its original outbreak to reach a current area of $150,000 km^2$. Disease incidence has tended to be initially high in the new areas, followed by a decline. Several possible explanations for the dynamics of this disease pattern have been discussed (ENRÍA and FEUILLADE 1998). Among these are an increase in seroprevalence and protective immunity in the human population, changing virulence of circulating virus over time, changes in agricultural practices, fluctuations in rodent populations and in virus prevalence in those populations, and rodent migration habits. GARCÍA et al. (2000) analyzed parts of the N and GP1 genes of isolates of Junín virus from different areas of the endemic region. Nucleotide sequence divergences up to 13% in the GP1 gene and 9% in the N gene were recorded, corresponding to amino acid sequence divergences of 9% and 4%, respectively. Phylogenetic analysis separated the isolates into three distinct clades, corresponding to the central part of the endemic area, its western part, and its far northeastern edge. Within these clades, isolates from neighboring areas tend to co-locate in the tree, reinforcing the picture of strong geographic clustering of genetic variants. The data provided little suggestion of any temporal correlation of divergence over the 35-year timespan covered in the study. Nor were there any indications that differences in virus virulence or human disease manifestation were reflected in the sequences examined.

6.2 Lassa Virus

The intraspecies variation in Lassa virus has also been the subject of discussion and investigation, since sequence analysis of the S segments of virus isolates from hemorrhagic fever patients infected in Sierra Leone and Nigeria demonstrated extensive divergence (AUPERIN and McCORMICK 1989; CLEGG et al. 1991b). At the nucleotide sequence level, divergence between the two strains occurred at 19%, 20%, and 22% in the sequences encoding G1, G2, and N, respectively. Much of this variation was in codon third base positions (up to 50%), and the amino acid sequences of G1, G2, and N retained 92%, 94%, and 91% similarity as a consequence (CLEGG et al. 1991b). This level of sequence divergence has prompted suggestions that the status of Lassa virus as a single species should be re-evaluated (LOZANO et al. 1997). Differing patterns of antigenicity using panels of monoclonal antibodies between virus isolates originating in Nigeria and Sierra Leone have also been documented (RUO et al. 1991), presumably a consequence of genetic variation, but there has been little suggestion that disease manifestations in human cases are virus-strain dependent. Difficulties in demonstrating in vitro neutralization have impeded most investigations of functional serological responses, but there have been reports of strain dependence of cross-neutralization sufficiently significant to impact on the selection of immune plasma for potential therapeutic application (JAHRLING 1983; JAHRLING and PETERS 1984; JAHRLING et al. 1985).

The virus is endemic in areas of Guinea, Sierra Leone, and Liberia in the west and in Nigeria in the east. In 1996–1997 in eastern Sierra Leone, over 1,000 cases of Lassa fever were reported, including 148 deaths (ANONYMOUS 1997). The frequently quoted estimate of 100,000 to 300,000 human cases of Lassa fever per year, with up to 5,000 deaths (McCORMICK et al. 1987), refers to the whole of sub-Saharan west Africa, but the situation in the intervening region of sub-Saharan west Africa remains unclear. There have been scant reports of Lassa fever-like illness from this region, no virus isolation from rodents, and little serological evidence of arenavirus circulation in the human or rodent population. However, the disease has been diagnosed serologically in a traveller returned from Burkina Faso (VAN DER HEIDE 1982), and more recently a German student who had visited Côte d'Ivoire, Ghana, and Burkina Faso died of Lassa fever after returning home, suggesting the virus is present in at least some part of this area (GÜNTHER et al. 2000).

Given the vast distance (approximately 1,800km) between the areas in which the virus is known to circulate and the potentially huge size of the endemic area, it would not be surprising if considerable diversity, already hinted at in the previously available genetic data, existed in the virus population. In order to provide some further evidence to test this hypothesis, we have amplified, cloned, and sequenced several hundred nucleotides from close to the 5'-terminus of the S RNA segment encoding the N-terminal of the G1 glycoprotein from a further six isolates of Lassa virus from human patients (including three who had returned to the UK from west Africa) and an additional isolate from the virus's reservoir host *Mastomys* (CLEGG et al. 1991a; J.C.S. Clegg, A.H. Demby, J. Chamberlain, G. Lloyd, unpublished results). We have also obtained sequences from two additional isolates of the related African arenavirus Mopeia for comparative purposes. Alignment of these sequences with those previously obtained from Old World arenaviruses and subsequent phylogenetic analysis confirm the existence of considerable divergence among Lassa virus isolates (Fig. 2). The isolates originating in Sierra Leone or Liberia form a very closely related group, together with the previously sequenced Josiah strain (AUPERIN and MCCORMICK 1989), also from Sierra Leone. In contrast, those originating in Nigeria all differ significantly from that group, from the previously sequenced Nigerian isolate (GA391; CLEGG et al. 1991b), and among themselves. Similar relationships among these virus nucleotide sequences have been found using distance-based or maximum parsimony phylogenetic methods or the amino acid sequences of the N-terminal G1 translation products.

Despite the observed sequence diversity, phylogenetic analyses indicate that the Lassa virus isolates all fall into a monophyletic group which is clearly distinguishable from the other Old World arenavirus species Mopeia virus and the prototype of the family, lymphocytic choriomeningitis virus. These results support

----

▶

Fig. 2A,B. Genetic diversity of Lassa virus. **A** Map of part of Africa, with countries with areas endemic for Lassa fever enclosed in *black outline*. **B** Nucleotide sequences corresponding to nt 8–382 of the S RNA of strain GA391 (GenBank accession no. X52400) from amplified, cloned, and sequenced materials were used. Sequences were aligned along with those of reference viruses in CLUSTAL W (THOMPSON et al. 1994) and the output adjusted manually where necessary to use gap positions found in alignments of corresponding translation products. Phylogenetic relationships were determined in PUZZLE (version 3.1; STRIMMER and VON HAESELER 1996) and the tree drawn with TREEVIEW (PAGE 1996). Support values (%) for internal branches are indicated. Lassa virus isolates originating in Sierra Leone or Liberia are enclosed in a *box*. Of the Lassa virus strains sequenced in this study, SA, PA, and PB1 (EMOND et al. 1982) were isolated from patients infected in Nigeria; strain 8189 was isolated from a patient in Sierra Leone (DEMBY et al. 1994), as was strain 331; LP is the prototype strain of Lassa virus, a patient isolate from Nigeria (BUCKLEY and CASALS 1970); strain 523 was isolated from *Mastomys* sp. in Liberia. Mopeia virus strains AN20410 and AN20615 were isolated from *Mastomys natalensis* in Mozambique (WULFF et al. 1977). Supply of virus strains not isolated at CAMR by CDC Atlanta is gratefully acknowledged. Other sequences were obtained from GenBank

the distinction currently made between Lassa virus and its closest relative, Mopeia virus, which is also based on geographical separation and pathogenic properties in humans. The striking and unexpected degree of sequence diversity among the Nigerian isolates also suggests that Lassa virus has been present in this part of west Africa for sufficient time to allow for evolutionary radiation, perhaps in rodent populations largely isolated from one another by geographical or other factors.

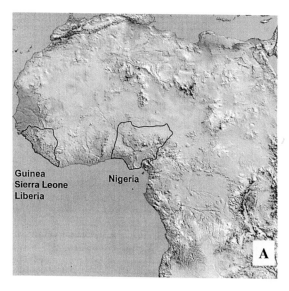

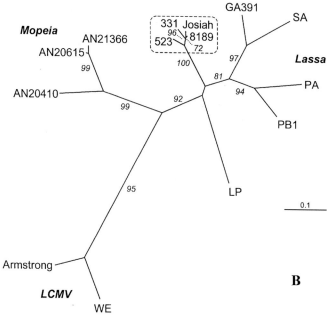

Conversely, the close genetic relationships between the isolates from Sierra Leone and Liberia suggests that Lassa virus is a relatively recent arrival in the western endemic area. This would imply a westward movement of the virus across west Africa. At a more practical level, the sequences from these diverse isolates have been used to identify PCR primers with enhanced capability of detecting virus RNA originating from anywhere in west Africa (DEMBY et al. 1994).

These results have been confirmed and extended in an exhaustive, large-scale study by BOWEN et al. (2000). Partial N gene sequences from a collection of 54 Lassa virus isolates from Nigeria, Sierra Leone, Liberia, and Guinea were determined. The extensive diversity of sequences from Nigeria was confirmed. In the N gene fragment analyzed, there was up to 27% variation at the nucleotide level and up to 15% at the amino acid sequence level. The scale of the study enabled phylogenetic analysis to demonstrate the existence of at least four virus lineages, three consisting of isolates originating in Nigeria, the other of isolates from Sierra Leone, Liberia, and Guinea. The variability correlated with geographical distance between isolates: lineage II was associated with southern central Nigeria, lineage III with northern central Nigeria, and lineage IV with the western endemic area of Sierra Leone, Liberia, and Guinea. Lineage I consisted of a single isolate, the prototype strain LP from Lassa in eastern Nigeria (BUCKLEY and CASALS 1970). Isolates taken directly from rodents were interspersed with those from human cases of Lassa fever, demonstrating genetic linkage between viruses circulating in rodents and humans in the same geographical area. No evidence for the occurrence of clock-like evolution was found in the dataset, which spanned a period of 28 years. This conclusion, that variation is a function of geographical rather than temporal separation, is similar to that of the Junín virus study (GARCÍA et al. 2000).

Full-length S RNA segment sequences were obtained from isolates representative of lineage I (the prototype LP strain) and lineage II, complementing the already available full-length sequences from lineages III and IV. Comparison of aligned GPC sequences demonstrated no evidence of recombination. Although the order of descent was not fully resolved, it was clear that the Nigerian lineages were ancestral to lineage IV, composed of viruses circulating in the western endemic region. Within this latter lineage, Guinean and Liberian strains appeared more basal than those from Sierra Leone. Both these findings are consistent with the notion of an ancestral virus population in Nigeria, which has moved westwards to occupy the endemic areas of Liberia, Guinea, and Sierra Leone. This might have happened by spread of the virus through the rodent population, or by movement of the virus-carrying rodents themselves. The situation in the intervening territory between Nigeria and Liberia remains unclear, although, as noted above, there is evidence of the presence of the virus (GÜNTHER et al. 2000) somewhere in this region.

6.3 Guanarito Virus

Parallel issues have emerged from a study of the diversity of Guanarito virus, and the distribution of the virus in relation to the Venezuelan hemorrhagic fever endemic area (WEAVER et al. 2000). Partial sequences of the N gene (as used in BOWEN et al. 1997) of isolates from within the endemic area and elsewhere from human infections and from rodents were analyzed. As with Junín virus and Lassa virus, considerable diversity among the virus isolates was found, with up to 17% nucleotide sequence differences and 9% at the amino acid sequence level, values perhaps surprisingly large given the rather small distances involved (up to a maximum of 300km between isolates). The 29 isolates analyzed fell into 9 well-supported genotypes. There was a very clear geographic component in the distribution of these genotypes. Most were strictly localized to a single discrete site, although one was much more widely distributed, being found in four of the five states included in the survey. It is notable that the most divergent genotype (genotype 1) was isolated from *Oligoryzomys fulvescens* trapped at the same site where genotypes 7 and 9 were isolated from *Zygodontomys brevicauda*, the major natural host. Although the difference in host species suggests a rationale for the separate existence of genotype 1, the mechanisms for maintenance of different virus lineages in close proximity in the same species remain a subject of speculation; these might include very limited mobility in rodent populations and consequent lack of virus mixing, or the existence of so far unrecognized ecological differences between virus or rodent lineages which provide for co-existence rather than competitive exclusion. Only two of the genotypes contained isolates from cases of human hemorrhagic disease. It is very clear that the virus is present in rodents of more than one species in areas outside the known endemic area. The factors which may contribute to the absence of discernable disease in these areas are not known, but may include the lower human population density or reduced levels of contact with rodents. It would be premature to conclude that only some genotypes were the etiological agents of human disease, in view of the relatively low numbers of some genotypes isolated.

6.4 Intraspecies Strain Variation: Conclusions

We can draw some general conclusions about strain variation and its correlates and consequences. Extensive sequence variation is the norm when arenaviruses are studied at the population level. This needs to be taken into account in setting criteria for the definition (and recognition) of virus species. The extent of sequence variation is related to geographical separation distance between isolates, and no correlation with date of isolation is apparent. This is similar to the situation previously found with vesicular stomatitis virus (NICHOL et al. 1993) and with the hantaviruses (PLYUSNIN et al. 1996). The geographical distance dependency seems to apply at all scales up to and including interspecies differences as instanced with Lassa virus and Mopeia virus. The absence of demonstrable clock-like evolution may be just a reflection of the limited time-span covered in these studies. Genetic variation in sequence among isolates does not have obvious consequences in terms of phenotype. In particular, human pathogenicity or variation in its clinical presentation does not seem to be associated with specific virus lineages.

7 Concluding Remarks

We are aware at present of 19 arenaviruses, infecting many rodent species in four continents, well-adapted to their natural hosts and causing them little harm. If and when transmission to humans occurs, severe and often fatal disease can ensue. There are many parallels in these and other respects with the hantaviruses. We now appreciate that both these groups of rodent-borne viruses are agents of severe, sometimes previously unrecognized diseases. Hantavirus pulmonary syndrome emerged in 1993 in the southwestern USA, and comparable diseases are being documented in South America today (JOHNSON et al. 1999; PADULA et al. 2000). Likewise, a fatal arenavirus disease may be presently emerging in California (BYRD et al. 2000), and the geographical range in which Lassa fever is recognized as a problem has increased (GÜNTHER et al. 2000). Our understanding of both these groups of viruses suggests that the viruses themselves are not changing in respect of their virulence for humans. However, fluctuations in the degree and nature of contact between human and rodent populations as a result of climatic, ecological, agricultural, or other changes can give rise to conditions in which the re-occurrence of recognized viruses and the emergence of new ones from their myriads of rodent hosts are facilitated. It is to be expected that this process will continue, and that molecular phylogenetic methods will be used to bring some order and understanding to the complexities of these interactions.

References

Ahmed R, Oldstone MB (1988) Organ-specific selection of viral variants during chronic infection. J Exp Med 167:1719–1724
Albariño CG, Posik DM, Ghiringhelli PD, Lozano ME, Romanowski V (1998) Arenavirus phylogeny: a new insight. Virus Genes 161:39–46
Anonymous (1997) Lassa fever. Wkly Epidemiol Rec 72:145–146
Auperin DD, McCormick JB (1989) Nucleotide sequence of the Lassa virus (Josiah strain) S genome RNA and amino acid sequence comparison of the N and GPC proteins to other arenaviruses. Virology 134:208–219
Auperin DD, Compans RW, Bishop DH (1982) Nucleotide sequence conservation at the 3' termini of the virion RNA species of New World and Old World arenaviruses. Virology 121:200–203
Benson SD, Bamford JK, Bamford DH, Burnett RM (1999) Viral evolution revealed by bacteriophage PRD1 and human adenovirus coat protein structures. Cell 98:825–833
Borrow P, Oldstone MB (1992) Characterization of lymphocytic choriomeningitis virus-binding protein(s): a candidate cellular receptor for the virus. J Virol 66:7270–7281
Bowen MD, Peters CJ, Mills JM, Nichol ST (1996a) Oliveros virus, a novel arenavirus from Argentina. Virology 217:262–266
Bowen MD, Peters CJ, Nichol ST (1996b) The phylogeny of New World (Tacaribe complex) arenaviruses. Virology 219:285–290
Bowen MD, Peters CJ, Nichol ST (1997) Phylogenetic analysis of the *Arenaviridae*: patterns of virus evolution and evidence for cospeciation between arenaviruses and their rodent hosts. Mol Phylogenet Evol 8:301–316
Bowen MD, Rollin PE, Ksiazek TG, Hustad HL, Bausch DG, Demby AH, Bajani MD, Peters CJ, Nichol ST (2000) Genetic diversity among Lassa virus strains. J Virol 74:6992–7004

Britton-Davidian J, Catalan J, Granjon L, DuPlantier J-M (1995) Chromosomal phylogeny and evolution of the genus *Mastomys* (Mammalia, Rodentia). J Mammol 76:248–262

Bruenn JA (1991) Relationships among the positive strand and double-strand RNA viruses as viewed through their RNA-dependent RNA polymerases. Nucl Acids Res 19:217–226

Buckley SM, Casals J (1970) Lassa fever, a new disease of man from West Africa. 3. Isolation and characterization of the virus. Am J Trop Med Hyg 19:680–691

Byrd RG, Cone LA, Commess BC, Williams-Herman D, Rowland JM, Lee B, Fitzgibbons MW, Glaser CA, Jay MT, Fritz C, Ascher MS, Cheung M, Kramer VL, Reilly K, Vugia DJ, Fulhorst CF, Milazzo ML, Charrel RN (2000) Fatal illnesses associated with a New World arenavirus – California, 1999–2000. MMWR 49:709–711

Cao W, Henry MD, Borrow P, Yamada H, Elder JH, Ravkov EV, Nichol ST, Compans RW, Campbell KP, Oldstone MB (1998) Identification of α-dystroglycan as a receptor for lymphocytic choriomeningitis virus and Lassa fever virus. Science 282:2079–2081

Cavanagh D (1997) *Nidovirales*: a new order comprising *Coronaviridae* and *Arteriviridae*. Arch Virol 142:629–633

Charrel RN, Lamballerie X de, Fulhorst CF (2001) The Whitewater Arroyo virus: natural evidence for genetic recombination among Tacaribe serocomplex viruses (family Arenaviridae). Virology 283:161–166

Chevret P, Granjon L, DuPlantier J-M, Denys C, Catzeflis FM (1994) Molecular phylogeny of the *Praomys* complex (Rodentia: Murinae): a study based on DNA/DNA hybridization experiments. Zool J Linnean Soc 112:425–442

Childs JE, Peters CJ (1993) Ecology and epidemiology of the arenaviruses and their hosts. In: Salvato MS (ed) The *Arenaviridae*. Plenum, New York

Clegg JCS (1993) Molecular phylogeny of the arenaviruses and guide to published sequence data. In: Salvato MS (ed) The *Arenaviridae*. Plenum, New York

Clegg JCS, Wilson SM, Lloyd G (1991a) Identification and analysis of African arenaviruses using the polymerase chain reaction. 8th International Conference on Negative Strand Viruses, Charleston, South Carolina

Clegg JCS, Wilson SM, Oram JD (1991b) Nucleotide sequence of the S RNA of Lassa virus (Nigerian strain) and comparative analysis of arenavirus gene products. Virus Res 18:151–164

Clegg JCS, Bowen MD, Buchmeier MJ, Gonzalez J-P, Lukashevich IS, Peters CJ, Rico-Hesse R, Romanowski V (2000). Family *Arenaviridae*. In: Regenmortel MHV van, Fauquet CM, Bishop DHL, Carstens EB, Estes MK, Lemon SM, Maniloff J, Mayo MA, McGeoch DJ, Pringle CR, Wickner RB (eds) *Virus taxonomy*. Seventh report of the International Committee on Taxonomy of Viruses. Academic, Orlando

Demby AH, Chamberlain J, Brown DWG, Clegg JCS (1994) Early diagnosis of Lassa fever by reverse transcription-PCR. J Clin Microbiol 32:2898–2903

Dickerman AW (1992) Molecular systematics of some New World muroid rodents. PhD dissertation, University of Wisconsin, Madison

Downs WG, Anderson CR, Spence L, Aitken THG, Greenhall AH (1963) Tacaribe virus, a new agent isolated from *Artibeus* bats and mosquitoes in Trinidad, West Indies. Am J Trop Med Hyg 12:640–646

Emond RT, Bannister B, Lloyd G, Southee TJ, Bowen ET (1982) A case of Lassa fever: clinical and virological findings. Br Med J (Clin Res Ed) 285:1001–1002

Engel SR, Hogan KM, Taylor JF, Davis SK (1998) Molecular systematics and paleobiogeography of the South American sigmodontine rodents. Mol Biol Evol 15:35–49

Enria D, Feuillade MR (1998) Argentine hemorrhagic fever (Junín virus – Arenaviridae): a review on clinical, epidemiological, ecological, treatment and preventive aspects of the disease. In: Travassos da Rosa APA, Vasconcelos PFC, Travassos da Rosa JFS (eds) An overview of arbovirology in Brazil and neighboring countries. Instituto Evandro Chagas, Belem

Fulhorst CF, Bowen MD, Ksiazek TG, Rollin PE, Nichol ST, Kosoy MY, Peters CJ (1996) Isolation and characterization of Whitewater Arroyo virus, a novel North American arenavirus. Virology 224:114–120

Fulhorst CE, Bowen MD, Salas RA, De Manzione NM, Duno G, Utrera A, Ksiazek TG, Peters CJ, Nichol ST, De Miller E, Tovar D, Ramos B, Vasquez C, Tesh RB (1997) Isolation and characterization of Pirital virus, a newly discovered South American arenavirus. Am J Trop Med Hyg 56:548–553

Fulhorst CF, Bowen MD, Salas RA, Duno G, Utrera A, Ksiazek TG, De Manzione NM, De Miller E, Vasquez C, Peters CJ, Tesh RB (1999a) Natural rodent host associations of Guanarito and Pirital viruses (family *Arenaviridae*) in central Venezuela. Am J Trop Med Hyg 61:325–330

Fulhorst CF, Ksiazek TG, Peters CJ, Tesh RB (1999b) Experimental infection of the cane mouse *Zygodontomys brevicauda* (family *Muridae*) with Guanarito virus (*Arenaviridae*), the etiologic agent of Venezuelan hemorrhagic fever. J Infect Dis 180:966–969

Gao F, Bailes E, Robertson DL, Chen Y, Rodenburg CM, Michael SF, Cummins LB, Arthur LO, Peeters M, Shaw GM, Sharp PM, Hahn BH (1999) Origin of HIV-1 in the chimpanzee *Pan troglodytes troglodytes*. Nature. 397:436–441

García JB, Morzunov SP, Levis S, Rowe J, Calderón G, Enría D, Sabattini M, Buchmeier MJ, Bowen MD, St Jeor SC (2000) Genetic diversity of the Junín virus in Argentina: geographic and temporal patterns. Virology 272:127–136

Goldbach R, Haan P de (1994) RNA virus supergroups and evolution of RNA viruses. In: Morse SS (ed) The evolutionary biology of viruses. Raven, New York

Gonzalez J-P, Georges AJ, Kiley MP, Meunier DM, Peters CJ, McCormick JB (1986) Evolutionary biology of a Lassa virus complex. Med Microbiol Immunol 175:157–159

Gonzalez J-P, Bowen MD, Nichol ST, Rico-Hesse R (1996) Genetic characterization and phylogeny of Sabiá virus, an emergent pathogen in Brazil. Virology 221:318–324

Griffiths CM, Wilson SM, Clegg JCS (1992) Sequence of the nucleocapsid protein gene of Machupo virus: close relationship with another South American pathogenic arenavirus, Junín. Arch Virol 124: 371–377

Günther S, Emmerich P, Laue T, Kühle O, Asper M, Jung A, Grewing T, ter Meulen J, Schmitz H (2000) Imported Lassa fever in Germany: molecular characterization of a new Lassa virus strain. Emerging Inf Dis 6 (in press)

Heide RM van der (1982) A patient with Lassa fever from the Upper Volta, diagnosed in the Netherlands. Ned Tijdschr Geneeskd 126:566–569

Henderson WW, Monroe MC, St Jeor SC, Thayer WP, Rowe JE, Peters CJ, Nichol ST (1995) Naturally occurring Sin Nombre virus genetic reassortants. Virology 214:602–610

Hendrix RW (1999) The long evolutionary reach of viruses. Current Biol 9:R914–R917

Holmes EC (1998) Molecular epidemiology and evolution of emerging infectious diseases. Br Med Bull 54:533–543

Howard CR (1993) Antigenic diversity among the arenaviruses. In: Salvato MS (ed) The *Arenaviridae*. Plenum, New York

Hungnes O, Jonassen TO, Jonassen CM, Grinde B (2000) Molecular epidemiology of viral infections. How sequence information helps us understand the evolution and dissemination of viruses. APMIS 108:81–97

Jahrling PB (1983) Protection of Lassa virus-infected guinea pigs with Lassa-immune plasma of guinea pig, primate, and human origin. J Med Virol 12:93–102

Jahrling PB, Peters CJ (1984) Passive antibody therapy of Lassa fever in cynomolgus monkeys: importance of neutralizing antibody and Lassa virus strain. Infect Immun 44:528–533

Jahrling PB, Frame JD, Rhoderick JB, Monson MH (1985) Endemic Lassa fever in Liberia. IV. Selection of optimally effective plasma for treatment by passive immunization. Trans R Soc Trop Med Hyg 79:380–384

Johnson AM, Souza LT de, Ferreira IB, Pereira LE, Ksiazek TG, Rollin PE, Peters CJ, Nichol ST (1999) Genetic investigation of novel hantaviruses causing fatal HPS in Brazil. J Med Virol 59:527–535

Johnson KM, Webb PA, Justines G (1973) Biology of Tacaribe-complex viruses. In: Lehmann-Grube F (ed) Lymphocytic chroriomeningitis virus and other arenaviruses. Springer, Berlin Heidelberg, New York

Kiley MP, Lange JV, Johnson KM (1979) Protection of rhesus monkeys from Lassa virus by immunisation with closely related arenavirus. Lancet 2:738

King CC, Fries R de, Kolhekar SR, Ahmed R (1990) *In vivo* selection of lymphocyte-tropic and macrophage-tropic variants of lymphocytic choriomeningitis virus during persistent infection. J Virol 64:5611–5616

Kirk WE, Cash P, Peters CJ, Bishop DH (1980) Formation and characterization of an intertypic lymphocytic choriomeningitis recombinant virus. J Gen Virol 51:213–218

Koonin EV (1991) The phylogeny of the RNA-dependent RNA polymerases of positive-strand RNA viruses. J Gen Virol 72:2197–2206

Koonin EV, Dolja VV (1993) Evolution and taxonomy of positive-strand RNA viruses: implication of comparative analysis of amino acid sequences. Crit Rev Biochem Mol Biol 28:373–430

Korber B, Muldoon M, Theiler J, Gao F, Gupta R, Lapedes A, Hahn BH, Wolinsky S, Bhattacharya T (2000) Timing the ancestor of the HIV-1 pandemic strains. Science 288:1789–1796

Lai MM (1995) Recombination and its evolutionary effect on viruses with RNA genomes. In: Gibbs A, Calisher CH, Garcia-Arenal F (eds) Molecular basis of virus evolution. Cambridge University, Cambridge, UK

Lisieux T, Coimbra M, Nassar ES, Burattini MN, Souza LT de, Ferreira I, Rocco IM, Rosa AP da, Vasconcelos PF, Pinheiro FP, LeDuc JW, Rico-Hesse R, Gonzalez J-P, Jahrling PB, Tesh RB (1994) New arenavirus isolated in Brazil. Lancet 343:391–392

Lozano ME, Posik DM, Albarino CG, Schujman G, Ghiringhelli PD, Calderon G, Sabattini M, Romanowski V (1997) Characterization of arenaviruses using a family-specific primer set for RT-PCR amplification and RFLP analysis. Its potential use for detection of uncharacterized arenaviruses. Virus Res 49:79–89

Lukashevich IS (1992) Generation of reassortants between African arenaviruses. Virology 188:600–605

Lukashevich IS, Djavani M, Shapiro K, Sanchez A, Ravkov E, Nichol ST, Salvato MS (1997) The Lassa fever virus L gene: nucleotide sequence, comparison, and precipitation of a predicted 250kDa protein with monospecific antiserum. J Gen Virol 78:547–551

Marriott AC, Nuttall PA (1996) Large segment of Dugbe nairovirus encodes the putative RNA polymerase. J Gen Virol 77:1775–1780

McCaughey C, Hart CA (2000) Hantaviruses. J Med Microbiol 49:587–599

McCormick JB, Webb PA, Krebs JW, Johnson KM, Smith ES (1987) A prospective study of the epidemiology and ecology of Lassa fever. J Infect Dis 155:437–444

McGeoch DJ, Cook S (1994) Molecular phylogeny of the *Alphaherpesvirinae* sub-family and a proposed evolutionary timescale. J Mol Biol 238:9–22

McGeoch DJ, Davison AJ (1999) The molecular evolutionary history of the herpesviruses. In: Domingo E, Webster RG, Holland J (eds) Origin and evolution of viruses. Academic, New York

McGeoch DJ, Cook S, Dolan A, Jamieson FE, Telford EA (1995) Molecular phylogeny and evolutionary timescale for the family of mammalian herpesviruses. J Mol Biol 247:443–458

Mills JN, Barrera Oro JG, Bressler DS, Childs JE, Tesh RB, Smith JF, Enria DA, Geisbert TW, McKee KT Jr, Bowen MD, Peters CJ, Jahrling PB (1996) Characterization of Oliveros virus, a new member of the Tacaribe complex (*Arenaviridae*: *Arenavirus*). Am J Trop Med Hyg 54:399–404

Monroe MC, Morzunov SP, Johnson AM, Bowen MD, Artsob H, Yates T, Peters CJ, Rollin PE, Ksiasek TG, Nichol ST (1999) Genetic diversity and distribution of *Peromyscus*-borne hantaviruses in North America and comparison with other hantaviruses. Emerging Infect Dis 5:75–86

Müller R, Poch O, Delarue M, Bishop DH, Bouloy M (1994) Rift Valley fever virus L segment: correction of the sequence and possible functional role of newly identified regions conserved in RNA-dependent polymerases. J Gen Virol 75:1345–1352

Musser GM, Carleton MD (1993) Family Muridae. In: Wilson DE, Reeder DM (eds) Mammal species of the world: a taxonomic and geographic reference (Smithsonian series in comparative evolutionary biology). Smithsonian Institution, Washington

Nichol ST, Rowe JE, Fitch WM (1993) Punctuated equilibrium and positive Darwinian evolution in vesicular stomatitis virus. Proc Natl Acad Sci USA 90:10424–10428

Nowak RM (1991) Walker's mammals of the world. Johns Hopkins University, Baltimore

Padula PJ, Colavecchia SB, Martinez VP, Gonzalez Della Valle MO, Edelstein A, Miguel SD, Russi J, Riquelme JM, Colucci N, Almiron M, Rabinovich RD (2000) Genetic diversity, distribution, and serological features of hantavirus infection in five countries in South America. J Clin Microbiol 38:3029–3035

Page RDM (1996) TREEVIEW: an application to display phylogenetic trees on personal computers. Comp Appl Biosci 12:357–358

Plyusnin A, Vapalahti O, Vaheri A (1996) Hantaviruses: genome structure, expression and evolution. J Gen Virol 77:2677–2687

Pringle CR (1997) The Order *Mononegavirales* – current status. Arch Virol 142:2321–2326

Pringle CR, Easton AJ (1997) Monopartite negative strand RNA genomes. Semin Virol 8:49–57

Poch O, Sauvaget I, Delarue M, Tordo N (1989) Identification of four conserved motifs among the RNA-dependent polymerase encoding elements. EMBO J 8:3867–3874

Regenmortel MH van (1992) What is a virus? Arch Virol Suppl 5:47–53

Rivière Y, Ahmed R, Southern PJ, Buchmeier MJ, Oldstone MB (1985) Genetic mapping of lymphocytic choriomeningitis virus pathogenicity: virulence in guinea pigs is associated with the L RNA segment. J Virol 55:704–709

Rowe JE, St Jeor SC, Riolo J, Otteson EW, Monroe MC, Henderson WW, Ksiazek TG, Rollin PE, Nichol ST (1995) Coexistence of several novel hantaviruses in rodents indigenous to North America. Virology 213:122–130

Ruo SL, Mitchell SW, Kiley MP, Roumillat LF, Fisher-Hoch SP, McCormick JB (1991) Antigenic relatedness between arenaviruses defined at the epitope level by monoclonal antibodies. J Gen Virol 72:549–555

Santti J, Harvala H, Kinnunen L, Hyypiä T (2000) Molecular epidemiology and evolution of coxsackievirus A9. J Gen Virol 81:1361–1372

Sibold C, Meisel H, Kruger DH, Labuda M, Lysy J, Kozuch O, Pejcoch M, Vaheri A, Plyusnin A (1999) Recombination in Tula hantavirus evolution: analysis of genetic lineages from Slovakia. J Virol 73:667–675

Steppan SJ (1995) Revision of the leaf-eared mice Phyllotini (Rodentia: Sigmodontinae) with a phylogenetic hypothesis for the Sigmodontinae. Fieldiana: Zool. n.s. 80:1–112

Strauss JH, Strauss EG (1997) Recombination in alphaviruses. Semin Virol 8:85–94

Strimmer K, Haeseler A von (1996) Quartet puzzling: a quartet maximum likelihood method for reconstructing tree topologies. Mol Biol Evol 13:964–969

Sullivan J, Holsinger KE, Simon C (1995) Among-site rate variation and phylogenetic analysis of 12S rRNA in Sigmondontine rodents. Mol Biol Evol 12:988–1001

Suzuki Y, Gojobori T, Nakagomi O (1998) Intragenic recombinations in rotaviruses. FEBS Lett 427: 183–187

Thompson JD, Higgins DG, Gibson TJ (1994) CLUSTAL W: improving the sensitivity of progressive multiple sequence alignment through sequence weighting, position-specific gap penalties and weight matrix choice. Nucleic Acids Res 22:4673–4680

Walker DH, Johnson KM, Lange JV, Gardner JJ, Kiley MP, McCormick JB (1982) Experimental infection of rhesus monkeys with Lassa virus and a closely related arenavirus, Mozambique virus. J Infect Dis 146:360–368

Ward CW (1993) Progress towards a higher taxonomy of viruses. Res Virol 144:419–453

Weaver SC, Kang W, Shirako Y, Rumenapf T, Strauss EG, Strauss JH (1997) Recombinational history and molecular evolution of western equine encephalomyelitis complex alphaviruses. J Virol 71: 613–623

Weaver SC, Salas RA, Manzione N de, Fulhorst CF, Duno G, Utrera A, Mills JN, Ksiazek TG, Tovar D, Tesh RB (2000) Guanarito virus (Arenaviridae) isolates from endemic and outlying localities in Venezuela: sequence comparisons among and within strains isolated from Venezuelan hemorrhagic fever patients and rodents. Virology 266:189–195

Weber EL, Buchmeier MJ (1988) Fine mapping of a peptide sequence containing an antigenic site conserved among arenaviruses. Virology 164:30–38

Wilson SM, Clegg JC (1991) Sequence analysis of the S RNA of the African arenavirus Mopeia: an unusual secondary structure feature in the intergenic region. Virology 180:543–552

Worobey M (2000) Extensive homologous recombination among widely divergent TT viruses. J Virol 74:7666–7670

Worobey M, Holmes EC (1999) Evolutionary aspects of recombination in RNA viruses. J Gen Virol 80:2535–2543

Worobey M, Rambaut A, Holmes EC (1999) Widespread intra-serotype recombination in natural populations of dengue virus. Proc Natl Acad Sci USA 96:7352–7357

Wulff H, McIntosh BM, Hamner DB, Johnson KM (1977) Isolation of an arenavirus closely related to Lassa virus from Mastomys natalensis in south-east Africa. Bull World Health Organ 55:441–444

Wulff H, Lange JV, Webb PA (1978) Interrelationships among arenaviruses measured by indirect immunofluorescence. Intervirology 9:344–350

Zanotto PM, Gibbs MJ, Gould EA, Holmes EC (1996) A reevaluation of the higher taxonomy of viruses based on RNA polymerases. J Virol 70:6083–6096

Zhu T, Korber BT, Nahmias AJ, Hooper E, Sharp PM, Ho DD (1998) An African HIV-1 sequence from 1959 and implications for the origin of the epidemic. Nature 391:594–597

Mammalian Reservoirs of Arenaviruses

J. Salazar-Bravo[1], L.A. Ruedas[2], and T.L. Yates[1,3]

[1] Department of Biology, and Museum of Southwestern Biology, University of New Mexico, Albuquerque, NM 87131, USA
[2] Department of Biology, Portland State University, Portland, OR 97207-0751, USA
[3] *Present address*: Office of the Vice-Provost for Research, The University of New Mexico, Scholes Hall 227A, Albuquerque, NM 87131, USA

1 Introduction

Arenaviruses are negative-stranded RNA viruses that have been isolated from several species of mammals in various parts of the world. With two exceptions, these viruses have all been isolated from rodents of the family Muridae – sensu MUSSER and CARLETON (1993). Tacaribe virus was originally isolated from fruit-eating bats of the genus *Artibeus*, while Sabiá virus has no known wild reservoir. Arenavirus infections in their rodent reservoirs are characterized by persistent shedding of infectious virus in the urine (JOHNSON 1970).

The history and classification of the virus species are treated elsewhere in this volume. Our purpose in this chapter is to present updated information on the identity of the various mammalian hosts of arenaviruses, reviewing aspects of their ecology, distribution, taxonomy, and systematics. In addition, we propose minimum standards we feel need to be considered when analyzing or reporting new species of viruses and their mammal hosts.

Because two serological groups of arenaviruses are recognized (PETERS 1997), this chapter on their mammal hosts is divided accordingly.

1.1 Zoonoses and Reservoir Species

Zoonoses, diseases transmitted between animals and humans, are of great public health importance. Although most occur only sporadically, some have been responsible for important epidemics. Most zoonotic diseases are derived from natural hosts that are any of a number of species or groups of mammals. ASHFORD (1997) suggested that four mammal orders (Artiodactyla, Carnivora, Primates, and Rodentia) are the most significant sources for zoonotic diseases, although it is becoming evident that other groups (e.g., Chiroptera, the bats) are also important (DASZAK et al. 2000).

Considerable contention currently surrounds the "proper way" of referring to the mammal host species from which a virus has been isolated; herein, we follow Benenson's recommendations and refer to these species as "reservoirs" (BENENSON 1995). A reservoir of infection is best identified as an ecological system in which the infectious agent survives indefinitely. Where a vertebrate host or group of hosts is essential to such a system, these are termed reservoir host(s) (ASHFORD 1997).

Mammal reservoir species and their viruses are nowadays the subject of intense study and scrutiny. This is not so much the result of the realization that certain diseases are "coming back", as it is that new diseases and disease-causing viruses are being discovered on a regular basis. It is therefore our contention that the appraisal of the mammal reservoirs' systematics and taxonomy is in a difficult position in this regard as several – if not most – of the rodent genera known to carry arenaviruses have yet to be revised critically. The precise identities of many hosts are therefore uncertain, with dire consequences for epidemiology or any prospects of disease control.

2 Mammal Hosts of Arenaviruses

Two serological groups of arenaviruses are recognized. This division is also present in their mammal reservoir species as most Old World arenaviruses have been recovered from Old World murid rodents. In contrast, New World arenaviruses (i.e., the Tacaribe complex) are found primarily in rodents of the New World.

2.1 Old World Arenaviruses

The known diversity of arenaviruses in the Old World is about one-third of that of the New World forms. The forms included in this group are: Lymphocytic choriomeningitis (LCM), Lassa (LAS), Mopeia (MOP), Mobala (MOB), and Ippy (IPP) viruses.

2.1.1 Lassa Fever Virus

The best known of the African arenaviruses is Lassa fever virus, having been described in a series of articles in *The American Journal of Tropical Medicine and Hygiene* in 1970 (BUCKLEY and CASALS 1970; FRAME et al. 1970; LEIFER et al. 1970; SPEIR et al. 1970; TROUP et al. 1970). It was 4 years later before a mammalian reservoir species (*Mastomys natalensis*) was associated with the disease (MONATH et al. 1974). The disease currently affects 300,000–500,000 cases annually, causing approximately 5,000 deaths per annum.

The virus and the disease it causes have thus been known for over 30 years; however, the taxonomy and systematics of the host remain problematic. Indeed, the systematic status of the rodent genus *Mastomys* may be succinctly summarized as confused and in a state of flux. Even the intrafamilial taxonomic status of *Mastomys* may be in doubt: traditionally classified as a genus in the subfamily Murinae of the rodent family Muridae, recent work by Catzeflis, Chevret, and collaborators (CATZEFLIS and DENYS 1992; CATZEFLIS et al. 1987, 1992; CHEVRET and HÄNNI 1994; CHEVRET et al. 1993a,b, 1994; DUBOIS et al. 1999; FURANO et al. 1994; HÄNNI et al. 1995; HUCHON et al. 1999; USDIN et al. 1995) has suggested that *Mastomys*, along with most African murids, may belong in a unique African subfamily of rodents allied to Murinae (see also GRAUR 1994).

Mastomys, described as a genus in 1915 by Oldfield Thomas, is currently thought to be constituted by eight species (MUSSER and CARLETON 1993): *M. angolensis* (Angola and southern Zaire), *M. coucha* (South Africa, southern and western Zimbabwe, and central Namibia), *M. erythroleucus* (a disjunct population in Morocco, and sub-Saharan Africa to Zaire), *M. hildebrandtii* (sub-Saharan Africa to Zaire; this name antedates *huberti*, hence references to *huberti* are, more properly, references to a species which should be called *hildebrandtii*), *M. natalensis* (South Africa, Zimbabwe, central and northeastern Namibia, east-central Tanzania, and a disjunct population in Senegal), *M. pernanus* (southwestern Kenya, northwestern Tanzania, and Rwanda), *M. shortridgei* (Okavango delta region between Botswana and Namibia), and *M. verheyeni* (Nigeria and Cameroun – and likely Chad – in the immediate vicinity of southern Lake Chad).

Lassa fever virus has been associated in the literature with the multimammate mouse, *M. natalensis* (MONATH et al. 1974). Although generally found in fields, the species reputedly is broadly distributed in all habitats from South Africa to sub-Saharan Africa. However, taxonomic problems exist associated with the assignation of LAS to *M. natalensis*. In fact, *M. natalensis* does not occur in the two disjunct hotbeds of Lassa fever in West Africa: Nigeria on the one hand, and Guinea, Sierra Leone, and Liberia on the other. The species potentially occurs in Senegal, although the taxonomic status of the Senegal population (and other populations) should be carefully scrutinized (WULFF et al. 1977; GORDON 1978; GREEN et al. 1978; GRANJON et al. 1996); GRANJON et al. (1996) hypothesized that the Sénégal and South African populations are conspecific and part of a single, continuous, panmictic population, but this hypothesis requires additional data and specimens from intervening areas in order to be rigorously tested. On the strength of these facts, namely absence from the Lassa fever zone of endemism, PETERS (1997) pointed out that it was more likely that the actual hosts of LAS were either *M. huberti* or *M. erythroleucus*; to our knowledge, there is no instance of a host with multiple arenaviruses, nor of multiple hosts with a single arenavirus (other than due to spillover, but see below).

Assignation of LAS to *M. huberti* and/or *M. erythroleucus* carries its own caveats, however. Indeed, like *M. natalensis*, these are more likely superspecies complexes, and constituted by a number of cryptic species. In fact, all *M. "huberti"* were, until recently, reported to have a diploid chromosome number ($2n$) of 32. However, VIEGAS-PÉQUIGNOT et al. (1983) and BASKEVICH and ORLOV (1993) reported on additional cytotypes, all $2n = 32$ but with radically differing fundamental numbers, which could not be considered conspecific with *M. huberti*. Thus, there exist (at least) four distinct $2n = 32$ cytotypes within *M. huberti*, no combinations of which should give rise to fertile F_1 hybrids given the nature of the chromosomal rearrangements between each possible pair. By the classical definition of species, failure to interbreed is *prima facie* evidence of non-conspecificity. These $2n = 32$ cytotypes, which may be considered full species, are distributed in Sénégal, Central African Republic, and the Central Ethiopian Rift Valley. LYONS et al. [(1977; "1978") – NB: LYONS et al. "1978" was seen cited in GORDON 1978 as "in press" in the journal *Heredity*; we have been unable to ascertain the existence of any such article in *Heredity* or any other journal; LYONS et al. 1977 mention that a "full report of the geographic distribution of the two species will appear at a later date (Lyons et al., in preparation)". It is possible that a manuscript circulated among certain individuals but was never published; we retain the citation herein for completeness] reported on additional chromosomal forms from Zimbabwe in what they considered *M. natalensis*, which they designate "species A" – $2n = 32$ – and "species B" – $2n = 36$. Based on chromosomal investigations undertaken at or near the type localities for some of these taxa (GREEN et al. 1978), it may be hypothesized that species A refers to a true *M. natalensis* type (as all *M. natalensis* are reputed to have $2n = 32$; MATTHEY 1965; VIEGAS-PEQUIGNOT et al. 1983, 1987; BASKEVICH and ORLOV 1993), while species B is assignable to *M. coucha*. To further complicate matters, *M. huberti* and *M. erythroleucus* have almost interchangeable ecologies, depending on geographic location: in West Africa, *M. huberti* is more aggressive, intra- and peridomestic, while in Central Africa, it is *M. erythroleucus* which takes over this role, relegating *M. huberti* to agricultural fields and forest edges.

The question of the taxonomic identity of the host of this disease, affecting 300,000–500,000 individuals annually, might have been satisfactorily resolved had the specimens upon which the MONATH et al. (1974) report is based been properly archived. However, they were not: Monath (T.P. Monath, personal communication) indicated that they were identified by Setzer (fourth author of the Monath et al. article), then transferred to Colorado State University for histological analyses (DeMARTINI et al. 1975). Subsequent to the latter publication, the carcasses used as a basis for the DeMartini et al. article were discarded. The track of the remaining specimens is lost: M.D. Carleton, current curator of mammals at the Smithsonian, reported (M.D. Carleton, personal communication) that there are no *Mastomys* from the original collection at the US National Museum, and only four from Panguma, collected in 1981 by C.J. Krebs; the original Monath collection consisted of 109 *Mastomys* (of a total of 475 rodents). Had the specimens been available for examination, their identity within the current – or any subsequent – taxonomic framework for *Mastomys* could have been determined. As MILLS and CHILDS (1998) stated, the imprecise taxonomy of the *Mastomys* species complex will result in "years before the geographic distributions of each species can be mapped and used to interpret the restricted distribution of Lassa fever".

2.1.2 Mobala

This arenavirus is relatively new, having been described in 1983 by Gonzalez et al. The host was reported by the authors as *Praomys* sp., which has since been restricted to *P. jacksoni* by PETERS (1997). The rodents were identified based on data in the literature, most notably ROSEVEAR's (1969) classic *Rodents of West Africa*, as well as data from PETTER (1977) and HUBERT et al. (1983).

Praomys, described by Oldfield Thomas in 1915, is another very problematic genus like *Mastomys*. *Praomys* is hypothesized to be closely allied to *Mastomys*, which latter genus has at various times been included within *Praomys* (e.g., DAVIS 1965; MISONNE 1974). In addition, at least one species formerly included at various times in *Praomys* and *Myomys* (*P. albipes*), has been excised from *Praomys* and placed in the Ethiopian endemic genus *Stenocephalemys* (LAVRACHENKO et al. 1999; these authors' data suggest that species limits in *Stenocephalemys* are problematic). *P. jacksoni* has variously been considered conspecific with *P. tullbergi*; however, as reviewed by VAN DER STRAETEN and DIETERLEN (1987), *P. jacksoni* was excised from *P. tullbergi*. Although antibodies to Mobala have been found in humans as well as nonhuman mammals in the Central African Republic (GEORGES et al. 1985), there does not appear to be any human disease caused by this virus.

The problems associated with the taxonomy of *Praomys* are as monumental as those described in the foregoing section on *Mastomys*; MUSSER and CARLETON (1993: p 642) summarize the situation as follows: "Not only do the contents of *Praomys* require careful systematic revision, but its phylogenetic relationships relative to *Mastomys*, *Myomys*, and *Hylomyscus* also needs resolution through revisionary studies". We further note that *P. jacksoni*, like most of the *Mastomys* species and, indeed, many of the remaining species of *Praomys*, likely is a composite that only will be defined through careful studies including morphology, karyology, and molecular data.

2.1.3 Ippy

Ippy virus first was described by Digoutte in 1970. However, it was not until 1985 that Swanepoel et al. identified Ippy as a virus in the Lassa fever group, closely followed by MEUNIER et al. (1985) who further cemented the association of Ippy as a LCM–LAS group virus. The host species was listed by DIGOUTTE (1970) as *Arvicanthis* sp. from the Central African Republic. However, the Institut Pasteur CRORA database lists as additional hosts the African murid rodents *Lemniscomys striatus*, *Praomys* sp., and *Mastomys* sp. Furthermore, of the 22 isolates (all from the Central African Republic), 16 are from *Praomys*. Thus, although the initial isolate was from *Arvicanthis*, the primary host is more likely *Praomys*. Only BISHOP (1990) lists *Praomys* as a potential host, citing unpublished data from Digoutte (likely data similar to that presently available in the Pasteur Institute's CRORA database). Other reviewers of arenaviruses (McCORMICK 1990: p 1246; PETERS 1997: p 974) all restrict Ippy to *Arvicanthis*. Data derived from micro-compliment fixation (as well as Digoutte, personal communication) are supportive of their being at least two distinct strains of Ippy virus which are not highly cross-reactive; it is possible that one of these is in *Arvicanthis*, while the other is from *Praomys*. Having discussed *Praomys* above (Mobala), we will restrict ourselves herein to *Arvicanthis*.

As currently understood (MUSSER and CARLETON 1993), *Arvicanthis* is comprised of five species, only one of which, *A. niloticus*, is distributed throughout the Central African Republic; however, there have been at least 44 named species in the genus (CAPANNA et al. 1996). In their review of murids, MUSSER and CARLETON (1993) further pointed out that more than one species likely is included in what is construed as *A. niloticus*. Ample chromosomal data exist in support of this hypothesis: for example, at least four distinct diploid numbers, with seven fundamental numbers (seven distinct karyotypes) have been documented within *A. niloticus*, some of which undoubtedly form panmictic populations, but others of which definitely cannot interbreed and therefore constitute distinct species (CAPANNA et al. 1996; CAPANNA and CIVITELLI 1988; CIVITELLI et al. 1995; GRANJON et al. 1992; MATTHEY 1965; VIEGAS-PEQUIGNOT et al. 1983; VOLOBOUEV et al. 1988).

Molecular data derived from sequences of the mitochondrial cytochrome *b* gene (DUCROZ et al. 1998) support the more extreme view of *Arvicanthis* as a more speciose genus than currently understood, with perhaps an additional 11 undescribed species. Their data suggest that the status *A. niloticus* as a single, unique species is not concordant with biological reality. We reanalyzed their sequence data in order to assess branch lengths among taxa. The results of our somewhat cursory analyses are not fully concordant with theirs, but we feel that the *A. niloticus* they sampled is best divided into at least three species: one sampled in Sénégal, one sampled in Niger, and one sampled in Egypt; the latter would be the sister species to *A. dembeensis*, which likely is a valid species, MUSSER and CARLTON (1993) and DUCROZ et al. (1998) notwithstanding: MUSSER and CARLETON (1993) relegate *A. dembeensis* to subspecific status within *A. niloticus*, albeit restricted to Ethiopia. DUCROZ et al. (1998) consider that the genetic divergence between *A. dembeensis* and *A. niloticus* does not warrant recognition of the former, however, that genetic divergence is equal to that between other sister species in *Arvicanthis*, suggesting that *A. dembeensis* is in fact a valid, species-level taxon. At very least, further studies are indicated to definitively clarify this question.

2.1.4 Mopeia

Two strains of Mopeia have been described: Mopeia Mozambique (WULFF et al. 1977) and Mopeia Zimbabwe (JOHNSON et al. 1981). Although antibodies have been detected in humans (K.M. Johnson, unpublished data), there is no evidence of pathogenicity to humans. As to reservoirs of MOP, WULFF et al. (1977) merely present *M. natalensis* as the mammal host species for the Mozambique strain. JOHNSON et al. (1981) brought captured and field-identified *M. natalensis* specimens back to the laboratory where further identifications (and confirmation) were undertaken based on electrophoresis of hemoglobin proteins after GREEN et al. (1978). SWANEPOEL (2001) reported that the WULFF et al. (1977) specimens were supplied in 1972 by a "long since retired" member of the South African National Institute for Virology; no tissues for these animals can currently be found, although sera may exist (SWANEPOEL 2001). As for the animals reported in JOHNSON et al. (1981), these were supplied by Paul Taylor of the Zimbabwe Department of Health Blair Laboratory. SWANEPOEL (2001) indicates that the specimens upon which the research of JOHNSON et al. (1981) was based may be at the National Museum in Harare, Zimbabwe. Our efforts to locate them there have come to naught.

We have already stressed above (see Sect. 2.1.1) the uncertainties regarding the taxonomic identifications of animals in the genus *Mastomys*, most specifically *M. natalensis*. In the case of specimens hosting Mopeia, some were identified using biochemical techniques; however, even these identifications were undertaken without the benefit of comparisons to type material, that is to say, the "name-bearing" specimen upon which the name *M. natalensis* is based. Accordingly, even these identifications remain suspect until a thorough review of *Mastomys* and *Praomys* is undertaken, leading to a clear understanding of species boundaries in this complex group.

2.1.5 Lymphocytic Choriomeningitis

Identification of lymphocytic choriomeningitis as a viral disease (LCM) was first done by Charles Armstrong and R.D. Lillie, of the US Public Health Service, in 1934 and further detailed by Armstrong and Dickens in 1935. The disease as such had previously been thoroughly described by Arvid Wallgren in 1924. WALLGREN (1924) noted, however, that cases likely referable to LCM were described in the literature as early as 1910, but none prior to 1906 (the nature of his method of citing precludes our investigation of the 1910 report). Apparently, identification of the disease as such, albeit not its viral association, was due to epidemics in France (1910–1913) and Scandinavia (1920–1923). Association of LCM with a mammal reservoir was reported soon thereafter: TRAUB (1935, 1936a,b) reported that LCM circulated in white laboratory mice. ARMSTRONG and SWEET (1939) first incriminated wild (i.e., peridomestic) *Mus musculus* as the reservoir species of LCM.

Although the genus *Mus* itself contains numerous species of nebulous validity, *Mus musculus* had previously been thought to be the one Old World host of an arenavirus wherein little if any taxonomic uncertainty exists. However, there in fact do remain substantive gaps in our knowledge of these organisms (BOURSOT et al. 1993) which may have a vital impact on the epidemiology of LCM: over 150 scientific names have been used for house mice (133 listed in BERRY and BRONSON 1992; more complete listing in Appendix I of MARSHALL 1998). The current scientific name of the house mouse, *Mus musculus*, is ascribable to LINNAEUS (1758). As with many of the species Linnaeus named, there is no holotype (vide MARSHALL 1977), that is to say, no specimen is available for examination and comparison as a basis for the nomenclature and taxonomy of *Mus musculus*. Although the genus *Mus* is clearly Asian in origin, *M. musculus* occurs worldwide, with a range habitually human abetted. The name *M. musculus*, as described by Linnaeus, refers to the taxon currently found in Sweden: *M. m. musculus*. Other former subspecies within *M. musculus* have been excised over time from that taxon, as the biological reality of their isolation has led to their recognition as a species distinct from *M. musculus*. Accordingly, our most recent understanding of the house mouse (BOURSOT et al. 1993; MARSHALL 1998) clearly indicates that the house mouse is a complex composed of at least three distinct valid species: *M. castaneus*, *M. domesticus*, and *M. musculus*.

The nominate subspecies of *M. musculus*, *Mus m. musculus*, ranges from far east Asia (Chukotskiy Peninsula) throughout Asia north of the Himalayas and Caucasus, to Central Europe, where it meets and hybridizes along a narrow band (30–40km) with *M. domesticus* (BOURSOT et al. 1993), the other potential host of LCM. *Mus domesticus* occurs in Western Europe, Africa, and the Middle East, including the Arabian Peninsula, to a band between the Persian Gulf and the Caspian Sea. The Caucasus forms the boundary between *M. musculus* and *M. domesticus* in this region, thereby affording little opportunity for hybridization. A broader zone of overlap, with some hybridization, exists in Asia between *M. musculus* and *M. castaneus*. This region of overlap and potential hybridization extends from the Sea of Okhotsk (Udskaya Guba, in Khabarovsk, Russia) to approximately the Tibetan Plateau (near the type locality for *M. m. gansuensis*). Nominally, *M. m. musculus* only occurs from the zone of hybridization in Central Europe (Denmark, then Mecklenburger Bucht in NE Germany, south along the Elbe and Danube, through eastern Austria, central Slovenia, interior Croatia and Bosnia-Herzegovina, and through Yugoslavia perhaps as far south as Macedonia to Bulgaria and the Black Sea; figured in BOURSOT et al. 1993 and MARSHALL 1998) to the Ural Mountains in the East. East of the Urals, *M. m. wagneri* is found.

Given that the predominant species in Western Europe is *M. domesticus*, we suspect that the host of LCM is, therefore, *M. domesticus*. Several lines of evidence point to that trend. In terms of indirect inference, most human immigration into North America historically has been from Western Europe. One might assume, therefore, that ships leaving western European ports would be occupied with the locally predominant species of mouse, that is: *M. domesticus*.

In addition, most (but not all) of the stocks of laboratory mice apparently are derived from *M. domesticus* (BOURSOT et al. 1993); it is possible, however, that these laboratory strains may all have been derived from *M. domesticus*, but from distinct geographic regions within the range of the species, hence from distinct demes, or gene pools, constituting the species. Given that no tests have been carried out on the susceptibility and transmission dynamics of LCM in wild *M. domesticus*, and that *Mus* species are notoriously variable at the molecular and morphological levels, different laboratory mouse strains with different origins even within a single species (be it *M. domesticus* or *M. musculus*) may very well display differing degrees of resistance, infectivity, and other host characteristics to LCM. The initial assessments by ARMSTRONG and LILLIE (1934) and TRAUB (1935) of the presence of a virus during some epidemics were undertaken post hoc the epidemic in laboratory strains of *Mus* species. None of these mouse specimens have been archived for subsequent identification, but all were susceptible to varying degrees. No figures are available in ARMSTRONG and LILLIE (1934); however, TRAUB (1935) reported a 13%–40% fatality rate in laboratory mice (intracerebral inoculation), while ARMSTRONG and SWEET (1939) reported a 100% fatality rate in mice also i.c. inoculated from a single infected mouse.

We point out as a cautionary note that certain populations of house mouse in the USA may indeed have a more likely origin in *M. musculus*, specifically *M. m. wagneri*. The tumbleweed, or Russian thistle (*Salsola* sp., generally *S. tragus* or *S. ibirica* or *S. kali*) has its origin in the Russian steppes east of the Urals. The invasion of *Salsola* is said to have been due to contaminated flax seeds brought to the USA (South Dakota) by Mennonite farmers (TELLMAN 1997), as well as in grain shipments from Russia. Given the current range of *Salsola* in Canada, México, and the USA, it would not be implausible to hypothesize that many populations of *Mus* in central and southwestern USA are derived not from *M. domesticus* (likely present in either coast), but rather from *M. m. wagneri* imported along with Russian grain shipments. Furthermore (and most critically), the epidemic of 1920–1923 took place in Scandinavia, where only *M. musculus* occurs. The 1910–1913 epidemic in France could have been due to either species, as both co-occur in parts of France.

Criteria to distinguish among the various species and subspecies have been established by Orsini et al. (1983), Gerasimov et al. (1990), Macholan (1996a,b), and most particularly Marshall (1998). The latter author particularly mentions (among pointed external differences) the difference in tail length between *M. domesticus* and *M. musculus*, and the difference in color of the underparts: white or whitish in *M. musculus* in contrast to the darker brownish-gray in *M. d. domesticus* (other subspecies of *M. domesticus* may have varying degrees of gray venter: from the brownish-gray of *M. d. domesticus*, through "sullied white" for Northern Mediterranean *M. d. brevirostris*, to white with gray bases in the Himalayan *M. d. humorous*, to the pure white North African, Middle Eastern, and Pakistani and Western Indian *M. d. praetextus*). Most populations of mice that we have observed in North America have had the gray or brown-gray venter characteristic of *M. d. domesticus*; careful and meticulous analysis nevertheless remains the order of the day. We have not touched upon the potential for *"bactrianus"* (Iran through India south of the Himalayas to Burma) being a valid species as well: Marshall (1998) considered *bactrianus* a synonym of *praetextus*, itself a subspecies of *M. domesticus*. However, genetic data from Bonhomme et al. (1984) indicate that it is almost certainly a distinct species, as *bactrianus* or *praetextus*, the latter being the oldest available name for the taxon.

From the foregoing discussion, it is clear that at present we simply do not nor cannot know what biological species of *Mus* constitutes the natural host of LCM. Association of an ongoing incidence of LCM to an indubitably identified host species is critical if we are to understand the dynamics of the disease. Accordingly, we recommend that specimens of *Mus* captured and tested in the course of LCM investigations should be deposited in museums (public, university, governmental, or private) and be identified by an expert in rodent taxonomy.

2.2 New World Arenaviruses

Members of this group are also known as members of the Tacaribe complex. This group includes the following viruses: Tacaribe (TCR), Junín (JUN), Machupo (MAC), Amaparí (AMA), Paraná (PAR), Tamiami (TAM), Latino (LAT), Pichindé (PIC), Flexal (FLE), Oliveros (OLV), Sabiá (SAB), Guanarito (GUA), Whitewater Arroyo (WWA), and Pirital (PIR), and Cupixi (CPX) (Tesh et al. 1999). One other virus (Pampa virus) is considered to be a strain of Oliveros (C.J. Peters, personal communication) and has as a putative reservoir an unrecognized species of *Bolomys* (Lozano et al. 1997). Consequently, we did not consider it further.

2.2.1 Tacaribe Virus

This virus was originally isolated by Downs et al. (1963) from tissues and salivary glands of two species of bats (*Artibeus lituratus palmarum* and *A. jamaicensis trinitatis*) captured between March 1956 and December 1958. Virus isolation from a mixed pool of mosquitoes collected in September 1956 was also reported.

No further isolation of virus from mosquito pools has been successful since although more than a million mosquitoes were processed in the ensuing 6 years; it is therefore unlikely that mosquitoes were ever involved in the circulation of Tacaribe.

The bat species reported by DOWNS et al. (1963) were identified by one of the most preeminent mammalogists of the first half of the century – G.G. Goodwin – who at the time was Associate Curator of Mammals at the American Museum of Natural History (AMNH). Voucher specimen numbers were reported in the original paper, and the voucher specimens are deposited in the collection of the Department of Mammalogy of that museum. In their monographic treatment of the bats of Trinidad and Tobago, GOODWIN and GREENHALL (1961) commented on the new viral strain isolated from these species.

The two bat subspecies *A. l. palmarum* and *A. j. trinitatis* are endemic to Trinidad and Tobago. The species *A. lituratus* and *A. jamaicensis*, however, range much more broadly: *A. jamaicensis* is distributed from Sinaloa and Tamaulipas (México) to Ecuador, Venezuela, the Greater and Lesser Antilles, and Trinidad and Tobago. *A. lituratus* ranges from Sinaloa and Tamaulipas (México) into southern Brazil, northern Argentina, and Bolivia. This species is also known from islands off the coast of South America (Trinidad and Tobago), the southern Lesser Antilles, and the Tres Marías Islands (KOOPMAN 1993; WILSON 1991) off the Pacific coast of México.

These two species are among the most common bats of the tropical environments they inhabit. Primarily frugivores, they feed principally on fruits of trees of the genus *Ficus* (HANDLEY et al. 1991). Both species exhibit a seasonal pattern in the timing of reproduction, which – at least in the case *of A. jamaicensis* – is highly coincident with the maximum abundance of fruit (WILSON 1979). GOODWIN and GREENHALL (1961) reported that both species shared roosting sites and dipteran streblid ectoparasites (*Pterellipis aranea*), as well as food items and general habits.

The fact that Tacaribe is the only arenavirus whose putative mammal host is not a rodent has provoked skepticism in the scientific community in light of recent works (e.g., BOWEN et al. 1997; MILLS et al. 1997) pointing to an appreciable degree of rodent–arenavirus co-evolution. At present, however, and based on the available evidence, Tacaribe remains known only from the aforementioned two species of bats. This is further supported by the fact that the virus was isolated from 11 animals collected over a span of 3 years (1956–1958), demonstrating that the virus was circulating in fruit-bats at least over that span of time.

Bats of the genera *Artibeus* and *Desmodus* infected with Tacaribe by inoculation in a laboratory setting did not circulate virus, and detectable antibodies were shown only in 1 of 39 bats studied (DOWNS et al. 1963). To our knowledge, no new attempts to isolate Tacaribe virus from other potential reservoirs have been undertaken since the original description of the virus in 1963.

2.2.2 Junín Virus

Junín virus, the etiological agent of Argentine hemorrhagic fever (AHF), has most commonly been isolated from the organs and body fluids of three species of rodents: *Calomys musculinus*, *C. laucha*, and *Akodon azarae*. In addition, the virus has been isolated from other rodent species such as *Mus musculus* (SABATTINI et al. 1977) and *Oligoryzomys flavescens* (MILLS et al. 1991a). The vesper mouse, *Calomys musculinus*, is considered the primary reservoir because it was the most commonly trapped rodent in the endemic area, and because persistent viremia and virus shedding via saliva was found both in naturally and laboratory-infected animals (CARBALLAL et al. 1986). Furthermore, in long-term studies of rodent populations in the greater risk area of AFH, MILLS et al. (1991a) found that *C. musculinus* comprised the bulk of the antigen-positive trapped rodents, thus confirming this species as the principal reservoir. In another study, (MILLS et al. 1992a) found 37 of 41 antigen-positive captures were individuals of *C. musculinus*, thereby lending support to the hypothesis that this species is the principal reservoir of JUN. Additional support comes from MILLS et al. (1994), who found that 89% of JUN-seropositive animals in two mark-recapture grids in the epidemic area of AHF were *C. musculinus*.

The type locality of *C. musculinus* is Jujuy, Province of Jujuy, Argentina, at an elevation of 1,200m, nearly 700 miles north of the area of distribution of AHF. The type specimen is British Museum (Natural History) number BMNH 20.1.7.46; it remains housed at the Natural History Museum in London. *C. musculinus* can be distinguished from all other species of the genus on the basis of the following characters: body size moderate (total length including tail of adults generally 155–200mm); tail long, equal to or slightly longer than head and body length; dorsum sandy brown, frequently lined with black hairs, venter white, hairs gray at base; skull medium in size, greatest length of skull in adults generally 22–26mm; auditory bullæ slightly inflated; maxillary toothrow moderately long (3.4–3.8mm; OLDS 1988).

As currently understood, this species ranges widely across South America, from central Bolivia at moderate to high elevations in the eastern slopes of the Andes (ANDERSON 1997), through the lowlands of central Argentina (in Chubut Province), to western Paraguay and possibly into Central Brazil. Obviously, such a variation in elevation and latitude encompasses a large number of habitats ranging from mesothermic valleys in southern Bolivia to subhumid tropical Chacoan forest in Paraguay and potentially Brazil.

MILLS et al. (1991b) have summarized some ecological information for *C. musculinus* near to or in the endo-epidemic zone of AHF. These authors found *C. musculinus* abundant in agricultural areas, especially corn and wheat fields, although linear habitats (fencerows, roadsides, and railroads) were also commonly occupied. Population densities for this species were described as relatively high in the spring and remaining so through the summer and early autumn from November to April (MILLS et al. 1991b). In another study, MILLS et al. (1992a) found that most *C. musculinus* that had tested positive for JUN antigen were statistically associated with linear habitats (roadsides and fence lines). Similar results were found by ELLIS et al. (1997), albeit contrasting with the results of BUSCH et al. (1997), who suggested that *C. musculinus* does not show habitat preference in any season, overlapping with both *C. laucha* and *Akodan azarae* in fields and linear habitats.

C. musculinus also appears to be relatively common in other habitats. For example, GONNET and OJEDA (1998) found this species to be one of the two most dominant species in the Andean foothills of the Monte Desert of Argentina. In that study, *C. musculinus* preferred grassy microhabitats within the most complex habitat (or undisturbed thicket). YAHNKE (1999) found that in the Paraguayan Chaco, *C. musculinus* occupied several habitats but showed a preference for microhabitats with low herbs and grassy vegetation.

The systematics of this species (and species-group) remains in need of a comprehensive revision. Our own work (SALAZAR-BRAVO et al. 2001) has shown that this species is a member of the "mountain clade" of the genus and closely related *to C. lepidus* and *C. sorellus*. What is not yet clear is whether more than one biological species is present in what we now understand as the singular *C. musculinus*. The species has been characterized chromosomally across a wide range of habitats and appears to present a relatively conserved karyotype throughout it range. The diploid chromosome number $2n = 38$ has been found in specimens from Córdoba and Buenos Aires provinces (Argentina). However, some chromosomal polymorphism has been detected, both in the morphology of the autosomes, as well as in the size and position of the centromere in the Y chromosome (CICCIOLI 1991; CICCIOLI and POGGIO 1993; LISANTI et al. 1996; MASSOIA et al. 1968). As a result, the fundamental number (FN) varies from 48 (MASSOIA et al. 1968) to 56 (LISANTI et al. 1996; CICCIOLI 1991). OLDS (1988) defined *C. musculinus* as present only in northwestern Argentina and southern Bolivia, and considered *C. murillus* a distinct species. However, in her concluding remarks (OLDS 1988: p 149), she acknowledged the potential for conspecificity of *C. musculinus* and *C. murillus*. SALAZAR-BRAVO et al. (2001) found no support for the recognition of *C. murillus*, although several specimens included in their analyses came from the province of Buenos Aires, and one from near the type locality of *C. murillus* (environs of La Plata).

2.2.3 Machupo Virus

Machupo virus, the etiological agent of Bolivian hemorrhagic fever (BHF), was isolated from the spleen, brain, and blood of a rodent species: *Calomys* cf. *callosus* (KUNS 1965; JOHNSON et al. 1966). WEBB et al. (1967) reported that 4 or 5 specimens of *Proechimys brevicauda* from the environs of San Joaquín also tested positive for neutralizing antibodies; this was the area of the endo-epidemic of BHF in 1963. Subsequent to these isolations, several attempts to isolate Machupo virus from *P. brevicauda* failed (JOHNSON et al. 1966; WEBB et al. 1975). This fact points to spill-over from *Calomys* as a contributing factor for the presence of Machupo in *Proechimys*.

The taxonomic status of *C.* cf. *callosus* remains nebulous (Salazar-Bravo et al., in preparation), but it now appears evident that this is a species separate from, yet morphologically similar to, *C. callosus* (*sensu stricto*). Following phylogenetic analysis based on genetic data (cytochrome *b* gene sequence of mitochondrial DNA), these authors suggested that *Calomys* spp. ex Beni (reservoir of MAC) is most closely related to *C. fecundus*, which is common to abundant in intermediate elevations (500–2,800m) on the eastern flank of the Andes in southern Bolivia and northern Argentina.

The distribution of *C.* cf. *callosus* appears to match closely the distribution of savannas in the northeastern Bolivian department of El Beni. These savanna plains lie east of the Andes in the Amazon basin and have a mean elevation of about 200m. The prevailing vegetation type "is that of a grassland broken occasionally with 'islands' of forest and laced with tree-lined rivers and streams" (KUNS 1965). A complete analysis of the vegetation, geography, and overview of the ecology of the savannas in northeastern Bolivia was presented in HANAGARTH (1993). The west-ernmost record of *C.* cf. *callosus.* is near the town of Reyes (PATTERSON 1992) on the border between Beni and La Paz departments (Bolivia). Although most cases of BHF have been reported from only a handful of localities, *C.* cf. *callosus* has been collected in other areas of the savannas where BHF is endemic.

Little is known or published about the ecology of this species. KUNS (1965) reported *C.* cf. *callosus* as a pastoral species often collected in grasslands and along forest edges around the town of San Joaquín. He also remarked on the comen-salism of this species with humans, as many individuals were trapped in and around houses. After the rodent control program was initiated in San Joaquín, almost 2,880 *C.* cf. *callosus* were recovered from the village, representing 96% of all rodents captured (KUNS 1965).

JUSTINES and JOHNSON (1970) summarized several years of data on laboratory rearing of this species. The colony, initiated with six animals, was still thriving after 5 years. Their report indicated that breeding was continuous throughout the year. Sexual maturity was attained at about 8 weeks, estrous cycle was 6 days, and gestation period was estimated as 21 days. Average litter size was approximately six, with high weaning ratios (ca. 97%).

2.2.4 Amaparí and Cupixi Virus

This arenavirus was originally isolated by PINHEIRO et al. (1966) from pools of tissues (liver, spleen, kidneys, and hearts) from spiny mice (*Neacomys guianae*), the rice rat (*Oryzomys* cf. *goeldi*), and a pool of mites (*n* = 199) combed from two infected *Oryzomys*. As suggested by BOWEN et al. (1998) it is likely that a second arenavirus (Cupixi) might have been responsible for the infection in *Oryzomys*, therefore here we follow their advice and treat Amapari as restricted to *Neacomys guianae*. The prototype strain of Amapari was isolated from an individual spiny mouse captured on 8 July 1964, near Serra do Navio in the northeastern Brazilian State of Amapa. Viruses were isolated only from one of seven animals tested. Later, PINHEIRO et al. (1977) reported on a long-term study during which the virus was isolated at the same locality from 145 *Neacomys* over a period of 7 years.

The spiny mouse (*Neacomys guianae*) is restricted to rainforest regions ranging throughout the Guianas and adjacent parts of northern Brazil, north of the Amazon and east of the Rio Negro (HUSSON 1978; EISENBERG and REDFORD 1999). As MUSSER and CARLETON (1993) stated, "traits for species recognition and distributional limits in this genus are poorly delineated". Furthermore, PATTON et al. (2000) showed levels of diversity in this genus that had previously been un-recognized. *Neacomys guianae* is recognized by a smaller size and darker coloration (ELLERMAN 1941; GYLDENSTOLPE 1932) compared with other species in the genus. Little is known of the ecology of this species. HUSSON (1978) reported that this species preferred dense, humid forests, and EMMONS and FEER (1999) reported that the animals favor areas of dense ground cover, travelling on the ground or on logs or vines near the ground. GUILLOTIN (1982) working in Guiana trapped more spiny mice between March and May in disturbed sites than in July and August in pristine forest. EMMONS and FEER (1999) reported that *N. guianae* is nocturnal, terrestrial, and solitary, and that the diet of this species was 60% insects and 40% fruit, seeds, and other plant material.

In contrast, successful isolation of an Arenavirus was accomplished from three individuals of *Oryzomys* cf. *goeldi* trapped between December 1964 and January 1965 at Sierra de Navio. Later, PINHEIRO et al. (1977) reported on a long-term study during which the virus was isolated at the same locality from 127 *Oryzomys*. It has been suggested by BOWEN et al. (1998) that this arenavirus is in fact different from Amapari and suggested the name Cupixi for it.

The species of *Oryzomys* implicated as a reservoir of Amaparí originally was identified as *O. goeldi*, although named *O. capito* in PINHEIRO et al. (1977). This incongruence is not actually so. The systematic knowledge of the genus *Oryzomys* has advanced greatly with recent work (e.g., MUSSER et al. 1998; Voss and CARLETON 1993; WEKSLER et al. 1999; BONVICINO and MARTINS 2001; PATTON et al. 2000). Recently, MUSSER et al. (1998) considered the two species synonymous with *O. megacephalus*. We note that differences in DNA sequence (PATTON et al. 1996, 2000; BONVICINO and MARTINS 2001) as well as chromosomal characters (summarized in MUSSER et al. 1998, Table 13) for geographic groups of populations (eastern vs. western Amazonian) point to the differentiation of *O. megacephalus* and *O. perennensis*, with *O. megacephalus* being restricted to eastern Amazonia.

But the problem with the identification of the reservoir of Cupixi does not end there. Sympatry and syntopy among three species of *Oryzomys* with similar mor-phological characteristics has been documented at Serra do Navio and the imme-diate area: *O. yunganus*, *O. megacephalus*, and *O. macconnelli* (cf. MUSSER et al. 1998). In the original publication describing Amaparí (PINHEIRO et al. 1966), only one species of *Oryzomys* was mentioned: *O. goeldi*. In PINHEIRO et al. (1977), two species were implicated: *O. capito* and *O. macconnelli*. If we accept the current taxonomy, both *O. capito* and *O. goeldi* are junior synonyms of *O. megacephalus*, and distinct from *O. yunganus*, a species also documented in the area. From which of these two species of *Oryzomys* was the virus isolated? Recent revisionary work on this group could easily allow us to answer that question. Unfortunately, we do not know which individual animals were the source of the virus. If we take the PINHEIRO et al. (1977) report at face value, the updated species name of the res-ervoir of Amaparí should be *O. megacephalus* – a course of action followed herein because this species appears to be more abundant at that locality – cf. MUSSER et al. (1998). We note, however, that further inquiry into the viral laboratory records may shed light on the positive identity of the mammal reservoir species.

The species *O. megacephalus* is broadly distributed and "occurs primarily in tropical evergreen rainforest formations (which include riverine or gallery forest in the Brazilian Cerrado) in the Orinoco basin in southern Venezuela, the Guiana Region (including the tepuis of eastern Venezuela), the island of Trinidad, and drainage basin of the Amazon River" (MUSSER et al. 1998).

The ecology of this species has been extensively studied (e.g., MARES et al. 1989; ALHO and PEREIRA 1985; LACHER et al. 1989; GUILLOTIN 1982). One study (GUILLOTIN 1982) reported this species (under the name *Oryzomys capito velutinus*) as nocturnal, terrestrial, found only in climax forest (not in secondary growth), and fairly abundant. She reported this species as the most abundant muroid rodent in the area.

2.2.5 Paraná Virus

WEBB et al. (1970) isolated this arenavirus from the kidneys of rodents collected in southern Paraguay, in the environs of the town of San Francisco, in the Department of Misiones. The virus was isolated from three specimens (of four collected) of *Oryzomys buccinatus*. No catalogue or accession numbers are presented in the paper, although it is likely that at least some of the specimens collected are now at the US National Museum (WEBB et al. 1970: p 380).

MUSSER et al. (1998) discussed the systematics and nomenclatural history of *O. buccinatus*, concluding that the name *O. angouya* has priority and should be used rather than *O. buccinatus*. According to these authors, the species *O. angouya* also includes *O. ratticeps*. Thus, the reservoir species of Paraná virus, as currently understood, is distributed from eastern Paraguay and northeastern Argentina to southeastern Brazil (MUSSER et al. 1998; REDFORD and EISENBERG 1992).

Not much has been published on the ecology of this species, but MYERS (1982) found it in the interface between forest and secondary vegetation. OLMOS (1991) during a 13-month capture–recapture study in the Atlantic forest in southern São Paulo found *O. ratticeps* in a 0.5-ha trapping-grid established within an old second growth forest. He also reported this species as terrestrial, but with the ability to climb well and exploit arboreal vegetation. The capture pattern suggested a general decrease in numbers towards the end of the year; reproduction appeared to occur outside winter (May–August).

2.2.6 Tamiami Virus

CALISHER et al. (1970) originally described this virus by isolating it from the heart tissue of an adult hispid cotton rat (*Sigmodon hispidus*) collected 5 January 1965 from Mahogany Hammock (latitude 26°17′N, longitude 81°05′W), Everglades National Park, Florida, USA. Further isolations were made from cotton rats collected just north of the park in or near the Big Cypress Seminole Indian Reservation in January 1964 and 1965. In addition, WELLINGS et al. (1972) reported isolation of Tamiami virus from rice rats (*Oryzomys palustris*), and BIGLER et al. (1975) reported antibodies in 4 of 27 rice rats (*O. palustris*) sampled from throughout Florida. Nevertheless, hispid cotton rats, *S. hispidus*, are considered the primary rodent host (cf. also KOSOY et al. 1996).

Cotton rats are distributed from about latitude 41° north (in Iowa and Nebraska) throughout most of the southern, southeastern, and southwestern USA, through Mexico and Central America, to northern South America. HALL (1981) mapped the ranges of all recognized subspecies within the taxon in his monumental work on North American mammals. Based on his maps, the specimens collected by CALISHER et al. (1970) are referable to the subspecies *S. hispidus spadicipygus*, originally described from Cape Sable, Florida, some 50miles southwest of the locality whence Tamiami virus was described (Mahogany Hammock).

The systematics of *Sigmodon* has received renewed attention since the early 1990s. Voss (1992), in reviewing the South American species of the genus, suggested that *S. hispidus* formed a morphologically cohesive group (including North American representatives in his study for comparison as well); but he also suggested that other methods of analysis be brought to bear to the study of this species. PEPPERS and BRADLEY (2000) analyzed several populations of hispid cotton rats from throughout the range of the species using sequence data from the cytochrome *b* gene. Their analyses showed that within the taxa sampled, at least three potential groups of species constituted the nominal "hispid group": *S. hispidus*, *S. toltecus*, and *S. hirsutus*. These authors confirmed the genetic identity of *spadicipygus* as a subspecies of *S. hispidus*, thus reinforcing the hypothesis that *S. hispidus* (*sensu stricto*) is the primary reservoir species of Tamiami.

The ecology of *S. hispidus* has been thoroughly studied since the pioneering work of Bangs (BANGS 1898). A summary of the ecological and life history aspects of the species is presented in CAMERON and SPENCER (1981). Only reports associated with *S. hispidus* (*s.s.*) are included herein.

S. hispidus exhibits bimodal population fluctuations annually in Texas and Georgia, with maximum densities occurring in the autumn and secondary peaks in the spring. Densities fluctuate depending on the study, with records of 25 animals/ha in Florida and 69/ha in Georgia to 10/ha and 8/ha at the low end, respectively. In the northern part of the range (Kansas), population densities were unimodal, with peaks in the autumn (20/ha) and lows in the spring (minimum densities 0.02/ha). Individual populations for which expectations of further life (average duration of local residence for all individuals) have been calculated indicate an average of 2 months for both sexes with longest periods of residence at 9.5 months (average for both sexes). This species prefers habitat dominated by grasses, mixed grass, and shrubs, or old fields in early stages to secondary succession. The diet is almost restricted to grasses but on occasion may include insects. Average home ranges for adults is 0.39ha for males and 0.22ha for females, although females have exclusive home ranges. Dispersal of *S. hispidus* is positively correlated with density, and the sex ratio and age structure of dispersers were similar to those of the source population. Males move longer distances within a day than females (17m vs. 6.6m on average), and reproductive males tend to move longer distances than nonreproductive males. Cotton rats are active at all hours of the day and night in coastal Texas, with two peaks of activity identified around 0900 and 1900 hours. Field and laboratory studies showed that *S. hispidus* are practically inactive between 2300 and 0500 hours. Although mostly ground-dwellers, they have also been caught along vines up to 2.7m above ground. *S. hispidus* is a solitary species as males build prolonged social contact (up to several days) only with females (depending on their reproductive status). This social contact is accompanied by frequent physical contact (i.e., sleeping, huddling, and mutual grooming), but males always remain dominant over females in these pairs.

2.2.7 Latino Virus

This virus has not been properly described, or at least not to the standards set in descriptions of remaining arenaviruses. Most of what has been recorded on the biology and reservoir of this virus was presented in WEBB et al. (1973). Later, WEBB et al. (1975) added some information on the subject. WEBB et al. (1973: p 315) referred to a paper to be published shortly thereafter where they intended to fully describe Latino virus; to our knowledge, that paper was never published. For our purposes however, WEBB et al. (1973) contains enough information on the rodent reservoir's geographic origin and putative identification.

Animals from localities in eastern Bolivia (towns of Juan Latino, San Ignacio) and neighboring Brazil (Corumbá) yielded 18 strains of Latino virus. It is unknown how many animals were tested or what proportion of all animals tested were positive. In the experimental work upon which these authors subsequently reported, a colony was founded with two breeding pairs captured in the town of Juan Latino (Santa Cruz Dept., Bolivia). These animals were free of virus as they were killed and tested after the second generation of breeders had matured.

WEBB et al. (1973) reported that the animals had been identified to the species level as *Calomys callosus* by Ronald H. Pine, then of the Smithsonian Institution. Chromosomal analysis on these animals was undertaken by Robert J. Baker at Texas Tech University. Some unpublished photographs of the karyotypes were later sent to NANCY OLDS from the American Museum of Natural History in New York, and material based on this work were included in her unpublished PhD dissertation (OLDS 1988). However, Pine (R. Pine, personal communication) was following HERSHKOVITZ (1962) in including within *C. callosus* all medium-sized species of *Calomys* with posteriorly divergent supraorbital regions.

Molecular analyses in our laboratory (Salazar-Bravo et al., in preparation) show that members of this population (and those of the semideciduous forest of southeastern Bolivia, extreme southwestern Brazil, western Paraguay, and northeastern Argentina) cluster outside the clade that includes other well differentiated taxa (e.g., *C. venustus*, *C. fecundus*, *Calomys* spp. ex Beni). This information helps to elucidate the biological properties of the virus-reservoir dynamics described by WEBB et al. (1973).

The proper name for the mammal reservoir species of Latino virus is therefore *C. callosus* (*s.s.*), the oldest name available for this clade. Recently, BONVICINO and ALMEIDA (2000) presented evidence that *C. expulsus* may have been confused in some instances with *C. callosus* in the literature on the ecology of small mammals in central Brazil. Thus, some of the information collated below may include aspects on the ecology of the former. Since most ecological studies fail to secure voucher specimens, it is impossible to confirm the identification of the species in these reports.

Several aspects of the ecology of *C. callosus* have been published. This species is found in thickets at the edge of pastures, ravines, and forest roads in the Pantanal of Brazil (SCHALLER 1983), in Caatinga, Cerrado (MARES et al. 1985, 1989; ENGEL and MELLO 1993; ALHO and PEREIRA 1985; ALHO et al. 1986), but not in Cerrado gallery forest of Brazil (NITIKMAN and MARES 1987; MARES and ERNEST 1995), in second growth habitats in mesic forested areas, such as stream areas, road cuts, old fields, grassy areas, sugar cane fields, and river banks of Chacoan thorn scrub, abandoned fields of Brazil (MARES et al. 1981a), and the Chaco of Paraguay (MYERS 1982). In the northeast of Brazil, KARIMI and PETTER (1976) and MARES et al. (1981b) found this species in piles of dried grass and later stages of oldfield succession in the Caatinga Baixa. *C. callosus* has been reported as rare in abandoned fields and the Caatinga Baixa of Brazil (MARES et al. 1981b); never in large numbers in Caatinga (STREILEIN 1982b), at low density in Pernambuco, Brazil (less than 1.7% of all rodents trapped in the study area in a 4 year period; KARIMI and PETTER 1976), low numbers in the Pantanal of Brazil (SCHALLER 1983), common in the Cerrado of Brazil and in Salta Province, Argentina (ALHO and PEREIRA 1985; ENGEL and MELLO 1993; MARES et al. 1981a).

MELLO (1980) found a population peak of *C. callosus* in July 1975, then another in August to November 1976, in the northern part of the state of Goias, Brazil. Out of a total of 963 captured rodents, individuals of *C. callosus* comprised about 41% (398/963) over 2.5 years; 44.2% were female and 55.8% male. Many of the females were immature. Density has been reported as 3–4 individuals per hectare (ALHO et al. 1986). Home range is about 100–1000m^2 according to ALHO et al. (1986).

The species is nocturnal and feeds on arachnids and seeds, moths, and beetles (KARIMI and PETTER 1976; STREILEIN 1982a). Contradictory reports on the arboreality of this species exist: *C. callosus* has been reported as not appearing to climb, but as an agile, active climber that uses its tail as a climbing aid, showing a tendency toward arboreal activity in the laboratory (STREILEIN 1982b; MARES et al. 1981b). STREILEIN (1982a) also noted that adults were capable of vertical leaps of 0.7–0.8m.

Nests have been described as made of dried grass (KARIMI and PETTER 1976) and as being spherical and made of "finely shredded, interwoven plant material found in depressions hollowed in the ground, camouflaged with twigs and leaves" (ALHO et al. 1986: p 453). Nests are generally above the ground in clumps of grass or in branches of dead trees (MELLO 1984). STREILEIN (1982a) found that nests in the laboratory were spherical, made of finely shredded, interwoven plant material, while those in the field were simple depressions hollowed in the ground 10–15cm deep and wide camouflaged with leaves. He noted that caches of seeds were occasionally found near the nests.

In a laboratory colony in Pernambuco, Brazil, PETTER et al. (1967) found the number of embryos ranged from 1 to 10, the newborn weight was 1.3–2.5g, more males were born than females (1.22:1), the gestation period was 19–22 days, adults weighed 35–45g, eyes opened in 7–8 days, the lower incisors erupted after 6–7 days, and the upper incisors erupted after 7–8 days. The dorsal pelage is gray by the third day and is about 2mm in length. MELLO (1978) reported the average litter size to be 4.5 (range 2–9) and the length of gestation to be 21.8 days, with a range of 20–23 days. The ratio at birth of males to females was 1.05:1. The eyes opened 6–7 days after birth, weaning occurred 15–17 days after birth, and pelage cover was complete on the sixth day.

MELLO (1980) reported gestation to require 21.8 days in the laboratory, intervals between matings to be 30–50 days, and the average number of embryos per litter to be 4.5. Animals were sexually mature at 22–23g, embryos were present in June (8 in a female), September (4 and 2, in two females), October (one female with 4), November (two females, both with 4), January (one female with 3), and April (two females, 4 and 7). She further noted that the reproductive periods were co-incident with the end of the rainy season. The average litter size in field studies in Brazil was 4.4, and the range was 2–8 (STREILEIN 1982a). Reproductive information from his study included a lactating female in September, two lactating females in October, one pregnant and one lactating female in November, two lactating females in February, one lactating female in April, and one female showing no reproductive activity in May. Little is known about the dispersal and population responses to disturbance and seasonal climate changes in this species.

2.2.8 Pichindé Virus

This virus, described by TRAPIDO and SANMARTIN (1971), was isolated from two species of sigmodontine rodents (*Oryzomys albigularis* and *Thomasomys fuscatus*) and from mites and ticks from viremic *O. albigularis*. This latter is considered the reservoir species because Pichindé was isolated from *T. fuscatus* only once and because *O. albigularis* showed the highest seroprevalence: 54 of 271 animals sampled from four different localities were positive for the virus. Interestingly, over a period of 2 years (March 1967 to December 1969), the authors isolated Pichindé several times from pools of mites of the species *Gigantolaelaps inca* and ticks of the species *Ixodes tropicalis* obtained from viremic *O. albigularis*. Moreover, virus isolation was successfully undertaken from a pool of four *I. tropicalis* individuals that had been maintained alive at ambient temperature 5–8 days after being recovered from an *O. albigularis*.

The range of *O. albigularis* as the species is currently understood from a taxonomic perspective (MUSSER and CARLETON 1993) includes the montane forests of north and western Venezuela, easternmost Panamá, Andes of Colombia and Ecuador, to northern Peru. The taxonomy of the species has recently been updated by the works of AGUILERA et al. (1995) and MARQUEZ et al. (2000). However, these two reports are based exclusively on specimens from Venezuela and did not include animals from Ecuador (wherein is the type locality) or from Colombia, where Pichindé was described. In an earlier report (GARDNER and PATTON 1976), animals were karyotyped from the same locality as those that had proven to be virulent in the valley of the Pichindé River. In that report, the karyotype of *O. albigularis* is presented as $2n = 66$, FN = 94. GARDNER and PATTON (1976) correctly argued that until chromosomal information of animals from the type locality is reported, the name *albigularis* likely was applicable to this chromosomal form. TRAPIDO and SANMARTIN (1971) argued that the identification of *O. albigularis* was warranted by the "distinctiveness" of this species. Although their report includes several individual rodent field numbers (e.g., HTC 1338, HTC 1341, etc. – probably Harold Trapido's field numbers) no reference in the paper is made as to where the voucher specimens were sent for identification, or where (and if) those animals are stored now. It is interesting that the more than 1,350 animals entered in their Table 4 are identified to the species level (representing 24 species), a fact implying that the specimens were handled and identified by a professional. It is possible that the specimens ensuing from this work were deposited in the Colección de Mamíferos of the Universidad del Valle.

The ecology of this species has been studied by BARNETT (1999) in Ecuador and by DIAZ DE PASCUAL (1994) and AAGARD (1982) in Venezuela. Ectoparasite associations of this species have been reported by TIMM and ASHE (1987) and ASHE and TIMM (1995). *O. albigularis* is among the largest rodent in the ecosystem in which it occurs (weighing up to 79g, total length of 330mm; BARNETT 1999). In Ecuador, specimens of *O. albigularis* were trapped only in cloud forest, a habitat preference also reported by HANDLEY (1976), ASHE and TIMM (1987), and EISENBERG and REDFORD (1999). The species appears to prefer dense cover. DURANT and DIAZ (1995) reported that this species was at its lowest density during the wet season. Such seasonal fluctuations may explain why it was reported by ZUÑIGA et al. (1983) as being the rarest species in northwest facing montane forest sites between 1,000 and 2,500m while PEFAUR and DIAZ DE PASCUAL (1985) reported *O. albigularis* as the numerically dominant species.

At Monte Zerpa's cloud forest in Mérida (Venezuela), DIAZ DE PASCUAL (1994) trapped *O. albigularis* with seven other species of rodents: *Microryzomys minutus*, *Aepeomys lugens*, *Thomasomys laniger*, *Rhipidomys venustus*, *Chilomys instans*, *Ichthyomys hydrobates*, and *Akodon urichi*. According to this author, *O. albigularis* lives in patchy environments which vary in space and time. Major inter- and intra-annual variation in relative abundance of this species was observed, potentially related to the availability of preferred food items for this species. It was suggested that *O. albigularis* are spatially structured as metapopulations, with food availability being the main factor determining dispersal between demes. AAGARD (1982) reported no significant seasonal differences in captures for this species in Mérida, Venezuela, and at the same time showed that most animals were trapped on the ground. Males were larger and heavier than females independently of season, and males were reproductively active all year round. A breeding peak in the wet season was indicated.

2.2.9 Flexal Virus

Flexal virus was presented in a paper by PINHEIRO et al. (1977) as a new type of arenavirus from a locality 212km S of Itaituba, in the Brazilian state of Pará. The authors made passing mention to the three specimens of *Oryzomys* from which the virus was isolated and that were captured between October and December 1975. No mention is made of field numbers identifying the rodent specimens nor whether the animals were sent to specialists for identification. As a consequence, the identification of the reservoir species of this virus remains highly suspect; we submit that the identity of the reservoir is not justified even at the generic level. In the text, the authors stated that "No antibodies were found in the sera of 3 *Oryzomys* that yielded the virus nor in the sera of the 8 *Oryzomys oecomys* [sic] captured in the area, including the two from which the virus was isolated" (PINHEIRO et al. 1977: p 179). This passage appears to suggest the reservoir is *O. oecomys*; however, that name combination does not exist (cf. MUSSER and CARLETON 1993). Both *Oryzomys* and *Oecomys* are distinct and equally valid taxa of genus level within the tribe Oryzomyini (VOSS and CARLETON 1993). Therefore, and since no voucher specimens exist with which to confirm identifications, we recommend that the reservoir of this arenavirus be restricted to a member of the Oryzomyini, with no specification as to generic identification. That being said, a cursory analysis of the primary and secondary literature suggests that the general area in which the Flexal virus was found harbors nowadays at least two species of *Oryzomys* and three to four species of *Oecomys* (VOSS and EMMONS 1996; EISENBERG and REDFORD 1999). Virologists and mammalogists working in that area would provide a great service by collecting and vouchering specimens of the Oryzomyini and having them tested for Flexal in order to identify the reservoir of this arenavirus properly.

2.2.10 Oliveros Virus

This arenavirus was characterized by MILLS et al. (1996) and its phylogenetic relationships explored by BOWEN et al. (1997). It was noted in central Argentina, a region described as "an area of intensive agriculture and cattle production" where "crop fields are bordered by fence lines, roadsides and railroads rights-of-ways" (MILLS et al. 1996). It is also one of the most populated areas in Argentina.

Although several species of sigmodontine rodents occur in the area (*Bolomys obscurus*, *Calomys musculinus*, *C. laucha*, *Akodon azarae*, and *Oligoryzomys flavescens*, as well as the murine *Mus musculus*), MILLS et al. (1996) concluded that *B. obscurus* was the reservoir of Oliveros because the virus was extracted from individuals of this species, and because about 25% of all *B. obscurus* were sero-positive as opposed to none or very few individuals from other species in the area.

The taxonomy of the genus *Bolomys* is currently in a state of flux. MASSOIA and PARDINAS (1993) suggested that *Necromys* is a senior synonym of *Bolomys*, an assertion that has received little support by most mammalogists (e.g., ANDERSON 1997; Salazar-Bravo and Yates, in preparation). On the other hand, GALLIARI and PARDINAS (2000) recently suggested that the Argentine Pampa is populated by *B. benefactus*, while populations in Uruguay and SE Buenos Aires province in contrast are referable to *B. obscurus*. Thus, based on geographic information and the identification of several specimens from the Mills et al. collections by one of us

(JSB), we suggest that the reservoir of Oliveros virus be restricted to *B. benefactus* rather than *B. obscurus*.

Several aspects of the ecology of *B. benefactus* have been studied extensively (MILLS et al. 1991b; FORNES and MASSOIA 1965, and references therein). The species appears to be restricted to the Pampa habitat of Argentina (GALLIARI and PARDINAS 2000).

ELLIS et al. (1997) found that *B. benefactus* (reported under the name of *B. obscurus*) primarily inhabited the more stable, weedy borders of cultivated fields, and MILLS et al. (1991b) showed peaks in relative densities in late autumn and early winter, with numbers more evenly distributed throughout the year. Also, MILLS et al. (1992b) reported that the breeding season – as assessed by pregnancies – was September or October through April or May. Although several reports (REIG 1987, and references therein) suggest that the species is mostly insectivorous, ELLIS et al. (1994, 1998) found that the diet corresponded more closely to that of an omnivorous species, with leaves forming a relatively minor proportion of the diet (average 16% for *Bolomys*) throughout the year. This species also consumed higher quantities of seeds (35%–60% of stomach volume) than arthropods (30%–35%) during the autumn and winter but switched to higher quantities of arthropods (30%–53%) in the spring and summer. No information is available on dispersal patterns.

2.2.11 Sabiá Virus

COIMBRA et al. (1994) described this virus from the Brazilian state of Saõ Paulo in a fatal case of hemorrhagic fever initially thought to be yellow fever. Antigenic and molecular analyses showed that this was a new arenavirus which they named Sabiá after the community wherein the index case was staying when she became ill. Sabiá is a small community in the southeastern part of the state. Several species of potential hosts occur in the area.

2.2.12 Guanarito Virus

Early reports on the etiology and characterization of Venezuelan hemorrhagic fever (VHF) implicated two rodents as reservoirs (TESH et al. 1993): *Zygodontomys brevicauda* and *Sigmodon alstoni*. As early as 1996, the possibility that two different arenaviruses were circulating in these two species of wild rodents in the same general area in Venezuela had been advanced. FULHORST et al. (1997) described a second arenavirus from *S. alstoni* (cf. below) and experimental work by FULHORST and colleagues (1999) clearly identified *Z. brevicauda* as the reservoir species of Guanarito, the etiological agent of VHF.

The taxonomic status of *Z. brevicauda* as well as some aspects of the natural history of this species were summarized in Voss (1991). This species ranges widely below 1,500m from the "Pacific littoral and foothills of eastern Costa Rica, through Panamá, Colombia (except the valleys of the upper Rio Cauca, Rio Patía and Rio Dagua), Venezuela, Guyana, Surinam, French Guiana, and Brazil north of the Amazon Basin". Voss (1991) further reported that *Z. brevicauda* inhabits a wide variety of lowland habitats with the exception of mature, closed-canopy rain forest. The species is nocturnal and terrestrial. In the agricultural and pastoral areas of the western Llanos of Venezuela, UTRERA et al. (2000) found that most habitat types, especially relatively uniform areas of mechanized agriculture, were numerically dominated by two rodents, *S. alstoni* and *Z. brevicauda*. The latter species has been said to be omnivorous (EINSENBERG 1989), but MARTINO and AGUILERA (1993) found that it is chiefly insectivorous (70.6%), although they also suggested that diet was dependent on resource availability. VOSS (1992) found that captive-bred litters typically consist of four or five pups each weighing 3–4g at birth. Adults 20–40 weeks old average 60–80g with some sexual dimorphism. Females are sexually mature at 3–4 weeks of age, males at 6–8 weeks. Ovulation is spontaneous, and gestation lasts 25 days. In the field, reproduction in *Z. brevicauda* appears to be continuous and aseasonal. Several reports indicated that *Z. brevicauda* are among the most abundant rodents in the areas where they occur. Densities reported for this species vary from "not very abundant" (MARTINO and AGUILERA 1993) to 40/ha or even 100/ha (summarized in VOSS 1992).

2.2.13 Whitewater Arroyo Virus

In 1996, Kosoy et al. reported an unexpectedly high level of prevalence of antibodies to arenaviruses in rodents from the southwestern USA, providing the first published evidence that these viruses infect individuals of the North American sigmodontine genus *Neotoma* (packrats). The same year, FULHORST et al. (1996) isolated and characterized three strains of Whitewater Arroyo virus from two individuals of *N. albigula* from Whitewater Arroyo in McKinley County, New Mexico. Other species of sigmodontine rodents also found to be antibody-positive to WWA were: *N. fuscipes*, *Peromyscus boylii*, *P. californicus*, *P. eremicus*, *P. maniculatus*, and *Reithrodontomys megalotis* (BENNET et al. 2000).

   N. albigula is nearly ubiquitous in western North America, occupying several habitat types throughout its geographic range (HALL 1981). It is found from southeastern California and southeastern Utah to central Texas, northeastern Michoacán, and Hidalgo, México (MACEDO and MARES 1988). The species is primarily found in arid regions and prefers areas where prickly pear (*Opuntia*) and piñon-juniper habitat are abundant. Shelter-site selection is influenced by the quantity of ground-level vegetation available for cover. *N. albigula* is nocturnal and terrestrial, although it has been trapped above the ground and been seen climbing in bushes and trees.

   The species is chiefly herbivorous. DIAL (1988) showed that in sympatry with congeners, *N. albigula* was found selectively to forage on *Yucca* while *N. devia* specialized on *Ephedra epidermis*, and *N. stephensi* on *Juniperus*. MACEDO and MARES (1988) reported that early accounts of the diet of this species showed up to 44% of the annual diet composed of cacti. Home-range estimates in this species vary with habitat but have been estimated to be $161 \pm 19m^2$ in Cholla-forest habitat. Nests are defended, but home ranges overlapped, at times by as much as 100% (BOGGS 1974). WHITFORD (1976) found that in southern New Mexico, *N. albigula* maintained stable and nearly constant population densities in a 4-year study at about 2/ha with a significant increase at the end of the third year. In analyzing 4 years of data from central New Mexico, PARMENTER et al. (1999) showed that *N. albigula* presented two distinct density patterns. In Placitas (at 2,200–2,300m in the foothills of the Sandia Mountains, Sandoval Co., north-central New Mexico), densities remained constant at 1–2/ha, whereas in the Sevilleta National Wildlife Refuge (high desert, 1,600–1,700m in central New Mexico) densities varied from 1–10/ha with population peaks in the late autumn. SERRANO (1987) showed that population densities in northern México varied from 10–46/ha in preferred habitat (*Opuntia* fields). BROWN and HESKE (1990) showed that at their study site in Arizona, *N. albigula* densities were relatively constant throughout their 10-year study period (~10/ha). MACEDO and MARES (1988) reported that reproduction occurred continuously through the year, gestation lasted 30–38 days, and pups were weaned at about 20–25 days.

2.2.14 Pirital Virus

This virus was isolated by FULHORST et al. (1997) from 10 of 46 *Sigmodon alstoni* rodents tested from the Venezuelan state of Portuguesa, a study subsequently expanded upon by FULHORST et al. (1999). These latter authors confirmed that *S. alstoni* is the reservoir of Pirital virus. No voucher specimens or museum names (where the animals may have been identified or are now deposited) are mentioned in the text.

   S. alstoni is common throughout unforested and deforested habitats below about 1,300m elevation east of the Andes and south of the coastal cordilleras, including all of the Llanos, some isolated savannas in the Venezuelan state of Amazonas, deforested regions in the northeastern Venezuelan highlands, the Gran Sabana in southeastern Venezuela, the savannas of the upper Rio Branco in Brazil, the Rupununi savannas of Guyana, the coastal and interior savannas of Suriname, and contiguous savannas in the upper Rio Parú drainage of the Brazilian state of Pará (Voss 1992). The species is said to be diurnal and nocturnal, and terrestrial.

   IBAÑEZ and MORENO (1982, cited in Voss 1992) concluded that this species is herbivorous based on the examination of stomach contents. Voss (1992) reported pregnancies throughout the annual cycle of flooding and drought that characterizes this extremely seasonal environment, but reproductive activity may be least in the dry season, based on autopsies of over 150 animals; the number of embryos counted *in utero* ranged from 2 to 8, with a mean of 4.4. VIVAS (1986) suggested that females of this species are reproductively active all year round in the Llanos of Venezuela.

3 A Synthesis of the Evolutionary History of Murid Rodents

The most obvious generalization that can be made about the mammal reservoir species of arenaviruses is that (with the exception of Tacaribe) they are all members of two groups (currently classified at the subfamilial level) of rodents in the family Muridae. These two groups (sometimes also treated as families) are the Murinae and Sigmodontinae. Primarily African and Asian, murine rodents are the ecological counterparts of the sigmodontine rodents of the Western Hemisphere. With close to 300 genera and over 1,300 species, murid rodents are the most speciose family of mammals (MUSSER and CARLETON 1993). This diversity is increasing at an accelerated pace: for example, PATTERSON (2000) has shown that 22 new species of murid rodents have been described in South America alone from 1992 to 1998. A detailed analysis of the evolution of murid rodents is beyond the scope of this chapter, but the following summary may contribute to an enhanced understanding of the evolutionary setting of Muridae–Arenavirus coevolution.

HARTENBERGER (1998) proposed that the lower Eocene (ca. 55Mya) form from Siberia, *Ivanantonia efremovi*, might represent the first murid rodent. Although the evolutionary history of murid rodents is probably more complex than the fossil record indicates, there appear to have been three major temporal climatically driven episodes that have defined the ecological success of this group. The first event probably occurred at the boundary between the Eocene and Oligocene, characterized by a dramatic climate change with a tendency to a major latitudinal zonation, an increase in seasonality, and a major faunal turnover, which has been designated in Asia as the Mongolian remodelling (MENG and McKENNA 1998), in Europe (e.g., CUENCA and CANUDO 1992) as the "Grande Coupure", and even extended into North America by HARTENBERGER (1998). The most dramatic cooling episode was at 33.5Mya, slightly subsequent to the Eocene/Oligocene boundary, and was characterized by a severe drop in mean annual temperature and changes in vegetation from Eocene dense forests to more open country during the Oligocene. In Mongolia and Europe, mammal faunae changed to be dominated by rodents and lagomorphs. This is the time of the split of the major groups of muroid rodents. At about the same time, hystricognath rodents (cavies, porcupines, and their allies) arrived in South America (FLYNN and WYSS 1998). As a result of these faunal turnovers, murid rodents arrive in Europe from Asia. Several forms may have made it to North America as well but went extinct ca. 16Mya [e.g., Eucricetodontinae, Eumyinae (FLYNN et al. 1985)].

The second major event is concurrent with the beginning of the Miocene (~23Mya) when the connections between Africa and Europe and North America and Asia were reestablished due to a reduction of sea level (HAMILTON 1983). RUEDAS and KIRSCH (1997) presented a constructive discussion of the timing and players of the murine evolution in Asia, and DENYS (1999) presented a complete analysis for Africa. The latter author suggested that the first true murine rodent from Africa is an undetermined *Praomys*-like genus from Chorora, Ethiopia (~10Mya) and *Karnimata* from Namibia (8–9Mya). In North America, the fossil record of ~16Mya is dominated by the presence of *Copemys*, a genus with obscure relationships to Old World forms that may have given rise to most contemporary genera of the tribal-level group Peromyscini (i.e., *Neotoma*, *Ochrotomys*, *Osgoodomys*, *Peromyscus*, etc.). Although current systematic treatments consider this tribe as part of the subfamily Sigmodontinae (cf. MUSSER and CARLETON 1993), recent molecular analysis (ENGEL et al. 1998) suggests that this subfamily may be polyphyletic. In this work, members of the North American Peromyscini and the (mostly) South American Sigmodontini are not sister to each other, indicating that they may have originated from separated lineages. BASKIN (1986) suggested that *Abelmoschomys* (from the Clarendonian of Florida, ~9Mya) is the first true sigmodontine. CZAPLEWSKI (1987) further recorded several forms assigned to Sigmodontinae from Arizona (ca. 4.5–5Mya), including members of the now exclusively South American tribe Akodontini and *Sigmodon* proper.

The beginning of the Pliocene was punctuated by the development of open environments which were apparently driven by a CO_2 starvation phenomenon (CERLING et al. 1997, 1998) documented in the tropical regions at around 8–7Mya. As a result, the number of rodent groups and genera increased, and most current-day associations were formed at that time. The connection of South America to North America with the establishment of the isthmus of Panama occurs at 3.5–7Mya, setting the scene for a full-scale Great American Biotic Interchange (GABI) that filtered representatives of South American forms from proceeding north while allowing the incursion of numerous northern taxa into South America. It is postulated, however, that the oldest sigmodontine rodent in South America (*Auliscomys formosus* from Argentina, ~4.5Mya) may predate the GABI (PARDINAS and TONNI 1998). Two lines of evidence are helpful to understand this conundrum. First, KNOWLTON and WEIGT (1998) proposed that the closure of the isthmus was gradual and may have started up to 7Mya before complete closure. Secondly, molecular phylogenies have proposed that the radiation of the Sigmodontinae may have been earlier than the fossil record suggests (SALAZAR-BRAVO et al. 2001; SMITH and PATTON 1999).

Of the major groups of murid rodents (murines, cricetines, arvicolines, and sigmodontines), only two are known to be reservoirs for arenavirus.

Considering that Murinae and Sigmodontinae are not sister taxons (cf. DICKERMAN 1992; ENGEL et al. 1998; CONROY and COOK 1999), it is tempting to suggest that early muroid rodents (like *Ivanantonia* or later forms) may have harbored arenaviruses or arenavirus-like forms well before the 30Mya figure mentioned elsewhere (e.g., BOWEN et al. 1997). Such a scenario results in a testable hypothesis: if arenaviruses had infected earlier forms, then all remaining murid subfamilies (cf. MUSSER and CARLETON 1993) should have genera that currently also harbor arenaviruses. Africa is the place to test this hypothesis as many subfamilies of Muridae – albeit not overly speciose – presently occur there. An alternative conclusion would suggest that arenaviruses might have infected the immediate ancestor of both Sigmodontinae and Murinae (which are not, however, each other's closest relatives). Since this putative ancestor must perforce also be ancestral to the Cricetinae, this latter subfamily must also have lineages infected with arenaviruses. A similar scenario has been proposed for hantaviruses (HJELLE and YATES 2001). These are all testable hypotheses and as such constitute a rich field for future research.

4 Ecological and Geographic Generalities of the Mammalian Reservoirs of Arenaviruses

A final important aspect to be considered is that, for the most part, the genera (and sometimes species) of rodents that are involved are among the most diverse and abundant elements of the ecosystems that occupy. *Oryzomys, Calomys, Mastomys, Bolomys, Arvicanthis*, etc. are highly abundant and considered by many to be akin to pest species. As ASHFORD (1997) suggested, the main population factor favoring a reservoir role are high density and longevity sufficient to provide a habitat for the parasite during any season or period of nontransmission (i.e., the ability of serving as "viral" refugia). Most rodent reservoirs identified thus far conform to this requisite.

Furthermore, there are some data that tend to indicate a certain level of "correlation" between population abundance and viral infection (or at least seroprevalence). In most epidemiological work ensuing from outbreak responses, rodent trapping usually results (depending on the geographic location) in the capture of one or two species of rodents in rather abundant numbers and a few more with lower levels of abundance. Usually, one of the more abundant species is also the reservoir species. In some extreme cases, if there are two "more abundant" species, each may harbor a different arenavirus (e.g., *Zygodontomys/Sigmodon* and Guanarito/Pirital or *Calomys/Bolomys* and Junín/Oliveros). There are, however, several other cases where even in relatively diverse and heterogeneous habitats (e.g., mountain forests in Colombia) and even after a large number of mammal species have been tested, only one (the most abundant) tests positive for the virus (e.g., Pichindé).

Another pattern is that most arenaviruses appear to use as reservoirs species that inhabit low to middle elevations. Certainly, no arenaviruses are known from elevations above 2,500m in the New World; Pichindé set the record, as it has been isolated from *O. albigularis* collected from a forest patch at Munchique (2,500m). In the Old World, with one possible exception, none of the mammal host species of arenaviruses occur above 2,000m. The one possible exception is *Mus domesticus*. This species can inhabit high elevations and does so in particular in the Pamir region of Pakistan and Kashmir, as well as in the Caucasus. However, as noted in the foregoing section on LCM, we cannot know with any degree of certainty whether it is *M. domesticus* or *M. musculus* (or both) which definitively hosts that virus. We might make a case, based on our hypothesis that if it is only species restricted to the lower elevations which host arenaviruses, that it is unlikely that *M. domesticus* is the host for LCM, which then would be restricted to *M. musculus*. This is a testable hypothesis that merits further investigation. Two further caveats conflate a tidy picture: (1) the most likely source for the émigré populations in the New World, that is Western Europe, is predominantly inhabited by *M. domesticus*; and (2) there exist populations of *M. musculus* in the Pamir (e.g., *M. m. theobaldi, M. m. pachycercus*) which also exist at high elevations. We suspect that the full extent of the biodiversity at present collectively amalgamated into *M. domesticus* and *M. musculus* far underdescribes the biological reality of their taxonomic distinctiveness.

The pattern holds even if species in arenavirus-infected genera are also "available" at higher elevations. For example, *Calomys lepidus* and *C. sorellus* are closely related to *C. musculinus* (SALAZAR-BRAVO et al. 2001), yet to date, no arenavirus has been described from either of the former species. Is this a sampling artifact? Perhaps. We submit that virologists should make use of phylogenetic analyses of those mammal genera known to serve as arenavirus reservoirs and test associated taxa for potential new species of arenaviruses.

It could be argued, moreover, that the patterns discerned here will change when and if more data are available. At present, it is clear that most arenaviruses have been discovered in the aftermath of outbreaks and therefore in a haphazard manner. A more systematic pursuit of arenaviruses in the freezers of mammalogists the world over will eventually show results one way or the other.

Lastly, one phenomenon evident in all of the species of disease-causing arenaviruses known to date is that there is an incomplete pattern of overlap between the distribution of the mammal species reservoir and that of the endo-epidemic zone of infection. This pattern is congruent with Pavloskii's concept of natural nidality (PAVLOSKII 1966). Pavloskii's definition is interpreted here as a dynamic process wherein several members (i.e., virus, reservoir, vectors) of an ecosystem in a particular geographic location (or biopathocenose) interact to promote the continuous circulation of the disease agent. Humans in the Pavloskii sense would then act as "sentinels" of these localized diseases. In Pavloskii's definition, the distribution of the disease does not necessarily correspond to the distribution of any element of the biopathocenose, a phenomenon distinctly observable in mammal host–arenavirus distributions.

5 Concluding Remarks and Recommendations

The underlying theme of the foregoing sections is uncertainty: there cannot be full knowledge of a zoonotic virus without knowledge of its reservoir; measures to attenuate the effects of viruses from a public health standpoint are doomed to failure if the host is unknown or, worse yet, if the host is misidentified. The basic alpha-level taxonomy of the mammalian hosts of arenaviruses is fluctuating so that at times a probable arenavirus host is subsumed as a subspecies within a broadly distributed species (although the virus itself may be geographically restricted). Other times, the taxonomy may be better known from a molecular or chromosomal perspective, but characters amenable to field identification of the mammal host species are few or nonexistent. The critical problem here is not so much the lack of a fundamental taxonomic framework for African or American murid rodents (although this does impede progress) as the lack of specimens upon which to undertake the research. Often, the initial research is undertaken, the animals given a cursory identification, and the specimens then disappear. The tools used by mammalogists to identify and further study the phylogenetic relationships of murid rodents are diverse. A perfunctory review of the current literature shows that characters ranging from general skull morphology and chromosomes to protein analyses and DNA sequencing are used to that effect. Thus, it is imperative that as much information as possible be obtained from the potential reservoirs. A potential – yet by no means exhaustive – list of ancillary material that should be obtained includes: chromosomes, cell suspensions, endoparasites, ectoparasites, stomach contents, tissues stored in alcohol and frozen, eye lenses, detailed information on habitat, trapping effort, etc. in addition to the voucher specimens, which usually consist of skins, skulls, whole body skeletons, or alcohol-preserved bodies. All of the ancillary materials need to be traceable to each other and to the voucher specimen by the assignation of an unique number that can serve as a link between them all. One such method is the New Mexico kryovoucher (NK) system used at the University of New Mexico. In this system, each specimen is assigned a unique NK number in the field at the beginning of the processing procedure. A wide variety of information is recorded on the NK data sheet, including the type of specimen prepared and the kind and amount of other materials (e.g., chromosomes, cell suspensions, tissues, parasites, etc.) that were taken from the specimen. Use of a single unique numbering system for tracking associated materials with a traditional voucher in the field has the advantage of allowing specimens to be given a number as soon as they are removed from the field. As a result, each worker in the process can label associated materials (e.g., parasites, tissues, etc.) with the same number and thus reduce confusion and errors that might occur using individual collector or preparator numbers. Such a system also has advantages for the storage and retrieval of these materials once they are in the collection. Because ancillary materials are stored numerically by NK number, the problem of wasted storage space common to taxonomically arranged collections is eliminated. Such a system is particularly valuable when ancillary materials and voucher specimens are deposited at different institutions. It also saves time once the collection is returned to the repository, because ancillary materials can be installed immediately without the need for "recataloguing" (YATES et al. 1996).

Deposition of specimens and their ancillary materials in a museum – where subsequent taxonomic work may be undertaken and the taxonomy constantly updated – is therefore more than a mere exercise in academic minutiae; rather, it is a *sine qua non* requirement of a research program wherein the outcome, human life and death, hangs in the balance.

N.B. While the manuscript was in revision, several papers pertinent to the ecology of mammalian reservoirs of Arenaviruses were published. Among them is the description of a new species of Arenavirus dubbed Allpahuayo by MONCAYO et al. (2001). This virus was isolated from two species of arboreal rice rats of the genus *Oecomys*. Although the authors refer to their identifications as preliminary, some of the original virus isolates were identified by field number (e.g., CLHP 2098, CLHP 2472), and being deposited at the Natural Science Research Laboratory of the Museum of Texas Tech are thus widely available for further taxonomic work. This Arenavirus was called PC-242 by Tesh et al. (1999).

Acknowledgements. The authors acknowledge helpful discussions with D. Bausch, J.N. Mills, C.J. Peters, K.M. Johnson, and R. Pine, as well as critical assistance in tracking down specimens from K.M. Johnson, R. Pine, N. Olds, S. Collins, and R. Swanepoel. Invaluable assistance with original citations, literature, and historical information on Ippy was received from JP Digoutte and personnel of Institut Pasteur. Thanks also to T. Monath for historical information regarding Lassa Fever specimens, and for assistance from MD Carleton (USNM) regarding the same specimens. C. Conroy read an earlier version of the manuscript and offered most valuable comments and suggestions.

References

Aagard EMJ (1982) Ecological distribution of mammals in the cloud forests and Páramos of the Andes, Mérida, Venezuela. PhD thesis, Colorado State University

Aguilera M, Perez Zapata A, Martino A (1995) Cytogenetics and karyosystematics of *Oryzomys albigularis* (Rodentia, Cricetidae) from Venezuela. Cytogenet Cell Genet 69:44–49

Alho CJR, Pereira LA (1985) Population ecology of a cerrado rodent community in central Brazil. Rev Bras Biol 45:597–608

Alho CJR, Pereira LA, Paula AC (1986) Patterns of habitat utilization by small mammal populations in Cerrado Biome of central Brazil. Mammalia 50:447–460

Anderson S (1997) Mammals of Bolivia: taxonomy and distribution. Bull Am Museum Natural History 231:652

Armstrong C, Dickens PF (1935) Benign lymphocytic choriomeningitis (acute aseptic meningitis). Public Health Rep 50:831–842

Armstrong C, Lillie RD (1934) Experimental lymphocytic choriomeningitis of monkeys and mice produced by a virus encountered in studies of the 1933 St. Louis encephalitis epidemic. Public Health Rep 49:1019–1027

Armstrong C, Sweet LK (1939) Lymphocytic choriomeningitis. Report of two cases, with recovery of virus from gray mice (*Mus musculus*) trapped in the two infected households. Public Health Rep 54:673–684

Ashe JS, Timm RM (1995) Systematics, distribution, and host specificity of *Amblyopinus* Solsky 1875 (Coleoptera Staphylinidae) in Mexico and Central America. Tropical Zool 8:373–399

Ashford AW (1997) What it takes to be a reservoir host. Belg J Zool 127 [Suppl]:85–90

Bangs O (1898) The lands mammals of peninsular Florida and the coastal region of Georgia. Proc Boston Soc Natural History 28:128

Barnett AA (1999) Small mammals of the Cajas Plateau, southern Ecuador: ecology and natural history. Bull Florida Museum Natural History 42:161–217

Baskevich MI, Orlov VN (1993) Karyological differentiation of rats of the genus *Mastomys* (Rodentia, Muridae) from the central part of Ethiopian Rift Valley. Zool Zhurnal 72:112–121

Baskin JA (1986) The late Miocene radiation of Neotropical sigmodontine rodents in North America. Contributions in Geology, University of Wyoming, Special Paper 3:287–303

Benenson AS (ed) (1995) Control of communicable diseases manual: an official report of the American Public Health Association, 16th edn. APHA,Washington, DC

Bennett SG, Milazzo ML, Webb JP, Fulhorst CF (2000) Arenavirus antibody in rodents indigenous to coastal southern California. Am J Trop Med Hyg 62:626–630

Berry RJ, Bronson FH (1992) Life history and bioeconomy of the house mouse. Biol Rev Camb Philos Soc 67:519–550

Bigler WJ, Lassing E, Buff E, Lewis AL, Hoff GL (1975) Arbovirus surveillance in Florida: wild vertebrate studies 1965–1974. J Wildl Dis 11:348–356

Bishop DHL (1990) Arenaviridae and their replication. In: Fields BN, Knipe DM, Chanock RM, Hirsch MS, Melnick JL, Monath TP, Roizman B (eds) Fields virology. Raven, New York

Boggs JR (1974) Social ecology of the white-throated woodrat (*Neotoma albigula*) in Arizona. PhD thesis, Arizona State University

Bonhomme F, Britton-Davidian J, Chapman VM, Moriwaki K, Nevo E, Thaler L (1984) Biochemical diversity and evolution in the genus *Mus*. Biochem Genet 22:275–303

Bonvicino C, Almeida FC (2000) Karyotype, morphology and taxonomic status of *Calomys expulsus* (Rodentia: Sigmodontinae). Mammalia 64:339–351

Bonvicino CR, Martins MA (2001) Molecular phylogeny of the genus *Oryzomys* (Rodentia: Sigmodontinae) based on cytochrome *b* DNA sequences. Mol Phylogenet Evol 18:282–292

Boursot P, Auffray J-C, Britton-Davidian J, Bonhomme F (1993) The evolution of house mice. Ann Rev Ecol Systematics 24:119–152

Bowen MD, Peters CJ, Nichol ST (1997) Phylogenetic analysis of the Arenaviridae: patterns of virus evolution and evidence for cospeciation between arenaviruses and their rodent hosts. Mol Phylogenet Evol 8:301–316

Bowen MD, Ksiazek TG, Rollin PE, Pinheiro FP, Goldsmith CS, Zaki SR, Nichol ST, Peters CJ, Travassos de Rosa AP (1998) Characterization of Cupixi virus, a newly recognized new world group B Arenavirus. Program and abstracts of the 47th annual meeting of the American Society of Tropical Medicine and Hygiene, San Juan, Puerto Rico. Abstract 429

Brown JH, Heske EJ (1990) Temporal changes in a Chihuahuan Desert rodent community. Oikos 59:290–302

Buckley SM, Casals J (1970) Lassa fever, a new virus disease of man from West Africa. III. Isolation and characterization of the virus. Am J Trop Med Hyg 19:680

Busch M, Alvarez MR, Cittadino EA, Kravetz FO (1997) Habitat selection and interspecific competition in rodents in pampean agroecosystems. Mammalia 61:167–184

Calisher CH, Tzianabos T, Lord RD, Coleman PH (1970) Tamiami virus, a new member of the Tacaribe group. Am J Trop Med Hyg 19:520–526

Cameron G, Spencer SR (1981) *Sigmodon hispidus*. Mammalian Species 158:1–9

Capanna E, Civitelli MV (1988) A cytotaxonomic approach to the systematics of *Arvicanthis niloticus* (Desmarest, 1822) (Mammalia Rodentia). Tropical Zool 1:29–37

Capanna E, Afework Bekele, Capula M, Castiglia R, Civitelli MV, Codjia JTCl, Corti M, Fadda C (1996) A multidisciplinary approach to the systematics of the genus *Arvicanthis* Lesson, 1842 (Rodentia, Murinae). Mammalia 60:677–696

Carballal G, Videla C, Dulout F, Cossio PM, Acuna AM, Bianchi NO (1986) Experimental infection of *Akodon molinae* (Rodentia, Cricetidae) with Junin virus. J Med Virol 19:47–54

Catzeflis FM, Denys C (1992) The African *Nannomys* (Muridae): an early offshoot from the *Mus* lineage: evidence from scnDNA hybridization experiments and compared morphology. Isr J Zool 38:219–231

Catzeflis FM, Sheldon FH, Ahlquist JE, Sibley CG (1987) DNA–DNA hybridization evidence of the rapid rate of muroid rodent DNA evolution. Mol Biol Evol 4:242–253

Catzeflis FM, Aguilar JP, Jaeger JJ (1992) Muroid rodents: phylogeny and evolution. Trends Ecol Evolution 7:122–126

Cerling TE, Harris JM, Macfadden BJ, Leakey MG, Quade J, Eisenmann V, Ehleringer JR (1997) Global vegetation change through the Miocene/Pliocene boundary. Nature 389:153–158

Cerling TE, Ehleringer JR, Harris JM (1998) Carbon dioxide starvation, the development of C4 ecosystems and mammalian evolution. Philos Trans R Soc Lond B Biol Sci 353:159–170

Chevret P, Hanni C (1994) Systematics of the spiny mouse (*Acomys*, Muroidea): molecular and biochemical evidence. Isr J Zool 40:247–254

Chevret P, Denys C, Jaeger JJ, Michaux J, Catzeflis FM (1993a) Molecular evidence that the spiny mouse (*Acomys*) is more closely related to gerbils (Gerbillinae) than to true mice (Murinae). Proc Natl Acad Sci USA 90:3433–3436

Chevret P, Denys C, Jaeger JJ, Michaux J, Catzeflis FM (1993b) Molecular and paleontological aspects of the tempo and mode of evolution in *Otomys* (Otomyinae, Muridae, Mammalia). Biochem Syst Ecol 21:123–131

Chevret P, Granjon L, Duplantier JM, Denys C, Catzeflis FM (1994) Molecular phylogeny of the *Praomys* complex (Rodentia, Murinae): a study based on DNA/DNA hybridization experiments. Zool J Linnean Soc 112:425–442

Ciccioli MA (1991) Classical; C-banding and Cd-banding karyotypes in mitotic and meiotic chromosomes of *Calomys musculinus* (Rodentia; Cricetidae). Caryologia 44:177–186

Ciccioli MA, Poggio L (1993) Genome size in *Calomys laucha* and *Calomys musculinus* (Rodentia; Cricetidae). Genetics Selection Evolution 25:109–119

Civitelli MV, Castiglia R, Codjia JCl, Capanna E (1995) Cytogenetics of the genus *Arvicanthis* (Rodentia, Muridae). 1. *Arvicanthis niloticus* from the Republic of Benin. Z Saugetierkd 60:215–225

Coimbra TLM, Nassar ES, Burattini MN, Souza LT de, Ferreira I, Rocco IM, Rosa AP da, Vasconcelos PF, Pinheiro FP, LeDuc J, et al. (1994) New arenavirus isolated in Brazil. Lancet 343:391–392

Conroy CJ, Cook JA (1999) MtDNA evidence for repeated pulses of speciation within Arvicoline and Murid rodents. J Mammalian Evolution 6:221–245

Cuenca G, Canudo JI (1992) The Sciuridae (Rodentia, Mammalia) from the Lower Oligocene of Montalban and Olalla (Teruel, Spain): some remarks on the origin of the sciurids. Boletin Real Sociedad Española Historia Natural Seccion Biol 87:155–169

Czaplewski NJ (1987) Sigmodont rodents (Mammalia; Muroidea; Sigmodontinae) from the Pliocene (early Blancan) Verde Formation, Arizona. J Vertebrate Paleontol 7:183–199

Daszak P, Cunningham AA, Hyatt AD (2000) Emerging infectious diseases of wildlife – threats to biodiversity and human health. Science 287:443–449

Davis DHS (1965) Classification problems of African Muridae. Zool Africana 1:121–145

DeMartini JC, Green DE, Monath TP (1975) Lassa virus infection in *Mastomys natalensis* in Sierra Leone. Gross and microscopic findings in infected and uninfected animals. Bull World Health Org 52:651–663

Denys C (1999) Of mice and men: evolution in East and South Africa during Plio-Pleistocene times. In: Bromage TG, Schrenk F (eds) African biogeography, climate change & human evolution.The human evolution series. Oxford University Press, New York, pp 226–252

Dial KP (1988) Three sympatric species of *Neotoma*: dietary specialization and coexistence. Oecologia 76:531–537

Diaz De Pascual A (1994) The rodent community of the Venezuelan cloud forest, Merida. Polish Ecol Stud 20:155–161

Dickerman AW (1992) Molecular systematics of some New World muroid rodents. PhD thesis, University of Wisconsin, Madison

Digoutte JP (1970) Ippy. In: Annuaire de l'Institut Pasteur, Bangui, République Centreafricaine

Downs WG, Anderson CR, Spence L, Aitken THG, Greenhall AH (1963) Tacaribe virus, a new agent isolated from *Artibeus* bats and mosquitos in Trinidad, West Indies. Am J Trop Med Hyg 12:640–646

Dubois JYF, Catzeflis FM, Beintema JJ (1999) The phylogenetic position of 'Acomyinae' (Rodentia, Mammalia) as sister group of a Murinae plus Gerbillinae clade: evidence from the nuclear ribonuclease gene. Mol Biol Evol 13:181–192

Ducroz JF, Volobouev V, Granjon L (1998) A molecular perspective on the systematics and evolution of the genus *Arvicanthis* (Rodentia, Muridae): inferences from complete cytochrome b gene sequences. Mol Phylogenet Evol 10:104–117

Durant P, Diaz A (1995) Aspectos de la ecologia de roedores y musarañas de las cuencas hidrográficas Andino-Venezolanas. Caribbean J Sci 31:83–94

Eisenberg J (1989) Mammals of the neotropics, Vol 1. The northern neotropics. University of Chicago Press, Chicago

Eisenberg J, Redford K (1999) Mammals of the neotropics, Vol 3. The central neotropics. University of Chicago Press, Chicago

Ellerman KR (1941) The families and genera of living rodents. Vol II. Muridae. British Museum (Natural History), London

Ellis BA, Mills JN, Kennedy EJT, Maiztegui JI, Childs JE (1994) The relationship among diet, alimentary-tract morphology, and life-history for 5 species of rodents from the central Argentine Pampa. Acta Theriol 39:345–355

Ellis BA, Mills JN, Childs JE, Muzzini MC, McKee KT Jr, Enria DA, Glass GE (1997) Structure and floristics of habitats associated with five rodent species in an agroecosystem in Central Argentina. J Zool Lond 243:437–460

Ellis BA, Mills JN, Glass GE, McKee KT, Enria DA, Childs JE (1998) Dietary habits of the common rodents in an agroecosystem in Argentina. J Mammal 79:1203–1220

Emmons L, Feer F (1999) Neotropical rainforest mammals, 2nd edn. University of Chicago Press, Chicago

Engel L, Mello Dalva A (1993) Rodents in agroecosystems in the Cerrado Province of the Federal District (Brasilia/DF, Brazil). Ciencia e Cultura Sao Paulo 45:128–133

Engel SR, Hogan KM, Taylor JF, Davis SK (1998) Molecular systematics and paleobiogeography of the South-American Sigmodontine rodents. Molecular Biol Evolution 15:35–49

Flynn JJ, Wyss AR (1998) Recent advances in South-American mammalian paleontology. Trends Ecol Evolution 13:449–454

Flynn LJ, Jacobs LL, Lindsay EH (1985) Problems in muroid phylogeny: relationships to other rodents and origins of major groups. In: Luckett WP, Hartenberger J-L (eds) Evolutionary relationships among rodents. A multidisciplinary analysis. NATO ASI Series A: Life Sciences 92:589–616. Plenum Press, New York

Fornes A, Massoia E (1965) Micromamiferos (Marsupialia y Rodentia) recolectados en la localidad Bonaerense de Miramar. Physis 25:99–108

Frame JD, Baldwin JM, Gocke DJ, Troup JM (1970) Lassa fever, a new virus disease of man from West Africa. I. Clinical description and pathological findings. Am J Trop Med Hyg 19:670–676

Fulhorst CF, Bowen MD, Ksiazek TG, Rollin PE, Nichol ST, Kosoy MY, Peters CJ (1996) Isolation and characterization of Whitewater Arroyo virus, a novel North American arenavirus. Virology 224: 114–120

Fulhorst CF, Bowen MD, Salas RA, Manzione NMCD, Duno G, Utrera A, Ksiazek Thomas G, Peters CJ, Nichol ST, De Miller E, Tovar D, Ramos B, Vasquez C, Tesh RB (1997) Isolation and characterization of Pirital virus, a newly discovered South American arenavirus. Am J Trop Med Hyg 56:548–553

Fulhorst CF, Bowen MD, Salas RA, Duno G, Utrera A, Ksiazek TG, Manzione NMC de, Miller E de, Vasquez C, Peters CJ, Tesh RB (1999) Natural rodent host associations of Guanarito and Pirital viruses (family Arenaviridae) in central Venezuela. Am J Trop Med Hyg 61:325–330

Furano AV, Hayward BE, Chevret P, Catzeflis F, Usdin K (1994) Amplification of the ancient murine Lx family of long interspersed repeated DNA occurred during the murine radiation. J Mol Evol 38:18–27

Galliari CA, Pardinas UFJ (2000) Taxonomy and distribution of the sigmodontine rodents of genus *Necromys* in central Argentina and Uruguay. Acta Theriol 45:211–232

Gardner AL, Patton JL (1976) Karyotypic variation in oryzomyine rodents (Cricetinae) with comments on chromosomal evolution in the neotropical cricetine complex. Occasional Papers, Museum of Zoology, Louisiana State University 49:1–48

Georges AJ, Gonzalez JP, Abdul-Wahid S, Saluzzo JF, Meunier DMY, McCormick JB (1985) Antibodies to Lassa and Lassa-like viruses in man and mammals in the Central African Republic. Trans R Soc Trop Med Hyg 79:78–79

Gerasimov S, Nikolov H, Mihailova V, Affray J-C, Bonhomme F (1990) Morphometric stepwise discriminant analysis of the five genetically determined European taxa of the genus *Mus*. Biol J Linnean Soc 41:47–64

Gonnet JM, Ojeda RA (1998) Habitat use by small mammals in the arid Andean foothills of the Monte desert of Mendoza; Argentina. J Arid Environments 38:349–357

Gonzalez JP, McCormick JB, Saluzzo JF, Hervé JP, Georges AJ, Johnson KM (1983) An arenavirus isolated from wild-caught rodents (*Praomys* species) in the Central African Republic. Intervirology 19:105–112

Goodwin GG, Greenhall AM (1961) A review of the bats of Trinidad and Tobago. Bull Am Museum Natural History 122:187–302

Gordon DH (1978) Distribution of the sibling species of the *Praomys* (*Mastomys*) *natalensis* group in Rhodesia (Mammalia: Rodentia). J Zool Lond 186:397–401

Granjon L, Duplantier JM, Catalan J, Britton-Davidian J (1992) Karyotypic data on rodents from Sénégal. Isr J Zool 38:263–276

Granjon L, Duplantier JM, Catalan J, Britton-Davidian J, Bronner GN (1996) Conspecificity of *Mastomys natalensis* (Rodentia: Muridae) from Sénégal and south Africa: evidence from experimental crosses, karyology and biometry. Mammalia 60:697–706

Graur D (1994) Molecular evidence concerning the phylogenetic integrity of the Murinae. Isr J Zool 40:255–264

Green CA, Gordon DH, Lyons NF (1978) Biological species in *Praomys* (*Mastomys*) *natalensis* (Smith), a rodent carrier of Lassa virus and bubonic plague in Africa. Am J Trop Med Hyg 27:627–629

Guillotin M (1982) *Proechimys cuvieri* (Rodentia, Echimyidae) in the terrestrial micro-mammals community of French Guyana forest. Mammalia 46:299–318

Gyldenstolpe N (1932) A manual of neotropical sigmodont rodents. Kunglika Svenska Vetenskapsakademiens Handlingar series 3, 11:1–164

Hall ER (1981) The mammals of North America, 2nd edn. John Wiley, New York 2:601–1181

Hamilton W (1983) Cretaceous and Cenozoic history of the northern continents. Ann Missouri Botanical Garden 70:440–458

Hanagarth W (1993) Acerca de la geoecologia de las sabanas del Beni en el noreste de Bolivia. Instituto de Ecologia, La Paz, Bolivia

Handley CO Jr (1976) Mammals of the Smithsonian Venezuelan project. Brigham Young University Science Bulletin, Biology Series 20:1–91

Handley COJ, Wilson DE, Gardner A (1991) Demography and natural history of the common fruit bat, *Artibeus jamaicensis* on Barro Colorado Island, Panama. Smithsonian Contributions to Zoology no. 511. Smithsonian Institution Press, Washington, DC

Hanni C, Laudet V, Barriel V, Catzeflis FM (1995) Evolutionary relationships of *Acomys* and other murids (Rodentia, Mammalia) based on complete 12s ribosomal–RNA mitochondrial gene-sequences. Isr J Zool 41:131–146

Hartenberger JL (1998) Description de la radiation des Rodentia (Mammalia) du Paléocène Superieur au Miocène: incidences phylogénétiques. Comptes rendus de l'Académie des sciences. Série II, Sciences de la terre et des planètes 326:439–444

Hershkovitz P (1962) Evolution of neotropical cricetine rodents (Muridae) with special reference to the Phyllotine group. Fieldiana: Zool 46:524

Hjelle B, Yates T (2001) Modeling Hantavirus maintenance and transmission in rodent communities. In: Schmaljohn C, Nichol S (eds) Hantaviruses. Curr Topics Microbiol Immunol 256. Springer Verlag, Berlin Heidelberg New York

Hubert B, Meylan A, Petter F, Poulet A, Trainer M (1983) Different species in the genus *Mastomys* from Western, Central and Southern Africa (Rodentia Muridae). Annales du musée royal du Congo belge. Série 8, Sciences Zoologiques 237:143–148

Huchon D, Catzeflis FM, Douzery EJP (1999) Molecular evolution of the nuclear von Willebrand factor gene in mammals and the phylogeny of rodents. Mol Biol Evol 16:577–589

Husson AM (1978) The mammals of Suriname. Rijkmuseum Natural History, Leiden

Ibañez C, Moreno S (1982) Ciclo reproductor de algunos cricetidos (Rodentia, Mammalia) de los Llanos de Apure (Venezuela). Actas, VIII Congreso Latino Americano de Zoologia. Tomo 1:471–480

Johnson K (1970) Fiebres Hemorrágicas de America del Sur. Adelantos en Medicina 30:99–110

Johnson KM, Kuns ML, Mackenzie RB, Webb PA, Yunker CE (1966) Isolation of Machupo virus from wild rodent *Calomys callosus*. Am J Trop Med Hyg 15:103–106

Johnson KM, Taylor P, Elliott LH, Tomori O (1981) Recovery of a Lassa-related arenavirus in Zimbabwe. Am J Trop Med Hyg 30:1291–1293

Justines G, Johnson KM (1970) Observations on the laboratory breeding of the cricetine rodent *Calomys callosus*. Lab Anim Care 20:57–60

Karimi CRA, Petter F (1976) Note sur les rongeurs du nord-est du Bresil. Mammalia 40:257–266

Knowlton N, Weigt LA (1998) New dates and new rates for divergence across the Isthmus of Panama. Proc R Soc Lond B Biol Sci 265:2257–2263

Koopman K (1993) Chiroptera. In: Wilson DE, Reeder D (eds) Mammal species of the world. A taxonomic and geographic reference, 2nd edn. Smithsonian Institution, Washington, DC, pp 137–241

Kosoy MY, Elliott LH, Ksiazek TG, Fulhorst CF, Rollin PE, Childs JE, Mills JN, Maupin GO, Peters CJ (1996) Prevalence of antibodies to arenaviruses in rodents from the southern and western United States: evidence for an arenavirus associated with the genus *Neotoma*. Am J Trop Med Hyg 54: 570–576

Kuns ML (1965) Epidemiology of Machupo virus infection. II. Ecological and control studies of hemorrhagic fever. Am J Trop Med Hyg 14:813–816

Lacher TE Jr, Mares MA, Alho CJR (1989) The structure of a small mammal community in a central Brazilian savanna. In: Redford KH, Eisenberg JF (eds) Advances in neotropical mammalogy. Sandhill Crane Press, Gainsville, pp 137–162

Lavrachenko LA, Milishnikov AN, Aniskin VM, Warshavsky AA (1999) Systematics and phylogeny of the genus *Stenocephalemys* Frick 1914 (Rodentia, Muridae): a multidisciplinary approach. Mammalia 63:475–494

Leifer E, Gocke DJ, Bourne H (1970) Lassa fever, a new virus disease of man from West Africa. II. Report of a laboratory-acquired infection treated with plasma from a person recently recovered from the disease. Am J Trop Med Hyg 19:677–679

Linnaeus C (1758) Systema Naturae per regna tria naturae, secundum classis, ordines, genera, species cum characteribus, differentiis, synonymis, locis. Laurentii Salvii, Stockholm

Lisanti J, Debarale GD, Senn EP, Bella JL (1996) Chromosomal characterization of *Calomys musculinus* (Rodentia; Cricetidae). Caryologia 49:327–334

Lozano ME, Posik DM, Albarino CG, Schujman G, Ghiringhelli PD, Calderon G, Sabattini M, Romanowski V (1997) Characterization of arenaviruses using a family-specific primer set for RT-PCR amplification and RFLP analysis. Its potential use for detection of uncharacterized arenaviruses. Virus Res 49:79–89

Lyons NF, Gordon DH, Green CA, Walters CR (1977) G-banding chromosome analysis of *Praomys natalensis* (Smith) (Rodentia: Muridae) from Rhodesia. 1. 36 chromosome population. Heredity 38:197–200

Lyons NF, Gordon DH, Green CA, Walters CR (1978) G-banding chromosome analysis of *Praomys natalensis* (Smith) (Rodentia: Muridae) from Rhodesia. 2. 32 chromosome population. Unpublished manuscript

Macedo R, Mares MA (1988) *Neotoma albigula*. Mammalian Species 310:1–7

Macholan M (1996a) Morphometric analysis of European house mice. Acta Theriol 61:255–275

Macholan M (1996b) Multivariate morphometric analysis of European species of the genus *Mus* (Mammalia, Muridae). Z Säugetierkd 61:304–319

Mares MA, Ernest KA (1995) Population and community ecology of small mammals in a gallery forest of central Brazil. J Mammal 76:750–768

Mares MA, Ojeda R, Kosko M (1981a) Observations on the distribution and ecology of the mammals of Salta Province, Argentina. Ann Carnegie Museum 50:151–206

Mares MA, Willig MR, Streilein KE, Lacher TT (1981b) The mammals of northeastern Brazil: a preliminary assessment. Ann Carnegie Museum 50:81–137

Mares MA, Willig M, Lacher TE (1985) The Brazilian Caatinga in South American zoogeography: tropical mammals in a dry region. J Biogeography 12:57–69

Mares MA, Braun JK, Gettinger D (1989) Observations on the distribution and ecology of the mammals of the cerrados of Central Brazil. Ann Carnegie Museum 58:1–60

Marquez EJ, Aguilera M, Corti M (2000) Morphometric and chromosomal variation in populations of *Oryzomys albigularis* (Muridae: Sigmodontinae) from Venezuela: multivariate aspects. Z Saugetierkd 65:84–99

Marshall JT (1977) A synopsis of Asian species of *Mus* (Rodentia, Muridae). Bull Am Museum Natural History 158:173–220

Marshall JT (1998) Identification and scientific names of Eurasian house mice and their European allies, subgenus *Mus* (Rodentia: Muridae). Privately printed, Springfield, Virgina

Martino AMG, Aguilera M (1993) Trophic relationships among four cricetid rodents in rice fields. Rev Biol Trop 41:131–141

Massoia E, Pardinas UFJ (1993) El estado sistematico de algunos muroideos estudiados por Ameghino en 1889. Revalidacion del genero *Necromys* (Mammalia, Rodentia, Cricetidae). Ameghiniana 30: 407–418

Massoia E, Fornes A, Wainberg R, Fronza TG (1968) Nuevos aportes al conocimiento de las especies bonaerenses del genero *Calomys* (Rodentia – Cricetidae). Rev Invest Agropecuarias 5:63–92

Matthey R (1965) Études de cytogénétique sur les Murinae africains appartenant aux genres *Arvicanthis*, *Praomys*, *Acomys* et *Mastomys* (Rodentia). Mammalia 29:228–249

McCormick JB (1990) Arenaviruses. In: Fields BN, Knipe DM, Chanock RM, Hirsch MS, Melnick JL, Monath TP, Roizman B (eds) Fields Virology. Raven, New York

Mello DA (1978) Biology of *Calomys callosus* (Rengger 1830) under laboratory conditions (Rodentia, Cricetinae). Rev Bras Biol 38:807–811

Mello DA (1980) Estudo populacional de algumas especies de roedores del cerrado (Norte do Municipio de Formosa, Goias. Rev Bras Biol 40:843–860

Mello DA (1984) *Calomys callosus* Rengger, 1830 (Rodentia-Cricetidae): its characterization, distribution, biology, breeding and management of a laboratory strain. Mem Inst Oswaldo Cruz 79:37–44

Meng J, McKenna MC (1998) Faunal turnovers of palaeogene mammals from the Mongolian Plateau. Nature 394:364–367

Meunier DY, McCormick JB, Georges AJ, Georges MC, Gonzalez JP (1985) Comparison of Lassa, Mobala, and Ippy virus reactions by immunofluorescence test. Lancet 8433:873–874

Mills JN, Childs JE (1998) Ecologic studies of rodent reservoirs: their relevance for human health. Emerg Infect Dis 4:529–537

Mills JN, Ellis BA, McKee KT, Ksiazek TG, Oro JGB, Maiztegui JI, Calderon GE, Peters CJ, Childs JE (1991a) Junin virus activity in rodents from endemic and nonendemic loci in Central Argentina. Am J Trop Med Hyg 44:589–597

Mills JN, Ellis BA, McKee KT, Maiztegui JI, Childs JE (1991b) Habitat associations and relative densities of rodent populations in cultivated areas of Central Argentina. J Mammal 72:470–479

Mills JN, Ellis BA, McKee KT, Calderon GE, Maiztegui JI, Nelson GO, Ksiazek TG, Peters CJ, Childs JE (1992a) A longitudinal study of Junín virus activity in the rodent reservoir of Argentine hemorrhagic fever. Am J Trop Med Hyg 47:749–763

Mills JN, Ellis BA, McKee KT, Maiztegui JI, Childs JE (1992b) Reproductive characteristics of rodent assemblages in cultivated regions of central Argentina. J Mammal 73:515–526

Mills JN, Ellis BA, Childs JE, McKee KT Jr, Maiztegui JI, Peters CJ, Ksiazek TG, Jahrling PB (1994) Prevalence of infection with Junín virus in rodent populations in the epidemic area of Argentine hemorrhagic fever. Am J Trop Med Hyg 51:554–562

Mills JN, Oro JGB, Bressler DS, Childs JE, Tesh RB, Smith JF, Enria DA, Geisbert TW, McKee KT, Bowen MD, Peters CJ, Jahrling PB (1996) Characterization of Oliveros virus, a new member of the Tacaribe complex (Arenaviridae, Arenavirus). Am J Trop Med Hyg 54:399–404

Mills JN, Bowen MD, Nichol ST (1997) African arenaviruses: coevolution between virus and murid host. Belg J Zool 127:19–28

Misonne X (1974) Order Rodentia. In: Meester J, Setzer HW (eds) The mammals of Africa: an identification manual. Smithsonian Institution, Washington, DC

Moncayo AC, Hice CL, Watts DM, Travassos de Rosa A, Guzman H, Russell KL, Calampa C, Gozalo A, Popov VT, Weaver SC, Tesh RB (2001) Allpahuayo virus: A newly recognized arenavirus (Arenaviridae) from arboreal rice rats (Oecomys bicolor and Oecomys paricola) in northeastern Peru. Virology 284:277–286s

Monath TP, Newhouse VF, Kemp GE, Setzer HW, Cacciapouti A (1974) Lassa virus isolation from Mastomys natalensis rodents during an epidemic in Sierra Leone. Science 185:263–265

Musser GG, Carleton MD (1993) Family Muridae. In: Wilson DE, Reeder DM (eds) Mammal species of the world: a taxonomic and geographic reference. Smithsonian Institute, Washington, DC

Musser GG, Carleton MD, Brothers EM, Gardner AL (1998) Systematic studies of oryzomyine rodents (Muridae, Sigmodontinae): diagnoses and distributions of species formerly assigned to Oryzomys 'capito'. Bull Am Museum Natural History 236:1–376

Myers P (1982) Origins and affinities of the mammal fauna of Paraguay. In: Mares MA, Genoways HH (eds) Mammalian biology in South America. The Pymatuning symposia in ecology, special publication series. Pymatuning Laboratory of Ecology, University of Pittsburgh, Linesville, Penn, v6:85–93

Nitikman LZ, Mares MA (1987) Ecology of small mammals in the gallery forest of central Brazil. Ann Carnegie Museum 56:75–95

Olds N (1988) A revision of the genus Calomys (Rodentia: Muridae). PhD thesis, City University of New York

Olmos F (1991) Observations on the behavior and population dynamics of some Brazilian Atlantic Forest rodents. Mammalia 55:555–565

Orsini P, Bonhomme F, Britton-Davidian J, Croset H, Gerasimov S, Thaler L (1983) Le complexe d'espèces du genre Mus en Europe Centrale et Orientale. II. Critères d'identification, repartition et caractéristiques écologiques. Z Säugetierkd 48:86–95

Pardinas UFJ, Tonni EP (1998) Stratigraphic provenance and age of the oldest muroids (Mammalia; Rodentia) in South America. Ameghiniana 35:473–475

Parmenter CA, Yates TL, Parmenter RR, Dunnum JL (1999) Statistical sensitivity for detection of spatial and temporal patterns in rodent population densities. Emerg Infect Dis 5:118–125

Patterson BD (1992) Mammals in the Royal Natural History Museum, Stockholm, collected in Brazil and Bolivia by A.M. Ollala during 1934–1938. Fieldiana Zool, new series, iii + 42

Patterson BD (2000) Patterns and trends in the discovery of new neotropical mammals. Diversity Distributions 6:145–151

Patton JL, Da Silva MNF, Malcolm JR (1996) Hierarchical genetic structure and gene flow in three sympatric species of Amazonian rodents. Mol Ecol 5:229–238

Patton JL, Da Silva MNF, Malcolm JR (2000) Mammals of the Rio Juruá and the evolutionary and ecological diversification of Amazonia. Bull Am Museum Natural History 244:1–306

Pavloskii EN (1966) Natural nidality of transmissible diseases, with special reference to the landscape epidemiology of zooanthroponoses. University of Illiniois Press, Urbana

Pefaur JE, Diaz De Pascual A (1985) Small mammal species diversity in the Venezuelan Andes. Acta Zool Fennica 173:57–59

Peppers LL, Bradley RD (2000) Cryptic species in Sigmodon hispidus: evidence from DNA sequences. J Mammal 81:332–343

Peters CJ (1997) Arenaviruses. In: Richman DD, Whitley RJ, Hayden FG (eds) Clinical virology. Churchill Livingstone, New York

Petter F (1977) Les rats à mammelles multiples d'Afrique occidentale et centrale: Mastomys erythroleucus (Temminck, 1853) et M. huberti (Wroughton, 1908). Mammalia 41:441–444

Petter F, Karimi Y, Almeida CR (1967) Un nouveau rongeur de laboratoire le cricetide Calomys callosus. C R Acad Sci Hebd Seances Acad Sci D 265:1974–1976

Pinheiro FP, Shope RE, Andrade AHP, Bensabath G, Cacios GV, Casals J (1966) Amaparí, a new virus of the Tacaribe group from rodents and mites of Amapa territory, Brazil. Proc Soc Exp Biol Med 122:531–535

Pinheiro FP, Woodall JP, Travassos da Rosa A, Travassos da Rosa JF (1977) Studies on arenavirus in Brazil. Medicina (Buenos Aires) 37 [Suppl 3]:175–181

Redford KH, Eisenberg JF (1992) Mammals of the neotropics, Vol 2. The southern cone. University of Chicago, Chicago

Reig OA (1987) An assessment of the systematics and evolution of the Akodontini, with the description of new fossil species of *Akodon* (Cricetidae, Sigmodontinae). Fieldiana Zool 39:347–399

Rosevear DR (1969) The rodents of West Africa. British Museum (Natural History), London

Ruedas LA, Kirsch JAW (1997) Systematics of *Maxomys* Sody, 1936 (Rodentia: Muridae: Murinae): DNA/DNA hybridization studies of some Borneo-Javan species and allied sundaic and Australo-Papuan genera. Biol J Linnean Soc 61:385–408

Sabattini MS, Gonzales de Rios LE, Diaz G, Vega VR (1977) Infeccion natural y experimental de roedores con virus Junin. Medicina (Buenos Aires) 37 [Suppl 3]:149–161

Salazar-Bravo J, Dragoo JW, Tinnin D, Yates TL (2001) Phylogeny and evolution of the neotropical rodent genus *Calomys*: inferences from mitochondrial DNA sequence data. Mol Phylogenet Evol (in press)

Schaller GB (1983) Mammals and their biomass in a Brazilian ranch. Arquivos Zool 31:1–36

Serrano V (1987) Desert-dwelling rodent communities of Bolson, Mapimi, and Durango (Mexico). Acta Zool Mexicana (n.s.) 20:1–25

Smith MF, Patton JL (1999) Phylogenetic relationships and the radiation of sigmodontine rodents in South America: evidence from cytochrome *b*. J Mammalian Evolution 6:89–128

Speir RW, Wood O, Liebhaber H, Buckley SM (1970) Lassa fever, a new virus disease of man from West Africa. IV. Electron microscopy of vero cell cultures infected with Lassa virus. Am J Trop Med Hyg 19:692–694

Streilein K (1982a) Ecology of small mammals in the semiarid Brazilian Caatinga. I. Climate and faunal composition. Ann Carnegie Museum 51:79–107

Streilein KE (1982b) Ecology of small mammals in the semiarid Brazilian Caatinga. III. Reproductive biology and population ecology. Ann Carnegie Museum 51:251–269

Swanepoel R, Leman PA, Shepherd AJ, Shepherd SP, Kiley MP, McCormick JB (1985) Identification of Ippy as a Lassa-fever-related virus. Lancet 8429:639

Tellman B (1997) Exotic pest plant introduction in the American Southwest. Desert Plants 13:3–10

Tesh RB, Wilson ML, Salas R, Manzione NMCD, Tovar D, Ksiazek Thomas G, Peters CJ (1993) Field studies on the epidemiology of Venezuelan hemorrhagic fever: implication of the cotton rat *Sigmodon alstoni* as the probable rodent reservoir. Am J Trop Med Hyg 49:227–235

Tesh R, Salas R, Fulhorst C, de Marzione N, Duno G, Weaver S, Utrera A, Paredes H, Ellis B, Mills J, Bowen M, Ksiazek T (1999) Epidemiology of Arenavirus in the Americas. In: Saluzzo J, Dodet B (eds) Emergence and control of rodent-borne viral diseases (Hantaviral and arenal diseases) Elsevier, Paris

Thomas O (1915) List of mammals (exclusive to Ungulata) collected on the Upper Congo by Dr Christy for the Congo Museum, Tervueren. Annals and Magazine of Natural History, Ser. 8, 16:465–481

Timm RM, Ashe JS (1987) Host and elevational specificity of parasitic beetles (*Amblyopinus* Solsky) (Coleoptera: Staphylinidae) in Panamá. Proc Biol Soc Washington 100:13–20

Trapido H, SanMartin C (1971) Pichinde virus. A new virus of the Tacaribe group from Colombia. Am J Trop Med Hyg 20:631–641

Traub E (1935) A filterable virus recovered from white mice. Science 81:298–299

Traub E (1936a) An epidemic in a mouse colony due to the virus of acute lymphocytic choriomeningitis. J Exp Med 63:533–546

Traub E (1936b) The epidemiology of lymphocytic choriomeningitis in white mice. J Exp Med 64:183–200

Troup JM, White HA, Fom ALMD, Carey DE (1970) An outbreak of Lassa fever on the Jos Plateau, Nigeria, in January–February 1970; a preliminary report. Am J Trop Med Hyg 19:695–696

Usdin K, Chevret P, Catzeflis FM, Verona R, Furano AV (1995) L1 (Line-1) retrotransposable elements provide a fossil record of the phylogenetic history of murid rodents. Mol Biol Evol 12:73–82

Utrera A, Duno G, Ellis BA, Salas RA, deManzione N, Fulhorst CF, Tesh RB, Mills JN (2000) Small mammals in agricultural areas of the western llanos of Venezuela: community structure, habitat associations, and relative densities. J Mammal 81:536–548

Van der Straeten E, Dieterlen F (1987) *Pramomys misonnei*, a new species of Muridae from Eastern Zaire (Mammalia). Stuttgart Beit Naturkd A (Biol) 402:1–40

Viegas-Pequignot E, Dutrillaux B, Prod'Homme M, Petter F (1983) Chromosomal phylogeny of Muridae: a study of 10 genera. Cytogenet Cell Genet 35:269–278

Viegas-Pequignot E, Petit D, Benazzou T, Prod'Homme M, Lombard M, Hoffshir S, Descailleaux G, Dutrillaux B (1986) Philogénie chromosomique chez les Sciuridae, Gerbillidae et Muridae et étude d'espèces appartenant a d'autres familles de Rongeurs. Mammalia 50:164–202

Vivas AM (1986) Population biology of *Sigmodon alstoni* (Rodentia, Cricetidae) in the Venezuelan llanos. Rev Chilena Historia Natural 59:179–192

Volobouev V, Viegas-Pequignot E, Lombard M, Petter F, Duplantier JM, Dutrillaux B (1988) Chromosomal evidence for a polytypic structure of *Arvicanthis niloticus* (Rodentia, Muridae). Z Zool System Evolution-forschung 26:276–285

Voss RS (1991) An introduction to the Neotropical muroid rodent genus *Zygodontomys*. Bull Am Museum Natural History 210:113

Voss RS (1992) A revision of the South American species of *Sigmodon* (Mammalia: Muridae) with notes on their natural history and biogeography. Am Museum Novitates 3050:1–56

Voss RS, Carleton MD (1993) A new genus for *Hesperomys molitor* Winge and *Holochilus magnus* Hershkovitz (Mammalia, Muridae) with an analysis of its phylogenetic relationships. Am Museum Novitates 3085:1–39

Voss RS, Emmons LH (1996) Mammalian diversity in neotropical lowland rainforests: a preliminary assessment. Bull Am Museum Natural History 230:5

Wallgren A (1924) Méningite aiguë; une nouvelle maladie infectieuse du système nerveux central? Acta Paediatr 4:158–181

Webb PA, Johnson KM, Mackenzie RB, Kuns ML (1967) Some characteristics of Machupo virus, causative agent of Bolivian hemorrhagic fever. Am J Trop Med Hyg 16:531–538

Webb PA, Johnson KM, Hibbs JB, Kuns ML (1970) Paraná, a new Tacaribe complex virus from Paraguay. Arch Gesamte Virusforschung 32:379–388

Webb PA, Johnson KM, Peters CJ, Justines G (1973) Behavior of Machupo and Latino viruses in *Calomys callosus* from two geographic areas in Bolivia. In: Lehmann-Grube F (ed) Lymphocytic choriomeningitis virus and other arenaviruses. Springer Verlag, Berlin Heidelberg New York, pp 313–322

Webb PA, Justines G, Johnson KM (1975) Infection of wild and laboratory animals with Machupo and Latino viruses. Bull World Health Org 52:493–499

Weksler M, Geise L, Cerqueira R (1999) A new species of *Oryzomys* (Rodentia, Sigmondontinae) from southeast Brazil, with comments on the classification of the *O. capito* species group. Zool J Linnean Soc 125:445–462

Wellings FM, Lewis AL, Pierce LV (1972) Agents encountered during arboviral ecological studies: Tampa Bay area, Florida, 1963 to 1970. Am J Trop Med Hyg 21:201–213

Whitford WG (1976) Temporal fluctuations in density and diversity of desert rodent populations. J Mammal 57:351–369

Wilson DE (1979) Reproductive patterns. In: Baker RJ, Jones JK, Carter DC (eds) Biology of bats of the new world family Phyllostomidae. Special publications of the Museum. Part III. Texas Tech University, Lubbock, pp 317–378

Wilson DE (1991) Mammals of the Tres Marias Islands. In: Griffiths T, Klingener D (eds) Contributions to mammalogy in honor of Karl F. Koopman. Bull Am Museum Natural History 206:214–250

Wulff H, McIntosh BM, Hamner DB, Johnson KM (1977) Isolation of an arenavirus closely related to Lassa virus from *Mastomys natalensis* in south-east Africa. Bull World Health Org 55:441–444

Yahnke C (1999) Community ecology of small mammals in the Paraguayan Chaco. PhD thesis, Northern Illinois University

Yates TL, Jones C, Cook JA (1996) Preservation of voucher specimens. In: Wilson DE, Cole FR, Nichols JD, Rudran R, Foster MS (eds) Measuring and monitoring biological diversity. Standard methods for mammals. Smithsonian Institution Press, Washington, DC

Zuñiga H, Rodriguez JR, Cadena A (1983) Densidad de población de pequeños mamíferos en dos comunidades del bosque Andino. Acta Biol Colombiana 1:85–93

Human Infection with Arenaviruses in the Americas

C.J. PETERS

1 Introduction

Numerous arenaviruses exist in the Americas as parasites of rodents belonging to the family Muridae, subfamily Sigmodontinae, 14 have been described (BUCHMEIER et al. 2001; BOWEN et al. 1997). Little is known about how these viruses interact with their rodent hosts and what diseases are caused when the viruses spill over into humans. In addition, the Americas host one Old World arenavirus, Lymphocytic choriomeningitis virus, which was introduced in post-Columbian times with its host, *Mus musculus*.

Human infection has been assessed by measuring antibody prevalence. Disease has been sought by anamnesis or by observing patients hospitalized in the region in question with attempts to identify characteristic hemorrhagic fever patients from records or actual observation. Virus infection is then confirmed by retrospective antibody studies or laboratory analysis of acute samples. When neither acute dis-

University of Texas Medical Branch, 301 University Blvd, Galveston, TX 77555-0609, USA

ease nor antibodies are found, it is not clear that this represents lack of human contact with the rodents, patterns of rodent virus excretion, human resistance to infection, or insensitivity of the laboratory tests for infection.

Most viruses have not been associated with extensive human infection or disease with the exception of Junin, Machupo, and Guanarito viruses, all three of which cause typical severe hemorrhagic fever (HF). Other viruses are known in a very fragmentary way and will be discussed below (Table 1).

2 Junin Virus

This virus was first recognized in the humid pampas of Argentina in the 1950s as the cause of a severe and highly characteristic clinical disease with high fever, thrombocytopenia, and shock (ARRIBALZAGA 1955). Isolation of the virus from humans and later rodents established the etiology (PARODI et al. 1958; PIROSKY et al. 1959), and numerous clinical, epidemiologic, and virologic studies followed from the endemic area over the next 40 years. Much has been written about the emergence of the disease and the relation of crops, herbicides, agricultural practices, and other factors, but there is no established reason for the appearance and progressive increase in incidence. What is well documented is that the disease area is increasing, the formerly "hot" areas are cooling off, and that measures of rodent infection correspond (D. Enria, personal communication).

The disease begins insidiously with fever, myalgia, and malaise after an incubation period of 1–2 weeks (perhaps as long as 3 weeks). Typically after 3–4 days the symptoms become increasingly severe and bring the patient to the physician

Table 1. Human arenavirus infection in the Americas

Virus	Geography	Number	Evidence
Junin	Argentina	100s to 1,000s annually	Virus isolation, seroconversion, immunohistochemistry
Machupo	Bolivia	Formerly 100s annually, now a handful	Virus isolation, seroconversion
Guanarito	Venezuela	100s to handful annually	Virus isolation, seroconversion
Sabia	Brazil	3	Virus isolation, seroconversion
Flexal	Brazil	2	Virus isolation, seroconversion
Whitewater Arroyo	Western USA	2	RT-PCR on postmortem tissue; awaiting confirmation
Pichinde	Colombia	~12	Seroconversion by IFA; lab infection
Tacaribe	Trinidad	1	Seroconversion by IFA; lab infection
Tamiami	USA	3/229	Seropositive in survey; no disease associated

IFA, indirect fluorescence antibody test; RT-PCR, reverse transcriptase polymerase chain reaction.

(ARRIBALZAGA 1955; MOLTENI et al. 1961; RUGGIERO et al. 1964; HARRISON et al. 1999; ENRIA et al. 1999). Multisystem involvement follows, particularly gastrointestinal distress with abdominal pain, nausea and vomiting, constipation or mild diarrhea. Dizziness, headache, photophobia, retroorbital pain, and disorientation occur commonly. Early findings include tachycardia, postural hypotension, petechiae, flushing over the face and thorax, and conjunctival injection (PETERS et al. 1997). Neurological signs may be prominent with tremor of the tongue and arms, coma, and convulsions.

The clinical laboratory is quite helpful. Leucopenia, thrombocytopenia, and proteinuria are virtually constant. Abnormal urinary sediment and slight hemoconcentration are common. The transaminases are usually normal. At times, the differential diagnosis involving hantavirus infection can be difficult (HARRISON et al. 1999; PARISI et al. 1996).

Later, hemorrhage becomes more prominent in the severe cases. This may be accompanied by shock, which is often fatal. Neurological disease can dominate the picture, and patients may die with progressive nervous system dysfunction and little in the way of hemorrhagic manifestations (RUGGIERO et al. 1960). Patients destined to recover generally develop antibodies and clear viremia in the second week of illness (DE BRACCO et al. 1978).

Treatment is achieved in the endemic area by use of convalescent plasma selected to provide an adequate dose of neutralizing antibodies given within the first week of disease (ENRIA and MAIZTEGUI 1994). Mortality is reduced from 25%–35% to under 1%, but about 10% of treated patients develop a transient cerebellar-cranial nerve syndrome (ENRIA et al. 1985). Ribavirin is likely to be effective therapy (ENRIA and MAIZTEGUI 1994). A safe, efficacious Junin vaccine has been developed (BARRERA-ORO and EDDY 1982; MAIZTEGUI et al. 1998) and is in use in risk groups to reduce disease in Argentina. Production of the vaccine is expected to begin soon in Argentina (D.A. Enria, personal communication).

3 Machupo Virus

This virus first appeared as a cause of occasional cases of "black typhus" in remote areas of the Bolivian Amazon basin. In the 1960s, Bolivian HF became a serious problem among the towns that were established in that region (JOHNSON et al. 1967). When it was established that the causative virus was rodent-borne (JOHNSON et al. 1966), the urban disease was controlled using rodent trappers immune from previous disease, and only occasional cases occurred subsequently (MERCADO 1975). High densities of the natural reservoir rodent develop in cleared fields in the Beni province and increase human risk in fields and isolated dwellings even when the rodents do not invade towns. Nosocomial (PETERS et al. 1971) and intrafamilial (KILGORE et al. 1995) interhuman transmission have occasionally occurred in small epidemics.

The clinical picture is similar to that of Argentine HF (JOHNSON et al. 1967; DOUGLAS et al. 1965; STINEBAUGH et al. 1966; PETERS et al. 1971; KILGORE et al. 1997). In an unusual nosocomial epidemic occurring at high altitude, jaundice was a feature.

Specific treatment has not been established, but animal studies and fragmentary clinical observations suggest that the antiviral drug ribavirin is efficacious (STEPHEN et al. 1980; KILGORE et al. 1997). The Junin vaccine protects experimental animals against Machupo challenge (BARRERA-ORO et al. 1988).

4 Guanarito Virus

As with Machupo virus, Guanarito virus emerged as the cause of Venezuelan HF when settlers moved into cleared forest areas. The disease was first recognized in 1989 and the virus isolated soon afterwards (SALAS et al. 1991; TESH et al. 1994). The disease incidence slacked but accelerated again soon afterwards (DE MANZIONE et al. 1998).

The clinical manifestations resemble those of Argentine HF, although deafness is mentioned as a finding in convalescence. There is no specific therapy established, but it is likely that ribavirin would have efficacy.

5 Sabia and Flexal Viruses

Sabia virus has been responsible for a fatal natural infection (COIMBRA et al. 1994), a moderately severe laboratory infection, and a laboratory infection aborted by ribavirin (BARRY et al. 1995). Flexal virus has caused two moderately severe laboratory infections and should be regarded as potentially dangerous (PINHEIRO et al. 1977; Pinheiro, personal communication). All these illnesses resemble Argentine HF to the degree one can ascertain from the small amount of data available. The fatal Sabia infection was also characterized by severe hepatic necrosis (COIMBRA et al. 1994).

6 Whitewater Arroyo Virus

In a search for new arenaviruses in North America, rodent sera were tested for antibodies to known arenaviruses. Wood rats had an encouragingly high prevalence of antibodies (KOSOY et al. 1996), and Whitewater Arroyo virus was isolated from them (FULHORST et al. 1996). This virus is widely distributed in the western USA. It has recently been implicated as a possible cause of severe human infection (CDC 2000).

7 Pichinde Virus

Pichinde virus was isolated from two different areas of Colombia, and the isolates differ in genetic sequences and in their ability to adapt to cause lethal guinea pig disease (PETERS et al. 1987). The adapted virus has proven to be a useful model for arenavirus HF, but apparently has no increased pathogenicity for nonhuman primates. Both these viral strains have caused a number of laboratory infections without any overt disease (BUCHMEIER et al. 1974; C.J. Peters, unpublished observations, 1991).

8 Other Viruses

Tacaribe virus has also resulted in a single example of febrile disease with mild central nervous symptomatology (J. Casals, personal communication). Antibodies to Tamiami virus have been found in serosurveys of apparently healthy humans without any disease association having been made (J. Nuckolls, unpublished data).

9 Diagnosis

Acute human infections are associated with viremia, and this can be detected by cultivation in VERO cells, inoculation of suckling mice, or occasionally by resorting to inoculation of suckling hamsters. Sometimes co-cultivation of blood mononuclear cells will allow the isolation of Junin virus when other methods fail (AMBROSIO et al. 1986). Other viral products can be sought. Viral RNA can be amplified by RT-PCR; there is some clinical experience (LOZANO et al. 1995; BARRY et al. 1995) and a general formulation of sensitive primers (BOWEN et al. 1996, 1997). Sufficient viral protein is present in acute phase sera to permit detection of either Junin or Machupo virus by antigen detection ELISA using Junin virus reagents (T.G. Ksiazek, unpublished observations).

Antibody tests become positive around the time of viral clearance and beginning recovery, typically in the second week of disease (DE BRACCO et al. 1978). Complement fixation tests are quite insensitive, and these antibodies wane quickly. Indirect fluorescent antibody (IFA) tests remain positive for several years and plaque reduction neutralizing (PRN) antibody or ELISA tests for decades (PETERS et al. 1972). Specificity of the PRN is thought to be quite high, perhaps less so for the ELISA.

10 Pathology and Pathogenesis of Arenavirus Hemorrhagic Fever

The pathogenesis of arenaviral HF is poorly understood, but a few facts are evident from consideration of both human and animal models. The virus presumably enters by inhalation in most cases and deposits in the terminal respiratory bronchiole. It gains entry to the lymphoid system and spreads systemically but does not leave a detectable pneumonic focus (KENYON et al. 1992). The virus is capable of infecting endothelium in culture (ANDREWS et al. 1978), and indeed some endothelial infection is seen in vivo (ZAKI and PETERS 1997). There is also prominent infection of mesothelial surfaces in vivo, perhaps the source of some of the effusions that are seen. Infection of parenchymal cells of several organs, particularly lymphoid tissues, occurs as well. Interestingly, the histopathological findings in humans and animal models do not reflect the severity of disease (ELSNER et al. 1973; CHILD et al. 1967; SALAS et al. 1991; PETERS et al. 1987; ARONSON et al. 1994; ZAKI and PETERS 1997).

Early investigations using the guinea pig-adapted Pichinde virus model of arenavirus HF explored soluble mediators of shock such as leukotrienes, platelet activating factor, and endorphins (LIU et al. 1986; PETERS et al. 1987; PETERS 1997) in an attempt to explain the resulting fatal disease. These substances were all activated, but the source of the activation was presumably tumor necrosis factor (TNF)-alpha which is increased in the guinea pigs (ARONSON et al. 1995). Patients with Argentine HF have extraordinarily high levels of interferon and also high levels of TNF-alpha, which correlate with a fatal outcome (LEVIS et al. 1985; HELLER et al. 1992). Indeed, more extensive cytokine measurements have shown extensive activation of inflammatory mediators in Argentine HF patients (MARTA et al. 1999).

Studies of the guinea pig model also revealed a markedly depressed cardiac contractility and output (QIAN et al. 1996). Such studies have not been done in patients with arenaviral HF, but this is a common observation in hantavirus disease and dengue HF. TNF-alpha has been suggested as the cause (PETERS et al. 1999). Given the ease of inducing pulmonary edema after fluid infusion in South American HF patients, myocardial depression may well be present there as well.

The profuse bleeding often seen is presumably a consequence of vascular damage by cytokines and virus combined with the marked thrombocytopenia commonly found. There is no evidence of disseminated intravascular coagulation, although there are several modest abnormalities of clotting factors and activation of fibrinolysis (MOLINAS et al. 1989; HELLER et al. 1995).

It is not known why the severity of infection varies from patient to patient. When Junin virus was studied in guinea pigs and in nonhuman primates, there was considerable variation among strains of virus with similar passage histories (McKee et al. 1985; Kenyon et al. 1986), and in the case of the monkeys, there was a correlation between the patterns seen in monkeys and those in the patients from whom the strains were derived. Host genetic factors are also involved in some models. The pathogenesis of Pichinde virus infection of inbred hamsters (and lymphocytic choriomeningitis, as well) depends on the hamster genotype and the delayed-type hypersensitivity response (Buchmeier et al. 1977; Genovesi and Peters 1987; Genovesi et al. 1989).

Recovery can be accomplished by passive antibody in patients and experimental animals (Enria and Maiztegui 1994; Peters et al. 1987). It is likely that T-cell immunity plays a large role as well, but this has not been well studied in the American arenaviruses. It is notable that the administration of Fab with virus-neutralizing capacity will not protect guinea pigs from fatal Junin virus infection (Kenyon et al. 1990). Antibody-dependent cellular cytotoxicity is active in this model and presumably is needed to eliminate cells infected with poorly cytopathic arenaviruses (Kenyon and Peters 1986), whereas in humans cytolytic T cells serve this function. Argentine HF patients have decreased circulating T cells (Vallejos et al. 1989), and fatal cases have lymphoid necrosis, both indicating an immuno-suppressive effect from the virus and/or from cytokines.

Interestingly, fetal invasion is common with both Argentine and Bolivian HF, reflecting the common fetal pathology seen with Lymphocytic choriomeningitis virus in humans (Briggiler et al. 1990; Barton and Hyndman 2000). The arenaviruses also readily pass into the pregnant rodent uterus in their natural hosts.

11 Conclusions

Human disease from arenaviruses is a major public health problem in the focal areas of South America where the human-rodent exposure leads to infection with pathogenic viruses. Fortunately, these areas are relatively small and isolated, and the overall problem is not large except in Argentina, where a successful vaccine has controlled the disease.

Supportive therapy is routinely administered in South American hospitals with little virus transmission, but occasionally a patient will disseminate to family and/or medical staff. Treatment with the antiviral drug ribavirin will likely allow the management of most arenavirus HF cases if therapy is initiated within the first few days of the illness.

Given the several hundred sigmodontine rodent species known to be present in the Americas, it is likely that there are numerous undiscovered arenaviruses. Continual habitat modification leading to conditions for emergence could lead to the appreciation of another arenaviral HF at any time. The North American arenavirus Whitewater Arroyo deserves further observation for its pathogenic proclivities.

References

Ambrosio AM, Enria DA, Maiztegui JI (1986) Junin virus isolation from lympho-mononuclear cells of patients with Argentine hemorrhagic fever. Intervirology 25:97–102

Andrews BS, Theofilopoulos AN, et al. (1978) Replication of dengue and Junin viruses in cultured rabbit and human endothelial cells. Infect Immun 20:776–781

Aronson JF, Herzog NK, Jerrells TR (1994) Pathological and virological features of arenavirus disease in guinea pigs – comparison of two Pichinde virus strains. Am J Pathol 145:228–235

Aronson JF, Herzog NK, Jerrells TR (1995) Tumor necrosis factor and the pathogenesis of Pichinde virus infection in guinea pigs. Am J Tropical Med Hyg 52:262–269

Arribalzaga RA (1955) Una nueva enfermedad epidemica a germen desconocido: hipertermia, nefrotoxica, leucopenica y enantematica. Dia Medico (Buenos Aires) 27:1204–1210

Barrera-Oro JG, Eddy GE (1982) Characteristics of candidate live attenuated Junin virus vaccine. In: Kurstak E, Marusyk RG, Maramorosch K (eds) Fourth International Conference on Comparative Virology, Banff, Canada, 17–22 October 1982 (abstract S4–10)

Barrera-Oro JG, Lupton HW, et al. (1988) Cross-protection against Machupo virus with Candid #1 live-attenuated Junin virus vaccine. I. The postvaccination prechallenge immune response. Second International Conference on the Impact of Viral Diseases on the Development of Latin American Countries and the Caribbean Region, Buenos Aires, Argentina, 20–26 March 1988

Barry M, Russi M, Armstrong L, Geller D, Tesh R, Dembry L, Gonzalez JP, Khan AS, Peters CJ (1995) Treatment of a laboratory-acquired Sabia virus infection. New Engl J Med 333:294–296

Barton LL, Hyndman NJ (2000) Lymphocytic choriomeningitis virus: reemerging central nervous system pathogen. Pediatrics. 105:E351-E352

Bowen MD, Peters CJ, Nichol ST (1996) The phylogeny of New World (Tacaribe complex) arenaviruses. Virology 219:285–290

Bowen MD, Peters CJ, Nichol ST (1997) Phylogenetic analysis of the Arenaviridae: patterns of virus evolution and evidence for cospeciation between arenaviruses and their rodent hosts. Mol Phylogenetics Evolution 8:301–316

Briggiler AM, Levis S, Enria D, Ambrosio AM, Maiztegui JI (1990) Argentine hemorrhagic fever in pregnant women. Medicina (Buenos Aires) 50:443

Buchmeier M, Rawls W (1977) Variation between strains of hamsters in the lethality of Pichinde virus infections. Infect Immun 16:413–421

Buchmeier MJ, Adam E, Rawls WE (1974) Serologic evidence of infection by Pichinde virus among laboratory workers. Infect Immun 9:821–823

Buchmeier MJ, Bowen MD, Peters CJ (2001) Arenaviridae: the viruses and their replication. In: Field Virology, 4th edn. (in press)

CDC (2000) Fatal illnesses associated with a New World arenavirus – California, 1999–2000. MMWR 49:709–711

Child PL, MacKenzie RB, Johnson KM (1967) Bolivian hemorrhagic fever. A pathologic description. Arch Pathol 83:434–445

Coimbra TLM, Nassar ES, Burattini MN, Souza LT de, Ferreira IB, Rocco IM, Travassos da Rosa AP, Vasconcelos PFC, Pinheiro FP, LeDuc JW, Rico-Hesse R, Gonzalez JP, Jahrling PB, Tesh RB (1994) New arenavirus isolated in Brazil. Lancet 343:391–392

De Bracco MME, Rimolldi MT, Cossio PM, Rabinovich A, Maiztegui J, Carballal G, Arana RM (1978) Argentine hemorrhagic fever. Alterations of the complement system and anti-Junin virus humoral response. N Engl J Med 209:216

Douglas RG, Wiebenga NH, Couch RB (1965) Bolivian hemorrhagic fever probably transmitted by personal contact. Am J Epidemiol 82:85–91

Elsner B, Schwarz ER, Mando OG, Maiztegui JI, Vilches AM (1973) Pathology of 12 fatal cases of Argentine hemorrhagic fever. Am J Trop Med Hyg 22:229–236

Enria D, Maiztegui JI (1994) Antiviral treatment of Argentine hemorrhagic fever. Antivir Res 23:23–31

Enria DA, Damilano AJ de, Briggiler AM, Ambrosio AM, Fernández NJ, Feuillade MR, Maiztegui JI (1985) Sindrome neurologico tardio en enfermos de fiebre hemorrágica Argentina tratados con plasma immune. Medicina (Buenos Aires) 45:615–620

Genovesi EV, Peters CJ (1987) Susceptibility of inbred Syrian hamsters (*Mesocricetus auratus*) to lethal disease by lymphocyte choriomeningitis virus (42541). Proc Soc Exp Biol Med 185:250–261

Harrison LH, Halsey NA, McKee KT Jr, Peters CJ, Barrera-Oro JG, Briggiler AM, Feuillade MR, Maiztegui JI (1999) Clinical case definitions for Argentine hemorrhagic fever. Clin Infect Dis 28:1091–1094

Heller MV, Saavedra MC, Falcoff R, Maiztegui JI, Molinas FC (1992) Increased tumor necrosis factor-alpha levels in Argentine hemorrhagic fever [letter]. J Infect Dis 166:1203–1204

Heller MV, Marta RF, Sturk A, Maiztegui JI, Hack CE, Cate JW ten, Molinas FC (1995) Early markers of blood coagulation and fibrinolysis activation in Argentine hemorrhagic fever. Thrombosis Hemostasis 73:368–373

Johnson KM, Kuns ML, Mackenzie RB, Webb PA, Yunker CE (1966) Isolation of Machupo virus from wild rodent *Calomys callosus*. Am J Trop Med Hyg 15:103–106

Johnson KM, Halstead SB, Cohen SN (1967) Hemorrhagic fevers of South-east Asia and South America: a comparative appraisal. Progr Med Virol 9:105–158

Kenyon RH, Peters CJ (1986) Cytolysis of Junin infected target cells by immune guinea pig spleen cells. Microbial Pathogenesis 1:453–464

Kenyon RH, McKee KT Jr, et al. (1986) Heterogeneity of Junin virus strains. Med Microbiol Immunol 175:165–167

Kenyon RH, Condie RM, et al. (1990) Protection of guinea pigs against experimental Argentine hemorrhagic fever by purified human IgG: importance of elimination of infected cells. Microbial Pathogenesis 9:219–226

Kenyon RH, McKee KT Jr, Zack PM, Rippy MK, Vogel AP, York C, Meegan J, Crabbs C, Peters CJ (1992) Aerosol infection of rhesus macaques with Junin virus. Intervirology 33:23–31

Kilgore PE, Peters CJ, Mills JN, Rollin PE, Armstrong L, Khan AS, Ksiazek TG (1995) Prospects for the control of Bolivian hemorrhagic fever. Emerg Infect Dis 1:97–100

Kilgore PE, Ksiazek TG, Rollin PE, Mills JN, Villagra MR, Montenegro MJ, Costales MA, Paredes LC, Peters CJ (1997) Treatment of Bolivian hemorrhagic fever with intravenous ribavirin. J Infect Dis 24:718–722

Kosoy MY, Elliott LH, Ksiazek TG, Fulhorst CF, Rollin PE, Childs JE, Mills JN, Maupin GO, Peters CJ (1996) Prevalence of antibodies to arenaviruses in rodents from the southern and western United States: evidence for an arenavirus associated with the genus *Neotoma*. Am J Trop Med Hyg 54: 570–576

Levis SC, Saavedra MC, Ceccoli C, Feuillade MR, Enria DA, Maiztegui JI, Falcoff R (1985) Correlation between endogenous interferon and the clinical evolution of patients with Argentine hemorrhagic fever. J Interferon Res 5:383–389

Liu CT, Jahrling PB, Peters CJ (1986) Evidence for the involvement of sulfidopeptide leukotrienes in the pathogenesis of Pichinde virus infection in strain 13 guinea pigs. Prostaglandins Leukotrienes Med 24:129–138

Lozano ME, Enria D, Maiztegui JI, Grau O, Romanowski V (1995) Rapid diagnosis of Argentine hemorrhagic fever by reverse transcriptase PCR-based assay. J Clin Microbiol 33:1327–1332

Maiztegui JI, McKee KT, Barrera-Oro JG, Harrison LH, Gibbs PH, Feuillade MR, Enria DA, Briggiler AM, Levis SC, Ambrosio AM, Halsey NA, Peters CJ, and the AHF Study Group (1998) Protective efficacy of a live attenuated vaccine against Argentine hemorrhagic fever. J Infect Dis 177:277–283

Manzione N de, Salas RA, Paredes H, Godoy O, Rojas L, Araoz F, Fulhorst CF, Ksiazek TG, Mills JN, Ellis BA, Peters CJ, Tesh RB (1998) Venezuelan hemorrhagic fever: clinical and epidemiologic studies of 165 cases. Clin Infect Dis 26:308–313

Marta RF, Montero VF, et al. (1999) Proinflammatory cytokines and elastase-alpha-1antitrypsin in Argentine hemorrhagic fever. Am J Trop Med Hyg 60:85–89

McKee KT, Mahlandt BG, et al. (1985) Experimental Argentine hemorrhagic fever in rhesus macaques: viral strain-dependent clinical response. J Infect Dis 152:218–221

Mercado RR (1975) Rodent control programmes in areas affected by Bolivian haemorrhagic fever. Bull World Health Org 52:691–696

Mills JN, Ellis BA, McKee KT, Calderon GE, Maiztegui JI, Nelson GO, Ksiazek TG, Peters CJ, Childs JE (1992) A longitudinal study of Junin virus activity in the rodent reservoir of Argentine hemorrhagic fever. Am J Trop Med Hyg 47:749–763

Mills JN, Ellis BA, et al. (1994) Prevalence of infection with Junin virus in rodent populations in the epidemic area of Argentine hemorrhagic fever. Am J Trop Med Hyg 51:554–562

Molinas FC, Bracco MME de, Maiztegui JI (1989) Hemostasis and the complement system in Argentine hemorrhagic fever. Rev Infect Dis 11 [Suppl 4]:762–767

Molteni HD, Guarinos HC, Petrillo CO, Jaschek FRJ (1961) Estudio clinico estadistico sobre 338 pacientes afectados por la fiebre hemorragica epidemica del Noroeste de la Provincia de Buenos Aires. Semana Méd 118:838–855, 878

Parisi MDN, Enria DA, Pini NC, Sabattini MS (1996) Retrospective detection of clinical infections caused by hantavirus in Argentina. Medicina (Buenos Aires) 56:1–13

Parodi AS, Greenway DJ, Rugiero HR, Rivero E, Frigerio MJ, Barrera JM de la, Mettler NE, Garzon F, Boxaca MC, Guerrero LB, Nota NR (1958) Sobre la etiología del brote epidémico de Junín (Nota previa). Dia Médico 30:62

Peters CJ (1997) Pathogenesis of viral hemorrhagic fevers. In: Nathanson N, Ahmed R, Gonzalez-Scarano F, Griffin D, Holmes KV, Murphy FA, Robinson HL (eds) Viral pathogenesis. Lippincott-Raven, Philadelphia, pp 779–799

Peters CJ, Webb PA, Johnson KM (1972) Measurement of antibodies to Machupo virus by the indirect fluorescent technique. Proc Soc Exp Biol Med 142:526–531

Peters CJ, Kuehne RW, et al. (1974) Hemorrhagic fever in Cochabamba, Bolivia, 1971. Am J Epidemiol 99:425–433

Peters CJ, Jahrling PB, et al. (1987) Experimental studies of arenaviral hemorrhagic fevers. In: Oldstone MB (ed) Current Topics in Microbiology and Immunology, Vol 134. Arenaviruses: epidemiology and immunotherapy. Springer Verlag, Berlin Heidelberg New York, pp 5–68

Peters CJ, Zaki SR, Rollin PE (1997) Viral hemorrhagic fevers. In: Fekety R (ed) Atlas of infectious diseases, Vol 8. External manifestations of systemic infections. Current Medicine, Philadelphia, pp 10.1–10.26

Peters CJ, Simpson GL, Levy H (1999) Spectrum of hantavirus infection: hemorrhagic fever with renal syndrome and hantavirus pulmonary syndrome. Annu Rev Med 50:531–545

Pinheiro FP, Woodall JP, Travassos da Rosa PA, Travassos da Rosa JF (1977) Studies on arenaviruses in Brazil. Medicina (Buenos Aires) 37:175–181

Pirosky I, Zuccarini J, Molinelli EA, Di Pietro A, Barrera-Oro JG, Martini P, Capello AR (1959) Virosis hemorrágica del noroeste bonaerense (endemo–epidémica, febril, enantemática y leucopenica). Buenos Aires Instituto Nacional de Microbiologia, Ministerio de Asistencia Social y Salud Publica

Qian C, Jahrling PB, Peters CJ, Liu CT (1994) Cardiovascular and pulmonary responses to Pichinde virus infection in strain 13 guinea pigs. Lab Animal Sci 44:600–607

Ruggiero HR, Cintora FA, Libonatti EJ, Magnoni CC, Castiglione EB, Locicero R (1960) Formas nerviosas de la fiebre hemorrágica epidemica. Prensa méd argent 47:1845–1849

Ruggiero HR, Ruggiero H, Gonzalez-Cambaceres C, Cintora FA, Maglio F, Magnoni CC, Astarloa LN, Squassi GJ, Giacosa A, Fernandez D (1964) Argentine hemorrhagic fever. II. Clinical studies. Rev Asoc Méd Argentina 78:281–294

Salas R, Manzione N de, Tesh RB, Rico-Hesse R, Shope RE, Betaucourt A, Godoy O, Bruzual R, Pacheco DE, Ramos B, Taibo ME, Tamayo JG, James E, Vasquez C, Araoz F, Querales J (1991) Venezuelan hemorrhagic fever. Lancet 338:1033–1036

Stephen EL, Jones DE, et al. (1980) Ribavirin treatment of toga-, arena-, and bunyavirus infections in subhuman primates and other laboratory animal species. In: Smith RA, Kirkpatrick W (eds) Ribavirin: a broad spectrum antiviral agent. Academic Press, New York, pp 169–183

Stinebaugh BJ, Schloeder FX, Johnson KM, et al. (1966) Bolivian hemorrhagic fever: a report of four cases. Am J Med 40:217

Tesh RB, Jahrling PB, Salas R, Shope RE (1994) Description of Guanarito virus (Arenaviridae: Arenavirus), the etiologic agent of Venezuelan hemorrhagic fever. Am J Trop Med Hyg 50:452–459

Vallejos DA, Ambrosio AM, Feuillade MR, Maiztegui JI (1989) Lymphocyte subsets alteration in patients with Argentine hemorrhagic fever. J Med Virol 27:160–163

Zaki SR, Peters CJ (1997) Viral hemorrhagic fevers. In: Connor DH, Chandler FW, Schwartz DA, Manz HJ, Lack EE (eds) The pathology of infectious diseases. Appleton and Lange, Norwalk, Conn., pp 347–364

Lassa Fever

J.B. McCormick and S.P. Fisher-Hoch

1 Background

Nineteen arenaviruses have been isolated in the Old and the New World, most of them identified in South or Central America. Current evidence suggests that arenaviruses have co-evolved along with their rodent hosts over a time scale of as

University of Texas, School of Public Health, Brownsville, TX, USA

much as 9 million years. Among six arenaviruses so far known to cause human illness, only one, Lassa virus, is from Africa. Three other arenaviruses have been isolated in Africa: Mopeia virus from *Mastomys natalensis* in southern Africa (WULFF et al. 1977; JOHNSON et al. 1981a) and two other viruses from two different rodent species, *Arvicanthus* and *Praomys* (GONZALEZ et al. 1983; SWANE-POEL et al. 1985) in the Central African Republic. None of them has been associated with human illness (GEORGES et al. 1985). Lassa fever was described as a clinical entity in the 1950s, well before the Lassa virus was identified in 1969, when it was isolated from febrile American missionaries working in northern Nigeria (FRAME et al. 1970; BUCKLEY and CASALS 1970). Further expansion of the family is to be anticipated with increased efforts at surveillance, including a possible a new North American arenavirus capable of causing fatal human disease.

Lassa virus is distributed throughout West Africa, where its reservoir is the ubiquitous rodent *Mastomys natalensis*. Serologic evidence of human infection has been identified in Senegal (SALUZZO et al. 1988), Guinea (KNOBLOCH et al. 1980), Sierra Leone (KNOBLOCH et al. 1980; FRASER et al. 1974), Liberia (MONATH et al. 1973; BLOCH 1978; MERTENS et al. 1973; YALLEY-OGUNRO et al. 1984; FRAME et al. 1979), Nigeria (FRAME et al. 1970, 1979; YALLEY-OGUNRO et al. 1984; BAJANI et al. 1997; TROUP et al. 1970; GRUNDY et al. 1980; FABIYI et al. 1979; BOWEN et al. 1975; WHITE 1972; CAREY et al. 1972; WULFF et al. 1975), and purportedly northern Cameroon (GONZALEZ et al. 1989). Among the arenaviruses, Lassa fever affects by far the largest number of humans, creating a geographic patchwork of endemic foci encompassing perhaps 180 million people from Guinea to eastern Nigeria (McCORMICK 1986, 1987; McCORMICK et al. 1987a) (Fig. 1). Over 200,000 infections are estimated to occur annually, with several thousand deaths

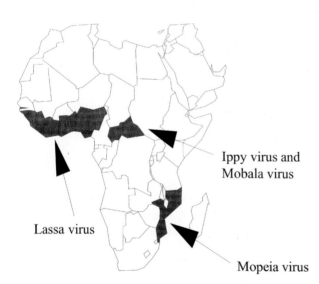

Ippy virus and
Mobala virus

Lassa virus

Mopeia virus

Fig. 1. Distribution of arenaviruses in Africa

(McCormick 1986, 1987). The only longitudinal study of Lassa fever in West Africa took place in eastern Sierra Leone from the late 1970s through 1990 (McCormick et al. 1987b). The Centers for Disease Control and Prevention (CDC) established and supported the study following repeated requests from the government of Sierra Leone to investigate epidemics in the eastern province. Over the years, many aspects of Lassa fever have been defined including the clinical presentation, epidemiology, immunology, pathophysiology, and therapy (McCormick et al. 1987b; Trappier et al. 1993; Fisher-Hoch and McCormick 1897). War and social chaos over the past decade have not only interrupted the ongoing studies and prevented new ones from taking place, but also probably increased the disease rates in these areas. Furthermore, the intervention in the war in Sierra Leone has resulted in the deaths of at least 4 expatriates working in Sierra Leone.

2 Lassa Fever: Clinical Disease and Sequelae

Lassa fever begins insidiously, after an incubation period of 7–18 days, with fever, weakness, malaise, severe headache, usually frontal, and a very painful sore throat (Fig. 2) (Knobloch et al. 1980; McCormick et al. 1987b; Monath et al. 1973, 1974; Mertens et al. 1973). More than 50% of patients then develop joint and lumbar pain, and 60% develop a nonproductive cough. Many also develop a severe

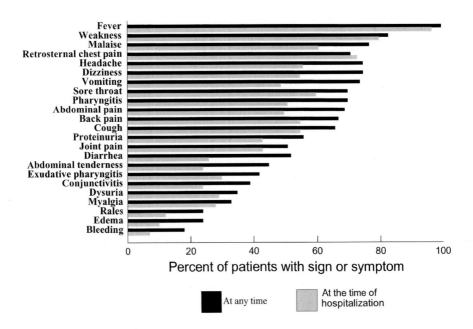

Fig. 2. Signs and symptoms in Lassa fever

retrosternal chest pain, and about half will have nausea with vomiting or diarrhea and abdominal pain. On physical examination, the respiratory rate, temperature, and pulse rate are elevated, and the blood pressure may be low. There is no characteristic skin rash in Lassa fever, and petechiae and ecchymoses are not seen. About a third of patients will have conjunctivitis; a few with conjunctival hemorrhages have a poor prognosis. More than two-thirds have pharyngitis, half with exudates, diffusely inflamed and swollen posterior pharynx and tonsils, but few if any ulcers or palatal petechiae. The abdomen is tender in 50% of patients, but bowel sounds are usually normal to marginally reduced. Neurological signs in the early stages are limited to a fine tremor, most marked in the lips and tongue (KNOBLOCH et al. 1980; McCORMICK 1986; McCORMICK et al. 1987b; CUMMINS et al. 1992; FISHER-HOCH et al. 1985).

Up to a third of hospitalized Lassa fever patients progress to a prostrating illness 6–8 days after onset of fever, usually with persistent vomiting and diarrhea. They are often dehydrated with elevated hematocrit. Proteinuria occurs in two-thirds of patients, and blood urea nitrogen may be moderately elevated. About half of Lassa fever patients will have diffuse abdominal tenderness but no localizing signs or loss of bowel sounds. The severe retrosternal or epigastric pain seen in many patients may be due to pleural or pericardial involvement. Bleeding is seen in only 15%–20% of patients, limited primarily to the mucosal surfaces or occasionally manifest as conjunctival hemorrhages or gastrointestinal or vaginal bleeding. Severe pulmonary edema and adult respiratory distress syndrome is common in fatal cases with gross head and neck edema, pharyngeal stridor, and hypovolemic shock (KNOBLOCH et al. 1980; McCORMICK et al. 1987b).

Over 70% of patients may have abnormal electrocardiograms including nonspecific ST-segment and T-wave abnormalities, ST-segment elevation, generalized low voltage complexes, and changes reflecting electrolyte disturbance, but none of these correlate with clinical or other measures of disease severity or outcome and are not associated with clinical manifestations of myocarditis (CUMMINS et al. 1989a). Neurological signs are infrequent, but carry a poor prognosis, ranging from confusion to severe encephalopathy with or without general seizures, but without focal signs (McCORMICK et al. 1987b; CUMMINS et al. 1992; FISHER-HOCH et al. 1985). Cerebrospinal fluid is usually normal, but with a few lymphocytes, and low titers of virus relative to serum. Interstitial crepitations indicative of pneumonitis, and pleural and pericardial rubs suggesting effusions, develop in early convalescence in about 20% of hospitalized patients, occasionally in association with congestive cardiac failure, perhaps as a result of pericardial tamponade (McCORMICK et al. 1987b; CUMMINS et al. 1989a; HIRABAYASHI et al. 1988).

Though the mean white blood cell count in Lassa fever on admission to hospital is normal ($6 \times 10^9/1$), this may mask marked lymphopenia and later relative or absolute neutrophilia, which may reach as much $30 \times 10^9/1$ in severely ill patients (McCORMICK et al. 1987b; FISHER-HOCH et al. 1988). Based on similar observations with Ebola virus, the lymphopenia of Lassa fever may be related to apoptosis of Lassa virus-specific CTL or CD4 lymphocytes, though objective evidence is required to confirm this hypothesis (BAIZE et al. 1999). Thrombocytopenia is moderate, even in severely ill patients, but platelet function is markedly depressed or even absent. This abnormality is usually maximal on admission to hospital and is present even when circulating platelet numbers remain above 100×10^9/l. A circulating inhibitor of platelet and neutrophil function has been described and will be discussed in detail in the section on pathogenesis (CUMMINS et al. 1989b).

A serum AST (aspartate transaminase, SGOT) level on admission of 150 or higher is associated with a high case fatality (Fig. 3a), and there is a correlation between an increasing level and a higher risk of fatal outcome (Fig. 3b). ALT (alanine transaminase, SGPT) is only marginally raised, and the ratio of AST:ALT in natural infections and in experimentally infected primates is as high as 11:1

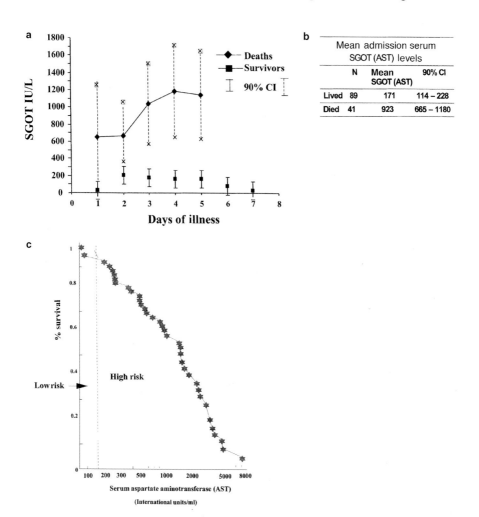

Fig. 3a–c. Survival in Lassa fever. Patients by outcome and interval of illness: mean serum AST levels in Lassa fever (**a**), cumulative survival in Lassa fever by level of AST (**b**), and mean admission serum AST levels (**c**)

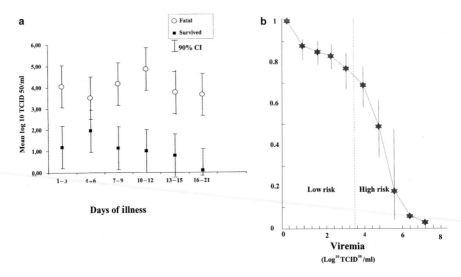

Fig. 4a,b. Survival in Lassa fever. **a** Titers of Lassa virus in serum of dying and surviving patients. **b** Cumulative survival in Lassa fever by viremia level (TCID$_{50}$). (McCORMICK et al. 1987b)

(McCORMICK et al. 1986, 1987b). The degree of hepatic damage observed clinically (no jaundice, prothrombin times, glucose and bilirubin levels are near normal) and in postmortem tissue in Lassa virus infection is limited and cannot account for the overall clinical picture, and certainly not for the severity of the disease observed (McCORMICK et al. 1986).

Viremia of $\geq 1 \times 10^{3.0}$ is associated with increasing case fatality (Fig. 4). High virus titers occur in the ovary, pancreas, uterus, and placenta in addition to the liver, but histological lesions are limited and not consistent with organ failure. Elevated viremia and AST together carry a risk of death of nearly 80% (Table 1) (McCORMICK et al. 1986, 1987b).

While the case fatality in hospitalized patients is about 16%, the death rate for all Lassa virus infections (nonhospitalized + hospitalized) may be as low as 2%–3% depending on the geographic and clinical setting (McCORMICK 1987, 1988). However, in recent outbreaks in Nigeria, much higher death rates have been observed in hospitalized patients possibly due to a variation in virus virulence or to parenteral transmission (FISHER-HOCH et al. 1995). Case fatality may be as much as 30% in the third trimester of pregnancy and exceeds 50% in patients with hemorrhage.

2.1 Complications and Convalescence

Infrequent complications, particularly in early convalescence, include uveitis, orchitis, and acute adrenal insufficiency. More commonly observed are pleural effusion with pleural rubs, clinical evidence of pericarditis with pericardial rubs,

Table 1. Outcome of Lassa fever by admission viremia and AST, Sierra Leone

Outcome	Viremia $< 10^{3.0}$		Viremia $\geq 10^{3.0}$	
	AST < 150	AST ≥ 150	AST < 150	AST ≥ 150
Survived	25	7	23	9
Died	4	1	6	31
Case fatality (%)	13.8	12.5	20.7	78

and ascites (McCORMICK et al. 1987b). Renal or hepatic failure is very rarely seen. A single case report described an interesting complex of hemorrhagic pericarditis and cardiac tamponade with pleural effusions and ascites 6 months after acute Lassa fever (HIRABAYASHI et al. 1988, 1989). Repeated cultures have failed to isolate virus from effusion fluids, but effusion specimens contained high titers of Lassa-specific IgG and numerous lymphocytes. Convalescence may be prolonged with periods of fatigue and weakness. Many patients also exhibit cerebellar signs during convalescence from severe disease, particularly tremors and ataxia, but the majority of these resolve with time (CUMMINS et al. 1992).

2.2 Deafness in Lassa Fever

Nearly 30% of patients with Lassa virus infection suffer an acute loss of hearing in one or both ears (CUMMINS et al. 1990a). The onset is nearly always during the convalescent phase of illness, and its development and degree are unrelated to the severity of the acute disease. It is unclear whether the damage is due to viral neurotropism, thrombosis, vasculitis, focal hemorrhage, or some other viral or immune response-related phenomenon. A sensorineural hearing deficit (SNHD) was detected in (29%) of confirmed hospitalized Lassa fever patients in Sierra Leone (compared to none in hospitalized febrile controls), and 50% had a bilateral deficit. A SNHD was detected in nearly 80% of those affected prior to a 2-week follow-up and in 21% of patients at the follow-up (all were symptomatic). The audiometric measurements of this deafness are found in Table 2; no patient gave a history of hearing difficulty prior to acute Lassa fever. The mean auditory threshold of these patients is 55dB (normal < 25dB), and the mean disability is over 20% consistent with substantial deafness (CUMMINS et al. 1990a). About half of the patients show a near or complete recovery by 3–4 months after onset, but the other half continue with significant sensorineural deafness, which becomes permanent if it does not resolve within about a year.

Table 2. Deafness in Lassa fever: epidemiology of acute deafness associated with Lassa fever (CUMMINS et al. 1990a)

Acute Lassa fever	Mean age and sex	Number acute deafness	Unilateral/ bilateral	Number permanent deficit	MAT
Yes (n = 49)	30.2 (18M/32F)	14 (29%)	7/7	9/14 (64%)	55dB (95%CI ± 7.1dB)
No (n = 20)	30.1 (10M/10F)	0 (0%)	–	–	–

The onset of hearing impairment in symptomatic patients may be instantaneous in some, while in others it may develop over a few hours. In patients with a hearing loss, antibody to Lassa virus is present before the clinical onset of their hearing loss, which occurs approximately 5–12 days after the fever subsides. Deafness is not associated with the level of AST or viremia and thus not with the degree of disease severity.

At final assessment, 60% of those with acute hearing loss also had a residual hearing loss about 1\3 unilateral and 2\3 bilateral. There was no obvious association between the percentage recovery and the severity of the initial deficit, peak AST recorded during admission, or antiviral therapy. In some patients with initial total bilateral deafness, the extent of spontaneous improvement was dramatic.

The overall prevalence of SNHD in a group of individuals seropositive to Lassa virus was 22% (Table 3). In this study 2\3 of those with hearing loss had a unilateral deficit, and 1\3 a bilateral deficit. The mean MAT of all affected ears in those with antibody and hearing loss was 43.7dB (90%CI = ±8.6dB), and the mean binaural disability, 30.5% (90%CI = ±9.7%). A group of seronegative controls from the local healthy adult population matched for age and sex and evaluated for sensorineural thresholds showed 97% of the ears had a MAT <25dB, and 100% had a MAT <27.5dB. Thus, the long-term proportion of all Lassa-infected patients with residual hearing loss is between 15% and 20%, and the hearing loss disability is over 30%, including some with complete deafness (CUMMINS et al. 1990a).

Individuals who had experienced deafness of sudden onset (mean duration 7.1 years), and controls were also evaluated (Table 4). All denied any hearing problem prior to their acute deafness, and all related its onset to an acute febrile illness. In 59%, this illness was severe (hospital admissions), in 16% moderate, and in 25% mild. Mild recovery of hearing occurs at least subjectively in about 40% of patients. Antibody to Lassa virus was present in 81% of deaf patients and 19% of controls. Positive serology was observed as frequently in those deaf patients who were unaware as those who were aware that Lassa fever may have been the illness associated with their deafness onset.

Table 3. Deafness in Lassa fever: prevalence of sensorineural hearing deficit (SNHD) in persons with previous Lassa virus infection (CUMMINS et al. 1990a)

Serology	Number	SNHD present	Mean MAT
Seropositive	51	11 (22%)	43.7db (90%CI ± 8.6dB)
Seronegative	92	2 (%)	≤27.5db

Table 4. Deafness in Lassa fever: evidence of Lassa virus infection in people with deafness (CUMMINS et al. 1990a)

Deafness of sudden onset	Prevalence of LF antibody	MAT	Bilateral/unilateral and mean disability
Yes ($n = 32$)	26/32 (81%)	90.1dB (90%CI +/− 4.0dB)	30/2 and 74% (+/−5.9%)
No ($n = 32$)	6/32 (19%)	NA	NA

In total, 94% of patients with a SNHD had a bilateral deficit. Severity ranged from a moderate unilateral deficit to total bilateral loss of hearing. Overall, the degree of impairment was substantial. Of these patients, 72% had a profound or total hearing loss in one or both ears. The mean MAT of all ears evaluated was 90.1dB (90%CI = ±4.0dB) and the mean binaural disability, 74% (±5.9%). This suggests that after the initial improvement seen in some with acute hearing loss, those with residual hearing loss have a profound deficit, which does not improve with time. No associations were observed between MAT values and age, sex, and severity of disease (mild vs. severe) associated with deafness onset. With bilateral impairment, there was a weak correlation between the severity of the deficit in each ear. This is one of the highest rates of sudden onset deafness associated with a single disease ever reported, and it further illustrates the large burden of acute and chronic illness from Lassa fever.

2.3 Lassa Fever in Pregnancy

Lassa fever may be a common cause of maternal mortality in many areas of West Africa, with case fatality about 20%. However, there is a nearly twofold increase in the number of third-trimester Lassa virus infections requiring hospitalization compared with the first two trimesters, and a corresponding two- to threefold risk of maternal death from infection in the third trimester (Table 5). Very high levels of virus replication have been found in placental tissue in third-trimester patients. A fourfold reduction was noted in case fatality among women who spontaneously or were therapeutically aborted compared with those who were not (odds ratio for fatality with pregnancy intact is 5.5 compared with after uterine evacuation) (Table 6). Fetal loss is near 90% and does not seem to vary by trimester. The excess maternal mortality in the third trimester may be related to the relative immuno-suppression of pregnancy at that time. Lassa virus is known to be present in the

Table 5. Lassa fever in pregnancy: mortality in pregnant and non-pregnant women with Lassa fever

Category of women	Patients	Deaths	Case fatality (%)
All pregnant	68	14	21
First trimester	6	1	18
Second trimester	22	1	5
Third trimester	40	12	30*
Not pregnant	79	10	13

Table 6. Lassa fever in pregnancy: case fatality in women with Lassa fever with and without uterine evacuation

Category	Number of women	Case fatality
No uterine evacuation	26	10/26 (38%)
Uterine evacuation	39	4/39 (10%)*

*$P = 0.05$ ($x^2 = 3.95$, DF = 1, odds ratio = 5.57) (95%CI 1.02–30.26).

breast milk of infected mothers, and neonates are therefore at risk of congenital, intrapartum, and puerperal infection with Lassa virus.

2.4 Lassa Fever in Children

Lassa fever is common in children, but may be difficult to diagnose because the clinical manifestations are so general (WEBB et al. 1986; MONSON et al. 1987). In very young babies, marked edema ("swollen baby syndrome") has been described in those with severe disease, and near uniform fatality. In both Sierra Leone and Liberia, fetal infection is nearly 100% fatal. In older children, the disease may manifest as diarrhea or pneumonia or simply as an unexplained, prolonged fever. In one hospital study in Sierra Leone, 21% of pediatric admissions had Lassa fever, with 12% fatality. Outpatient studies in the same hospital found 4% with evidence of previous Lassa infection and a further 10% with febrile illness who seroconverted (Table 7).

3 Diagnosis

The laboratory diagnosis of Lassa virus infections is based on isolation of virus from serum, demonstration of a fourfold rise in IgG antibody titer, or virus-specific IgG and/or IgM antibody in association with compatible clinical disease (MCCORMICK et al. 1987b). Routine virus isolation may be accomplished easily from serum or tissues in cell cultures, but should be performed in BSL4 laboratory facilities (JOHNSON et al. 1987). Specimens should be drawn preferably into a vacuum tube system to minimize the risk of infection. Virus has also been isolated from urine, throat swabs, breast milk, spinal fluid, pleural and pericardial transudate, and autopsy material (Table 8). Virus may be recovered for 1–2 months in urine, but its detection in urine during acute disease is intermittent (MCCORMICK et al. 1987b). Given the technical and safety considerations for virus isolation, other techniques should be considered for most laboratories, particularly in endemic areas, where the diagnostic need is the greatest. The most reliable and safe routine method for the laboratory at present is detection of virus-specific antibody by IFA (JOHNSON et al. 1981b) or ELISA (BAUSCH et al. 2000). At present, no commercial diagnostic reagents are available. All reagents must come from a

Table 7. Lassa fever in children, Eastern Province, Sierra Leone (WEBB et al. 1986)

Age (years)	Number	Seroconversion	Past infection
< 1	80	3/80 (3.8%)	0
1–5	121	15/121 (12.4%)	3/121 (2.5%)
6–10	92	12/95 (12.6%)	6/95 (6.3%)
11–14	63	6/63 (9.5%)	6/63 (9.5%)
Total	356	36/356 (10.1%)	15/356 (4.2%)

Table 8. Isolation of Lassa virus from sites other than blood in hospitalized patients, Sierra Leone (J.B. McCormick, unpublished data)

Days of illness	Urine	Throat	CSF	Breast milk
0–5	0/10	1/3	1/3	NA
6–10	2/43	5/11	2/2	2/7
11–15	1/26	0/1	0/1	2/7
16–20	0/8	1/3	NA	1/4
21+	0/9	NA	NA	NA
Total (% positive)	3/96 (3.1)	7/18 (39)	3/6 (50)	5/18 (28)

handful of laboratories able to produce them under safe conditions. Many of these BSL 4 laboratories cannot, or do not, produce noninfectious reagents for use by other laboratories.

In most situations, the critical issue is rapid and accurate diagnosis. The ideal situation would be the detection of RNA by RT-PCR, since it would detect replicating virus, rapidly allowing for appropriate treatment and barrier nursing measures. RT-PCR is highly sensitive compared with virus isolation, and of course much more rapid (TRAPPIER et al. 1993) (Fig. 5 and Tables 9–11). Despite the recent advances in simplifying RT-PCR, it is not yet generally available and would only be applicable in situations where the quality control of the test is assured. Recently, a paper was published regarding Lassa viral antigen detection by ELISA (BAUSCH et al. 2000) in which the authors state that in only 1 out of 590 specimens did they find antigen in the presence of IgM antibody. The authors speculate that the virus might be cleared and thus not present or that the antigen is masked. This is surprising since a study published more than 10 years ago shows clearly the

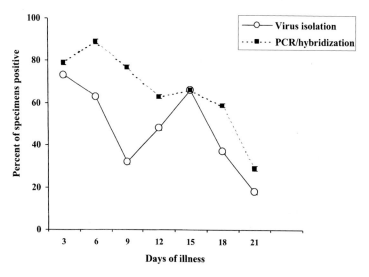

Fig. 5. Percentage of positive isolation and reverse transcriptase polymerase chain reaction (RT-PCR)/hybridization in serum of patients with laboratory-confirmed Lassa fever, by day of illness. (TRAPPIER et al. 1993)

Table 9. Lassa virus detection in Lassa fever: virus isolation and PCR/hybridization for Lassa virus (Trappier et al. 1993)

Virus isolation	PCR			Hybridization		
	+	–	Total	+	–	Total
Positive	84	44	128	108	20	128
Negative	39	126	165	63	102	165
Total	123	170	293	171	122	293
Sensitivity[a]			66 (57–74)			84 (77–90)
Specificity[a]			76 (69–83)			62 (54–69)

[a] 95% confidence intervals in parentheses.

Table 10. Lassa virus detection in Lassa fever: sensitivity and specificity for PCR/hybridization diagnosis of a patient with Lassa fever compared with those without Lassa fever (Trappier et al. 1993)

PCR/hybridization	Patients with Lassa fever	Patients without Lassa fever	Undiagnosed illness
Positive	76	0	8
Negative	22	42	2
Total	98	42	10

Sensitivity for correct diagnosis of Lassa fever: 78% (95%CI 68–85).
Specificity for identifying patients without Lassa fever: 100 (95%CI 89–100).
Predictive value for Lassa fever if the test is positive 100% (95%CI 94–100).
Predictive value for identifying a patient without Lassa fever if test is negative 66% (95%CI 53–77).

Table 11. Lassa virus detection in Lassa fever: relationship between Lassa virus titers and frequency of positive PCR and PCR/hybridization in the diagnosis of Lassa fever (Trappier et al. 1993)

Serum virus titer (TCID$_{50}$)	PCR alone		PCR/hybridization	
	PCR positive	PCR negative	Both positive	Both negative
Virus negative	35	99	22	54
Positive titers				
1.2	0	1	0	0
1.6	9	12	7	6
2.1	4	13	4	8
2.6	6	4	1	0
3.1	17	4	6	0
3.6	5	1	4	1
4.1	14	1	6	0
4.6	5	0	2	0
5.1	5	1	3	0
5.5	1	0	0	0

simultaneous presence of antibody and virus throughout the course of illness (seen in over a hundred specimens from proven cases of Lassa fever; Table 12). Thus, the problem is clearly the masking of antigen by IgM rendering antigen detection as currently practised virtually useless for early diagnosis. Antigen detection ELISA and ELISA for IgM have recently been reported to have a specificity of 90% and a sensitivity of 88% compared with RT-PCR (Bausch et al. 2000). It would appear

Table 12. The simulation presence of virus and specific antibodies to Lassa virus in patients

Interval[a]	Total no. of samples	No. positive for		
		Virus	Virus and antibody	Percent positive for virus and antibody
1–6	117	87	23	26
7–12	199	114	63	51
13–18	93	28	25	89
19–24	18	2	2	100

[a] The disease interval is the number of days that clinical symptoms lasted before specimens were taken.

that the critical part of this is IgM, since antigen detection seems to add very little to the two.

The most widely available, simplest, and safest tests are the serological ones (BAUSCH et al. 2000). There are generally two types of tests available, the older and well tried immunofluorescent antibody assay (IFA) and the enzyme-linked immunosorbent assay (ELISA). Each test has advantages and disadvantages depending on the situation and the information that is needed. The advantages of IFA are its simplicity, low cost, ease of manipulation, its ability to control the background reaction, its overall reliability, and its flexibility, since it allows screening for several antigens in one test (JOHNSON et al. 1981a; ELLIOTT et al. 1982). Its disadvantages are a slightly, but not significantly, lower sensitivity than ELISA (BAUSCH et al. 2000), its modest subjectivity for the complete novice, and the cross-reactivity of the reagents with IgM, IgG, and IgA. In earlier studies, confirmed by virus isolation, an IFA IgG titer of at least 16 and an IgM titer of ≥4, both by IFA, in a patient with clinically compatible disease are highly specific for Lassa infection. Similarly, an ELISA IgM positive early in disease is highly correlated with the presence of virus and predicative of acute infection (Table 8). IFA IgM antibody appears early in infection (53% positive in the first 6 days of illness, and 76% in the first 12 days of illness (Table 13). Clearly, therefore, IgM by any method is highly associated with acute infection, particularly in a patient with clinically compatible illness (BAUSCH et al. 2000). The use of ELISA in Africa is replete with problems resulting in a significant misrepresentation of reality (BIGGAR 1986; BIGGAR et al. 1985, 1986). While testing the background of each serum has resolved many of these problems, the advantage of IFA is that all positive and negative cells are on the

Table 13. The correlation between IgM and IgG antibodies to Lassa virus in hospitalized patients

Interval	Total no. of specimens	No. of specimens				
		IgM–, IgG–	IgM+, IgG–	IgM–, IgG+	IgM+, IgG+	Percent positive for any class of antibody
1–6	128	57	16	3	48/128 53%	55
7–12	136	30	10	3	103/136 76%	78
13–18	71	8	1	4	58/71 83%	89

same spot on the slide, and they can be compared with each other in the same field. Indeed, with a minimum of experience, one can judge immediately the specificity by the appearance of the cells. Furthermore, cells with antigens from multiple viruses can be put on the same spot for the purposes of screening for several viruses at once (JOHNSON et al. 1981b; ELLIOTT et al. 1982).

While newer reagents make the cross-reactivity of IFA with IgG, IgM, and IgA less of a problem than previously, nevertheless current technology suggests that under optimal conditions, ELISA is slightly more sensitive than the older IFA, which is not surprising. However, it may also provide different information. Where the conditions are optimal and reagents are available, ELISA should be used. Where the simplicity and reliability of IFA are advantageous, it remains a functional and reasonable alternative.

4 Pathogenesis of Lassa Fever

4.1 Route of Infection and Early Events

Natural infection from Lassa virus in the endemic areas of West Africa has two primary sources, infected rodents and infected patients (see Sect. 5 for details). The primary route of virus entry is through cuts or abrasions on the skin, or in some instances mucosal surfaces, such as conjunctiva. A second source of direct entry is close contact with secretions or blood from patients infected with Lassa virus, particularly in the household setting. In these circumstances, infection is due to direct contact with infected blood, vomitus, urine, or secretions, or from contaminated needles or instruments.

Needle injection may carry a very high risk of mortality (FISHER-HOCH et al. 1995). Otherwise, there are no data that allow us to distinguish between pathogenic processes resulting from direct entry of virus into cuts and scratches or mucosal surfaces. Subcutaneous or mucosal inoculation of virus probably allows direct entry into the peripheral capillary system, and easy access to the lymphatics and the bloodstream. We can speculate that dendritic cells – antigen-presenting cells – become infected or take up viral antigen at the site of entry at an early stage, and then participate in the disease process and immune response. The ubiquitous presence of the putative Lassa receptor, alpha-dystroglycan, particularly on dendritic cells, undoubtedly facilitates viral entry into endothelial or dendritic cells at the site of primary infection (CAO et al. 1998). However, it is not yet clear whether this receptor is the only receptor component required for viral entry into cells. Infection of these initial sites facilitates access to and subsequent dissemination of the virus throughout the reticuloendothelial system, for which Lassa virus has tropism. The presence of alpha-dystroglycan in cells in many organs may also explain why Lassa virus eventually enters and replicates in a wide array of cells and organs (CAO et al. 1998).

4.2 Viral Replication

Other than an early antibody response to the viral proteins, we know little about the early host response to infection, but we do know that the severity of the disease is related to the level of viremia, and therefore presumably the level of virus replication (Fig. 4 and Tables 14, 15). It is worth noting that studies of genetic control of LCM virulence in mice suggest that the L gene plays a central role in pathogenesis (RIVIERE et al. 1985), and therefore it is interesting to speculate that even in Lassa fever the control of replication, and therefore pathogenesis, may depend in part on the polymerase gene. A single such observation with a reassortant of Mopeia virus L gene and Lassa virus S gene showed a reduced pathogenicity in mice compared with a recombinant with the Lassa L gene (LUKASHEVICH 1992; LUKASHEVICH et al. 1991). Thus, the situation with African arenaviruses may well be similar to that of LCMV in that the L gene, and presumably the polymerase gene, holds the key to virus replication and ultimately pathogenesis.

4.3 Persistence

There is some evidence that Lassa virus may persist, albeit at low titer, and for a limited period of time in primates. For example, virus may be detected intermittently in human urine for up to 60 days, and in monkeys viral RNA was detected in postmortem and biopsy material when examined by RT-PCR up to 112 days after challenge (FISHER-HOCH et al. 2000). Unlike in rodents, persistent virus is sequestered, and contamination of the environment with secondary infections is unlikely. Furthermore, virus is not recoverable in tissue culture from serum or blood of vaccinated and subsequently challenged primates after 14 days, or from tissues after 21 days even by co-cultivation.

Table 14. Viremia in Lassa fever: mean concentration of Lassa virus in blood of hospitalized patients by outcome

	Number	Mean day of illness	Mean viremia titer
Survived	315	11.1	$10^{1.3}$
Died	77	8.0	$10^{3.9}$

Table 15. Viremia in Lassa fever: isolation of Lassa virus from blood of hospitalized patients by illness interval and outcome

	Days of clinical symptoms						
	1–3	4–6	7–9	10–12	13–15	16–21	Total
Survived (n)	19	58	84	63	50	64	338
% positive	33	67	54	35	28	3	38
Died (n)	8	30	29	19	11	5	103
% positive	88	90	90	100	82	100	91

4.4 Lymphopenia and Neutrophilia

The lymphopenia observed in Lassa virus infection in humans is compatible with B cells being a prime target of Lassa virus, as they are in LCMV infection; however, against this is the observation of a reasonably early antibody response to all of the viral proteins. The fact that these antibodies do not neutralize the virus might be attributed to antigen-specific B cell destruction, but this is speculation at present. The lymphocyte depletion is most marked in severe and fatal infections (Fig. 6). In human and non-human primate infections, this early lymphopenia is accompanied by pathological evidence of areas of necrosis in lymphatic organs, compatible with acute destruction of immune cells (WINN and WALKER 1975). The processes leading to cell death in these organs could be due to a combination of lytic infection, and bystander, apoptotic cell death, which depletes both T and B cell populations. This kind of process has recently been shown to be important in another viral hemorrhagic fever, Ebola hemorrhagic fever in humans (Baize et al. 1999). In vitro many cell lines can be infected with Lassa virus with the important exception of T cells and nonactivated mononuclear cells (activated mononuclear/macrophage cells can be easily infected). Lassa is not lytic in these cells in vitro (LUKASHEVICH et al. 1999). Thus, lymphopenia is a prime feature of moderate and severe Lassa fever, but the details of why it occurs remain unclear.

The occurrence of neutrophilia in severe disease is largely unexplained. It may reach as high as 20×10^5 cells per milliliter (FISHER-HOCH et al. 1987, 1988). Furthermore, there is some evidence that neutrophil function may be impaired or deranged in the observation that acute Lassa plasma is able to inhibit degranulation. Sera from Lassa fever patients inhibit the amount of superoxide generated by normal neutrophils in response to the chemotactic peptide f-met-leu-phe (FMLP). In fact, sera from Lassa patients that inhibited the ADP-induced aggregation responses of normal platelets also inhibit the neutrophil response to FMLP. The inhibition of neutrophils is not due to either interference with FMLP-neutrophil binding or an effect on the NADPH-oxidase, suggesting a suppression of signal

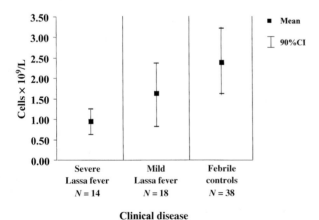

Fig. 6. Minimum mean lymphocyte counts in patients with Lassa fever (normal range of lymphocytes $1.5–3.5 \times 10^9$/l). (FISHER-HOCH et al. 1988)

transduction (ROBERTS et al. 1989). Thus, the inhibitory factor in Lassa plasma has global effects on cellular function beyond that of platelets and may play a central role in the pathogenesis.

4.5 Host Inflammatory Response

In contrast to the spleen, infection in solid organs (liver, kidney) involves only modest cell damage or death compared with, for example, acute fulminating hepatitis B, and this difference may be explained by the poor cellular inflammatory response observed in tissues from patients with Lassa fever (McCORMICK et al. 1986; WALKER et al. 1982). Data on this issue are conflicting, as in vitro suppression of IL-8, a molecule critically central to inflammatory cell migration, is consistent with the in vivo picture of a low inflammatory cell response (LUKASHEVICH et al. 1999). This process could be part of a larger set of events precipitated by the infection of central inflammatory cells such as macrophages, but once again further data are not available. However, since elevation of IL-8 has been observed in Argentinian hemorrhagic fever, caution must be exercised in over-interpreting these data, particularly since more extensive studies of the broader inflammatory response have not been done (MARTA et al. 1999).

4.6 Host Control of Virus Replication

It is clear that failure to control viral replication is associated with severe disease. The viral control, as discussed above, is likely to reside in the L segment polymerase gene. The host's control of replication is determined mostly by the T-cell response, based on the observations that early antibody responses in humans do not correlate with outcome (Fig. 7) or with reduced virus replication, and that primates with high levels of antibody to all viral proteins induced by killed vaccine are not protected, and experience no limitation of viral replication (McCORMICK et al. 1992). Little is known about the T-cell response to Lassa in humans, other than that it occurs, as would be predicted (TER MEULEN et al. 2000). Animals vaccinated with Lassa glycoprotein expressed in vaccinia virus have virtually no detectable antibody response, but they have solid immunity from the same challenge of Lassa virus (FISHER-HOCH et al. 1989, 2000) and are clearly able to control virus replication (see Sect. 9).

4.7 Shock and Vascular Leakage

During the progression to severe Lassa fever disease, there is ample clinical evidence of vascular leakage, which may be quite dramatic. There are effusions in the peritoneum, pleura, and pericardia, progressing to facial (but not lower extremity) edema, pulmonary edema with adult respiratory distress syndrome (ARDS), and hypovolemic shock. While in vitro human endothelial cells can be productively infected to high titer with no apparent cellular damage (LUKASHEVICH et al. 1999),

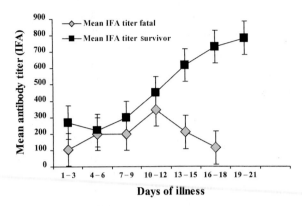

Fig. 7. Antibody (*IFA*) to Lassa virus and outcome of patients with acute Lassa fever

there is no evidence to support a similar process in vivo (FISHER-HOCH et al. 1987). Similar studies of filoviruses have also had mixed results. Infection of endothelial cells in vitro by filoviruses is possible (FELDMANN et al. 1996; SCHNITTLER et al. 1993), even though there is little evidence of this in vivo. However, recent data suggest that just the presence of Ebola transmembrane glycoprotein may adversely affect endothelial cells (YANG et al. 2000), perhaps through binding of the endothelial cell by a mucin site on the Ebola glycoprotein (YANG et al. 2000). There are currently no data for or against such a process in Lassa infection, but it is worth bearing in mind that the clinical evidence of capillary leak is much more marked in Lassa than Ebola infection. ARDS, the frequent cause of death in Lassa infection, has never been reported in Ebola. Encephalopathy, but not encephalitis, is prominent in some patients with Lassa fever, but there is little or no virus found in CNS free of blood contamination and no evidence of parenchymal damage in the brain. Leaky capillaries and edema may well explain this process. Essentially, there are two major choices for initiating the process of vascular leakage: one is the direct effect of the virus, and the second is the host response to the virus infection. In neither instance is actual host cell destruction an attractive hypothesis, since the processes are readily and rapidly reversible if the patient recovers. Unfortunately, there has been no opportunity to observe patients in places where such a study could be done, for instance we do not even have pulmonary X-ray data from West Africa. However, in early primate studies, a marked decrease in prostacyclin production by endothelium has been documented in primates experimentally infected by Lassa virus (FISHER-HOCH et al. 1987). This observation is just a small part of the complex process involving cytokines, chemokines, and other cellular products not yet studied in this disease.

4.8 Hemorrhage and Platelet Function

Another important clinical manifestation in this infection is that patients begin to bleed. The bleeding is usually oozing from the mucosal surfaces, and not petechiae or ecchymoses as seen with some of the other viral hemorrhagic fevers (FISHER-HOCH et al. 1988; McCORMICK 1986). Platelets are modestly reduced in number (range of $1 \times 10^5/\text{ml}$), but this drop is insufficient in itself to explain the bleeding (Fig. 8a). An inhibitor of platelet function has been identified in the plasma of nonhuman primates and patients with severe Lassa fever which appears to be a protein of undetermined molecular weight which is heat stable and highly bioactive (Fig. 8b). Its origin is presumably the host since this phenomenon cannot be reproduced with viral material nor can it be blocked by antibodies to Lassa virus (McCormick 1990). A similar inhibitory effect has also been observed with Junin virus-infected serum (Cummins et al. 1990b). The effect of the Lassa fever platelet inhibitor has been shown to involve interference with the second messenger mechanisms, not through the thromboxane synthetase pathway but through the calcium calmodulin pathway, which leads to ATP release. This has already been described in an earlier section. This effect is manifest by inhibition of the secondary, irreversible wave of platelet aggregation (Fig. 8c,d). It is possible that this host-derived factor may well have a significant effect on other cells besides platelets and endothelial cells. Platelet and fibrinogen turnover are normal, and there is no increase in fibrinogen breakdown products nor evidence of platelet consumption, so that disseminated intravascular coagulation (DIC) is not a significant component of Lassa fever (Fisher-Hoch et al. 1987, 1988).

More insight into the pathophysiology of zoonotic diseases such as Lassa fever may come from considering the very marked species differences in response to infection. How a virus that can silently and persistently infect rodents with no adverse effects can produce a fulminating, highly fatal infection in higher mammals (primates) with no evidence of persistence is an important biological issue that is worth exploration. Since there is no evolutionary adaptation of the virus to primates, and indeed no advantage to the virus, we have to assume that the dramatic events of Lassa fever are a biological 'accident'.

5 Epidemiology of Lassa Fever

One of the first prospective studies conducted established the frequency of patients admitted with confirmed Lassa fever to hospitals in eastern Sierra Leone. As many as 13% of all medical admissions to two study hospitals were acute Lassa virus infections, and 27 percent of medical deaths in the same two hospitals were attributable to laboratory-confirmed Lassa virus infections (Table 16). Hospital admissions of Lassa virus-infected patients were observed to have a seasonal pattern, with the highest number of cases admitted during the dry season months from February through April or May, but patients were seen at all times of year (Fig. 9). The proportion of deaths among hospitalized patients did not vary by season. The explanation for the seasonality of Lassa fever is not entirely understood, but it may relate to the stability of the virus during the dry season (December to May) and therefore increased availability of infectious virus in village homes where the rodent reservoir is found or to the dynamics of local rodent infestations.

94   J.B. McCormick and S.P. Fisher-Hoch

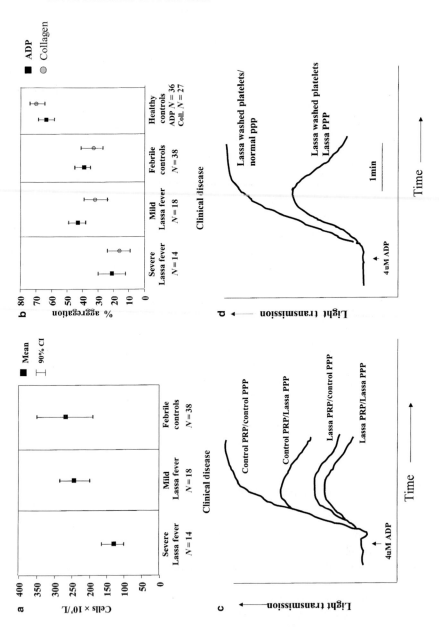

Fig. 8a–d. Platelets in Lassa fever. **a** Mean minimum platelets in patients with Lassa fever. **b** Reversibility of depressed ADP-induced aggregation responses in Lassa fever. Platelets from a patient with severe Lassa fever show a depressed aggregation response mixed 1:1 with autologous plasma compared with the response of control platelets mixed 1:1 with control plasma. Platelets from a healthy person show a depressed response in plasma from a Lassa fever patient. **c,d** Platelets of the Lassa fever patient respond normally after washing and resuspension in normal plasma. Similar improvement is not seen when the Lassa platelets are washed and resuspended in autologous plasma or where PRP from the Lassa fever patient is mixed with control plasma (**c**). (FISHER-HOCH et al. 1988)

Table 16. Lassa fever in adult medical services of two hospitals, Eastern Province, Sierra Leone

Medical admissions in two hospitals (1 year)	3,473
Patients with Lassa fever	444 (13%)
Medical deaths	281
Deaths from Lassa fever	71 (27%)

6 Transmission

6.1 Rodent to Humans

The transmission of Lassa virus to humans is directly related to contact between the rodent reservoir *Mastomys natalensis* and humans living in villages of West Africa

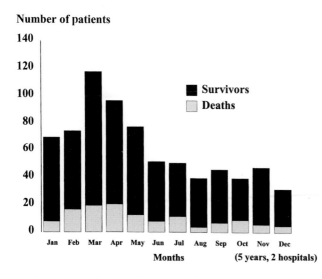

Fig. 9. Lassa fever hospital admissions and deaths, eastern Sierra Leone

Table 17. Studies of the natural host of Lassa virus, *Mastomys natalensis*: distribution of *M. natalensis* in villages in Sierra Leone (McCORMICK et al. 1987a)

Distribution	Domestic (in village)	Agriculture (village fields)
Mastomys (%)	846 (57)	52 (14)
Other species	645 (43)	315 (86)
Total	1491	367

(FRASER et al. 1974; KEENLYSIDE et al. 1983). Systematic longitudinal studies of rodents in villages in Sierra Leone demonstrated that the rodents prefer to occupy human habitats (Table 17) (ROBBINS et al. 1983). These observations suggested that Lassa fever should occur in all age groups given that exposure is primarily in and around village houses. Numerous serologic surveys were carried out in villages of the eastern province. *Mastomys natalensis* is peridomestic in habit. Rodents are infected in utero and remain infective throughout life, excreting between 1000 and 10,000 infectious viral particles per milliliter of urine (Table 18). The average number of *Mastomys* per village house is below 10, with only 5%–10% infected, but in some houses as many as 50–75 rodents have been found and as many as 50% of those may excrete Lassa virus. Experimental data show that virtually all *Mastomys* excrete virus once infected (Table 19). The level of infection in families is related to the number of rodents in the house and the level of infection. The average number of *Mastomys* rodents in the houses was 2.4, and the total proportion infected was about 30% (Table 19). *Mastomys* do not tend to move far from the houses (average distance between sites of capture and recapture was 22m (Table 19). Those houses with a larger proportion of *Mastomys* infected ($>25\%$) were associated with human populations with higher rates of infection as well (Table 20). Thus, this is an infection spread primarily by rodent contact with humans in houses that afford the ideal environment for the rodent, namely, water, food, and darkness much of the time; because the houses are often shut up during the day, the rodents are able to circulate in darkness even during the day and deposit virus-laden urine on surfaces including tables, floors, beds, and even eating

Table 18. Studies of the natural host of Lassa virus, *Mastomys natalensis*: biology of Lassa virus in *M. natalensis* (McCORMICK et al. 1987a)

Virus infection		Virus concentration	
Viremia	33/34	Blood ($n = 85$)	$10^{3.06}$
Viruria	31/34	Urine ($n = 55$)	$10^{3.32}$

Virus titers $= \text{TCID}_{50}$.

Table 19. Studies of the natural host of Lassa virus, *Mastomys natalensis*: dynamics of *M. natalensis* in a west African village in Sierra Leone (McCORMICK et al. 1987a)

No. of *Mastomys*/house	2.4
Virus-infected (%)	84/736 (11)
Antibody (%)	217/720 (30)
Movement	$22.3 + 39.6$m (mean 50 recaptures)
Life span	150–180 days (based on 50 recaptures)

Table 20. Studies of the natural host of Lassa virus, *Mastomys natalensis*: prevalence of human antibody to Lassa virus in households correlated with prevalence of antibody in rodents (McCormick et al. 1987a)

Human antibody prevalences	Rodents with antibody	Rodents with no antibody
<10%	5 (20%)	20
>10%	40 (45%)	48

$P = 0.038$ (Fisher's exact test, two-tailed), odds ratio 3.3 (1.1–10.5).

utensils. Locally made straw mattresses are common in poor rural homes, and the rodents burrow inside these. Contact with infected surfaces by individuals with cuts and scratches on their hands and feet and perhaps even contact with contaminated food may result in infection. In some instances, the stirring of dust containing urine may result in virus entry into the respiratory system, but epidemiological evidence (secondary attack rates in households) does not support aerosol infection as a frequent event (Keenlyside et al. 1983). Recent civil disturbances have resulted in the destruction of the more solid, concrete, tin-roofed housing in the endemic areas of Sierra Leone and Liberia, and villagers who are not in refugee camps have to reconstruct with local materials such as mud, reeds, and palm leaves. This is an ideal habitat for *Mastomys* and will naturally predispose to a greater frequency of contact of humans with infected animals.

There are other risk factors, including catching and cooking rats for eating, which result in even more substantial contact with infected rodents (Table 21) (Ter Meulen et al. 1996). Consumption of rodents is common in the areas endemic for Lassa fever, and although the frequency is difficult to estimate accurately, its importance appears to be substantial.

6.2 Transmission from Person to Person: Hospital and Household

The earliest reported cases of Lassa fever were associated with hospital transmission, and the history of the infection since its discovery is associated with nosocomial transmission (Fraser et al. 1974; Monath et al. 1973, 1974; Mertens et al. 1973; Troup et al. 1970; Bowen et al. 1975; Carey et al. 1972; Fisher-Hoch et al. 1995; Frame et al. 1984).This observation is most likely the result of visibility, that is, infection of expatriates or of hospital staff. The disease has clearly been endemic for centuries, probably much longer. Transmission to hospital staff

Table 21. Risk factors associated with Lassa virus infection, Sierra Leone (D. Bennett and J.B. McCormick, unpublished study)

Activity	Risk
Catching rats	$p<0.001$
Eating rats	$p<0.001$
Rats in house	$p<0.009$
Caring for ill person	$p<0.001$
Touching ill person	$p<0.026$
Sexual intercourse with ill person	$p<0.001$

Stepwise logistic regression of a prospective study of 20 infections among 381 villagers.

98   J.B. McCormick and S.P. Fisher-Hoch

or other patients occurs following close contact with infected secretions, blood, or tissues from hospitalized patients with Lassa fever. There is no credible epidemiological evidence of airborne person-to-person transmission of Lassa virus, and much evidence to suggest that this is not an important mode of transmission since attack rates are low, sporadic in fact, even in crowded lodgings. It is much clearer that close contact with infected secretions from a person ill from Lassa fever in the household is a significant risk factor (KEENLYSIDE et al. 1983) (Table 21). It is also well documented that that person-to-person transmission in a hospital setting may be effectively prevented with simple barrier nursing techniques, available to most hospitals or clinics (FISHER-HOCH 1993; FISHER-HOCH et al. 1985; COOPER et al. 1982; CDC 1988; HELMICK et al. 1986). Indeed, even procedures such as intubation and surgery have been safely performed following basic guidelines (CDC 1988; HELMICK et al. 1986; HOLMES et al. 1990).

Contact in households with persons ill, or recently ill with Lassa fever, as well as sexual contact with someone convalescent with Lassa fever also appear to be significant risk factors (Table 21). It has long been known that Lassa virus may persist at low levels in the urine of humans after infection for up to 2 months (without evidence of circulation in the blood) (EMOND et al. 1982). The source of this virus has not been determined, and in particular there are no studies of the presence of Lassa virus in semen. Thus, the epidemiological implications need follow up to determine, as with Marburg virus (SIEGERT et al. 1968; MARTINI and SCHMIDT 1968; ROWE et al. 1999), if sequestration of the virus in semen is a common biologic event in human infection from Lassa virus.

The case fatality in Lassa fever may vary with geographic location, presumably because of variations in virus virulence. In the western part of West Africa (Liberia, Guinea, Sierra Leone), the case fatality of hospitalized, untreated patients appears to be around 16% and does not vary significantly according to the patient's age (Table 22). There is evidence, however, that the case fatality of hospitalized patients may be somewhat higher in Nigeria, where in some outbreaks mortality of about 50% has been reported (TROUP et al. 1970; BOWEN et al. 1975; CAREY et al. 1972). More recently, the case fatality in a community outbreak was also about 50%, but in two nosocomial outbreaks, it was above 70% (HOLMES et al. 1990). Since there are differences in the dose and route of infection between person-to-person spread

Table 22. Case fatality of hospitalized patients with Lassa fever by age and sex, Sierra Leone (JOHNSON et al. 1987)

Age (years)	Cases	% total	Case fatality (%)
10–19	60	14	20
20–29	204	48	16
30–39	105	24	16
≥40	43	10	16
Unknown	18	4	22
Total	430	100	16
Female	243	57	18
Male	187	43	15

Patients seen prior to availability of antiviral treatment.

in the community and nosocomial spread from needles and direct inoculation in hospitals, all of these factors will influence the outcome, and therefore the direct comparison of case fatality is problematic. The role of virus strain or genotype in severity is not known. It is known, however, that other arenaviruses in Africa appear not to be pathogenic and indeed protect from subsequent illness with the pathogenic ones. As discussed earlier, LCMV varies in virulence in large measure due to its polymerase gene, and similar variation within the African arenaviruses, and indeed within the family of Lassa strains, is quite conceivable.

7 Burden of Infection and Disease in West Africa

In Sierra Leone, human antibody prevalence ranges from around 5% in coastal villages to 40% in secondary forest and savannah (average of 18%) (Table 23). In some highly endemic villages, 5%–20% of susceptible (antibody-negative) persons are infected per year, and seroconversion to Lassa virus antigen has been observed in 5%–13% of all febrile illnesses in these villages (Table 24) (McCormick 1987). Antibody levels to Lassa virus may decline to unmeasurable levels after 3–5 years, and re-infection, with mild or no illness, appears to occur, based on the dynamics of antibody change in populations and the frequency of silent infections (defined by fourfold antibody rise) in adults (Table 24) (McCormick 1987). Antibody is found in patients of all ages, and the prevalence increases with age, suggesting consistent, relatively uniform exposure during life in endemic areas, as one would expect with an environmental pathogen associated with rodent-infested housing (Table 25).

The prevalence of infection in Liberia and Guinea also range from a low of 1% to highs of on average 5%–6% (Yalley-Ogunro et al. 1984) (Table 25)

Table 23. Prevalence of antibody to Lassa virus by age, Sierra Leone

Age (years)	Village A		Village B	
	Pos/total	% Pos	Pos/total	% Pos
<1	1/20	5	1/24	4
1–4	6/50	12	8/79	10
5–9	31/76	29	23/82	28
10–19	50/113	44	19/69	28
20–39	121/245	49	90/212	42
40+	91/200	45	11/24	45
Total	301/737	41	145/434	31

Table 24. Lassa fever illness to infection and case fatality ratios, West Africa

Illness to infection ratio	9%–50% (5 studies)
% Febrile illness	5%–14% (4 studies)
Case fatality ratio (hospitalized, untreated)	16% (? higher in Nigeria)
Case fatality all infections (estimated)	2%–4%

Table 25. Prevalence of antibody to Lassa virus in West Africa

Country	Antibody	Pos/tested	Village range
Nigeria	21	357/1677	5%–25%
Sierra Leone	18	684/2601	6%–40%
Guinea	6	61/1152	0%–20%
Liberia	5	68/1432	1%–14%

(A. Demby and J.B. McCormick, unpublished observations). In Nigeria, there are fewer studies of the prevalence, but in those areas surveyed, the prevalence of antibody ranges from 5% to 25%, and the average prevalence was 21% (BAJANI et al. 1997; TOMORI et al. 1988). We know that in Nigeria infections occur not just in the rural village population, but also in the larger towns and cities, even state capitals (BAJANI et al. 1997; BOWEN et al. 1975). Wealthier patients falling sick in rural areas are brought to hospitals in urban centers, where poor hygiene leads to nosocomial transmission. These hospital outbreaks cause alarm and bring attention to the disease. During three such outbreaks in1989, a systematic search in all hospitals and clinics revealed several unconnected and undiagnosed cases, suggesting the disease is there all the time, and only special events bring it to the public's attention (FISHER-HOCH et al. 1995). The prevalence of Lassa virus antibody in the geographic areas between Nigeria and Liberia and beyond is not known, but it has never been looked for systematically. All we do know is that a German art student returned to Europe and died of Lassa fever in 2000 and that she had visited the Ivory Coast and Ghana, both countries which report no Lassa fever (ANONYMOUS 2000). The West African area known to contain Lassa fever now comprises a population of some 180 million people, and even assuming only half to one-third (a conservative estimate) are in areas of risk for Lassa fever, this results in a population of 90–120 million people living in areas endemic for Lassa virus. If the dynamics of antibody loss and acquisition are approximately those that have been observed in prospective studies in Sierra Leone, we can estimate that as many as 20% of the observed prevalence of past infection may occur each year. These estimates mean that of 90–120 million people in endemic areas for Lassa virus in West Africa, about 15%–20% have antibody to Lassa virus (15–20 million). If 1/5 of those infections occur in any given year, then that would be an infection in 3–4 million people per year. If 10% are symptomatic (a highly conservative estimate based on published data), then there are well over 200,000 symptomatic Lassa virus infections in West Africa each year. We have estimated based on previous data that as many as 5% of all Lassa symptomatic infections may be fatal, so can estimate that there are at least 10,000 deaths per year in all of West Africa due to Lassa fever. Since we have had the experience of finding a laboratory confirmed case of Lassa fever in virtually every hospital and clinic in one area of Nigeria on a brief (afternoon) visit to the areas, these numbers do not appear to be unrealistic, indeed they may well underestimate the overall problem. In the year 2000, deaths of peacekeepers and medical personnel working in areas of civil strife have begun to draw attention to this ill appreciated, emerging disease. The war has uprooted people and is undoubtedly creating conditions for more human contact with the virus, especially in the cities. If Lassa fever were a developed world problem, there would be vociferous demands for control and vaccine.

8 Prevention and Control

8.1 Rodent Control

The key to prevention and control is either to interrupt the contact between infectious source and susceptible persons or to avoid disease in the event of infection. The ideal method of prevention for these rodent-borne diseases is to prevent contact between rodents and humans. The effectiveness of this has been admirably shown in the outbreaks of the arenavirus disease, Bolivian hemorrhagic fever, in Bolivia in the 1960s when rodent control programs in the villages were highly successful in eliminating the epidemic (JOHNSON et al. 1967). Under current social circumstances, the control of rodents as a broad approach to preventing Lassa fever is not realistic. The improvement of housing and food storage might reduce the domestic rodent population, but such changes are not easily made. Rodent trapping in an individual village where transmission is high has demonstrated as much as a fivefold reduction in the rate of virus transmission (Table 26). However, such a program is only applicable in villages with exceptional transmission rates and stable social conditions, and would certainly not be applicable to large areas. Furthermore, without a sustained program of rodent control, the rodents return after a period of a few months (Table 21).

9 Vaccine

Studies of potential vaccines to Lassa virus began in the 1980s when Clegg expressed the nucleocapsid protein of Lassa virus in vaccinia and was able to show the recombinant vaccine protected guinea pigs, but not primates, from subsequent challenge of 10^2 of virus (CLEGG and LLOYD 1987). Further work showed that both

Table 26. Seroconversion rates to Lassa virus, illness to infection ratios, and febrile illness due to Lassa fever in five Sierra Leone villages (McCORMICK et al. 1987a)

Seroconversion before trapout	6.9/100 susceptibles/year
Seroconversion after trapout	1.3/100 susceptibles/year
Relative risk of infection	5.3 before compared to after
Seroconversion in control villages:	
Village A	10/100 susceptibles/year
Village B	34/100 susceptibles/year

NP and glycoprotein expressed in vaccinia could protect guinea pigs, but that only the glycoprotein protected primates (MORRISON et al. 1989). The protection of guinea pigs was not related to antibody levels, so it was concluded that cellular immune responses were more important than antibody. Subsequently, immunization of primates with inactivated (gamma-irradiated) whole Lassa virus resulted in antibody responses to both NP and GPC, and a brisk booster response following challenge (Table 27) (Fig. 10). However despite this impressive antibody memory response, the animals all died with serum virus titers equal to unvaccinated controls (Table 28) (McCORMICK et al. 1992). Data from field studies in the late 1970s and early 1980s in humans and further experimental studies in primates suggested that

Table 27. Antibody titers to Lassa virus in monkeys after vaccination and challenge

	Vaccinated			Unvaccinated	
Day post-vaccine:					
0	0	0	0	0	0
14	64	16	256	0	0
35	32	32	128	0	0
71	64	64	256	0	0
101	64	64	64	0	0
108	256	64	64	0	0
Day post-challenge:					
4	256	64	256	0	0
8	1,024	256	1,024	0	0
10	4,096	1,024	4,096	0	4
12	1,639	4,096	4,096	64	256

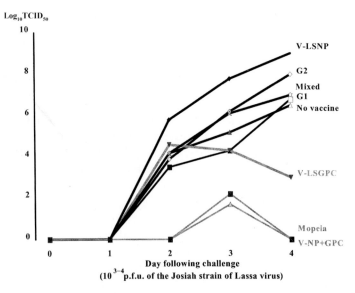

Fig. 10. Viremias in primates by day after vaccination and challenge with 10^{3-4} pfu Lassa virus. (FISHER-HOCH et al. 2000)

Table 28. Postmortem Lassa virus titers ($log_{10}TCID_{50}$)

Site	Vaccinated monkeys			Unvaccinated monkeys	
Liver	8.5	7.9	6.6	8.0	7.3
Spleen	7.5	7.2	6.3	7.3	6.9
Kidney	6.8	6.7	6.2	6.6	6.9
Lung	7.4	7.4	6.0	6.8	6.6
Adrenal	8.1	7.8	8.1	8.0	7.5
Spinal fluid	5.0	4.2	3.4	3.1	4.3
Serum	6.1	5.7	5.2	6.1	6.1

the immune response to NP is not protective and furthermore that the presence of antibody to either glycoprotein or nucleoprotein at the time of hospital admission was not associated with increased survival or even severity of disease. A more recent study suggests the antibody (for NP) may be a marker for severe or fatal disease (BAUSCH et al. 2000). Since a similar observation was made in primates given NP vaccine and then challenged with lethal virus (e.g., the disease appeared worse) (FISHER-HOCH et al. 2000), the biology of this phenomenon merits further study.

The latter is a more recent, broader study of protection by recombinant expressions of NP, GPC, and combinations of the two involved nonhuman primates; 28 *Macaca mulatta* (rhesus) and 16 *M. fascicularis* (cynomolgus) (FISHER-HOCH et al. 2000) (Table 29). The vaccinia viruses expressed S-segment Lassa structural proteins, the full-length glycoprotein (V-LSG), the nucleoprotein (V-LSN), the full-length glycoprotein and nucleoprotein in the same construct (V-LSG/N), and the single glycoproteins (V-LSG1, residues 1–296, and V-LSG2, deletion of residues 67–234) (MORRISON et al. 1989, 1991). All animals were challenged subcutaneously with 10^3–10^4 pfu of the Josiah strain of Lassa virus. Following Lassa virus challenge, all unvaccinated animals died (0% survival), while 9/10 animals vaccinated with all proteins survived (90% survival). Although no animals that received full-length glycoprotein alone had a high titer of antibody prior to challenge, 17/19

Table 29. Outcome of challenge of nonhuman primates vaccinated with Lassa virus vaccinia recombinants and challenged with virulent Lassa virus CITER (YANG et al. 2000)

Virion protein expression	Protection	Vaccine	n	Survivors	Median day of death (range)	Mean viremia at death (log_{10})
None	0%	NTBH vaccinia	3	0	15 (15–19)	5.7
		None	7	0	12 (10–15)	
Single glycoproteins	0%	V-LSG1	2	0	15 (14–16)	6.8
		V-LSG2	2	0	12.5 (12–13)	
Nucleoprotein	27%	V-LSN	11	3	11.5 (9–13)	6.7
Full glycoprotein	88%	V-LSG	7	6	21[a] (21)	2.5
		V-LSG1 + V-LSG2	2	2		
Full S-segment	90%	Mopeia virus	2	2		
		V-LSG + V-LSN	6	5	11[a] (11)	7.0
		V-LSG/N	2	2		
Total			44	20		

[a] These two animals were challenged 488 and 700 days post-vaccination. All protected animals were challenged between 38 and 354 days post-vaccination.

survived (88%). In contrast, all animals vaccinated with nucleoprotein developed a high titer of antibody, but 12/15 died (20% survival). All animals vaccinated with single glycoproteins (G1 or G2) died, but all those that received both single glycoproteins (G1 + G2) at separate sites survived, showing that both glycoproteins are independently important in protection. Neither group had demonstrable antibody prior to challenge.

The two deaths among the glycoprotein-vaccinated animals were associated with the longest vaccine to challenge intervals (488 and 700 days, range 36–700 days, mean 319 days). Survival diminished as the vaccine to challenge interval extended. A trend towards lengthening the duration of challenge viremia (days) was also observed with an increased interval between vaccination and challenge. The three animals that were vaccinated with the nucleoprotein that survived inadvertently received a lower challenge dose (10^3pfu compared with 10^4pfu), showing that the challenge dose also has a bearing on the outcome. Nevertheless, clearly the nucleoprotein vaccine is not protective compared with the glycoprotein.

None of the protective vaccines provided sterilizing immunity, since almost all surviving, asymptomatic animals experienced viremia, even those vaccinated with Mopeia virus (essentially a live attenuated Lassa virus). This is consistent with the hypothesis that virus replication is controlled by CTL responses and not antibody responses. In general, however, the outcome correlates with the level of viremia, and thus protection with limitation of viremia (Table 29). The highest virus titers were seen in the animals that had received the V-LSN recombinant vaccine (higher than in unvaccinated animals). This difference was not statistically significant, possible due to the small sample size, and a larger study is needed to settle the issue of whether this vaccine actually potentiates viremia following challenge. What is clear is that animals that received the entire glycoprotein (V-LSG) or all the S-segment proteins (V-LSG/N or V-LSG + V-LSN) showed significantly diminished mean virus titers compared with unvaccinated animals, and that these animals, with two exceptions, were not sick and did not die. These data show that the GPC gene is necessary and sufficient to protect primates against a large parenteral challenge dose. In contrast, the NP gene provides little if any protection, casting doubt on the need for, and indeed the safety of, using an NP gene as part of the vaccine for primates or humans (FISHER-HOCH et al. 2000).

A lack of correlation between the titer of antibody (IFA) to whole Lassa virus antigens prior to challenge and any level of protection has been observed in human disease. Following vaccination and prior to challenge, IFA antibody could be detected in V-LSN/V-LSG and V-LSN vaccinated animals, with titers ranging from 4 to 256. Nor are antibodies neutralizing. Multiple efforts failed to demonstrate the presence of plaque reduction neutralization in serum from vaccinated animals after vaccination and before challenge, as well as in the serum of animals after recovery from challenge (despite very high titer fluorescent antibody) (FISHER-HOCH et al. 1989, 2000). What we can now conclude is that epitopes on both glycoproteins are needed for protection, and that these are apparently able to induce immunity in concert, but not independently (FISHER-HOCH et al. 2000; WRIGHT et al. 1989,

1990; Di Simone and Buchmeier 1995). Despite the strong evidence implicating cell-mediated immunity, we still think we have to keep an open mind about some contribution to protective processes by antibodies, particularly ones induced in novel ways.

Mopeia virus is an obvious candidate for an effective live attenuated vaccine, with the advantage that a single administration might induce life-long protection. Mopeia virus is presently classified as a BSL3 pathogen, even though data from Mozambique suggest that this virus is not pathogenic for humans. There are major sequence differences in the S segments of Lassa and Mopeia viruses, but no sites associated with virulence have been genetically mapped. Vaccine candidates expressing the Lassa glycoprotein gene will therefore have to be sought that are likely to pass the stringent requirements for safety needed for a human use vaccine.

Cross-protection against other West African strains of Lassa virus remains to be addressed. The protection afforded by Mopeia virus from Southern Africa certainly supports the idea that broad protection is achievable and desirable, particularly since some Nigerian strains may induce more severe and fatal illnesses than strains from further west (Troup et al. 1970; Bowen et al. 1975; Carey et al. 1972; Fisher-Hoch et al. 1995; Keenlyside et al. 1983). Monoclonal antibody mapping and molecular studies of the glycoproteins of African arenaviruses show a conserved B-cell epitope on G2 across all of the known African arenaviruses including Mopeia and most South American arenaviruses. However, both G1 and G2 recognition is necessary for protection based on our primate studies. We concluded from continuous observations over 14 years in Sierra Leone that a single natural infection provides long-term protective immunity against disease, and therefore we believe that a single vaccination will provide lengthy protection, and given the virus circulation in the endemic area, the opportunity for natural boosting from infection is substantial.

The need for a vaccine is clear. The sizeable disease burden, a high frequency of hospitalization and death, with severe sequelae from cardiac disease to deafness, make a compelling case for application of a vaccine. Furthermore, the evidence of an effective vaccine has been published. Similar situations in developed countries would have long ago resulted in a vaccine effort. This is a disease that something can be done about, and it is unacceptable not to act.

References

Anonymous (2000) Lassa fever, case imported to Germany. Wkly Epidemiol Rec 75:8–17

Baize S, Leroy EM, Georges-Courbot MC, Capron M, Lansoud-Soukate J, Debre P, et al. (1999) Defective humoral responses and extensive intravascular apoptosis are associated with fatal outcome in Ebola virus-infected patients [see comments]. Nat Med 5:423–426

Bajani MD, Tomori O, Rollin PE, Harry TO, Bukbuk ND, Wilson L, et al. (1997) A survey for antibodies to Lassa virus among health workers in Nigeria. Trans R Soc Trop Med Hyg 91:379–381

Bausch DG, Rollin PE, Demby AH, Coulibaly M, Kanu J, Conteh AS, et al. (2000) Diagnosis and clinical virology of Lassa fever as evaluated by enzyme-linked immunosorbent assay, indirect fluorescent-antibody test, and virus isolation. J Clin Microbiol 38:2670–2677

Biggar RJ (1986) Possible nonspecific association between malaria and HTLV-III/LAV [letter]. N Engl J Med 315:457–458

Biggar RJ, Gigase PL, Melbye M, Kestens L, Sarin PS, Bodner AJ, et al. (1985) ELISA HTLV retrovirus antibody reactivity associated with malaria and immune complexes in healthy Africans. Lancet 2:520–523

Biggar RJ, Saxinger C, Sarin P, Blattner WA (1986) Non-specificity of HTLV-III reactivity in sera from rural Kenya and eastern Zaire [letter]. East Afr Med J 63:683–684

Bloch A (1978) A serological survey of Lassa fever in Liberia. Bull World Health Org 56:811–813

Bowen GS, Tomori O, Wulff H, Casals J, Noonan A, Downs WG (1975) Lassa fever in Onitsha, East Central State, Nigeria in 1974. Bull World Health Org 52:599–604

Buckley SM, Casals J (1970) Lassa fever, a new virus disease of man from West Africa. 3. Isolation and characterization of the virus. Am J Trop Med Hyg 19:680–691

Cao W, Henry MD, Borrow P, Yamada H, Elder JH, Ravkov EV, et al. (1998) Identification of alpha-dystroglycan as a receptor for lymphocytic choriomeningitis virus and Lassa fever virus [see comments]. Science 282:2079–2081

Carey DE, Kemp GE, White HA, Pinneo L, Addy RF, Fom AL, et al. (1972) Lassa fever. Epidemiological aspects of the 1970 epidemic, Jos, Nigeria. Trans R Soc Trop Med Hyg 66:402–408

Centers for Disease Control (1988) Management of patients with suspected viral hemorrhagic fever. MMWR 37:S1–S15

Fraser DW, Campbell CC, Monath TP, Goff PA, Gregg MB (1974) Lassa fever in the Eastern Province of Sierra Leone, 1970–1972. I. Epidemiologic studies. Am J Trop Med Hyg 23:1131–1139

Clegg JC, Lloyd G (1987) Vaccinia recombinant expressing Lassa-virus internal nucleocapsid protein protects guineapigs against Lassa fever. Lancet 2:186–188

Cooper CB, Gransden WR, Webster M, King M, O'Mahony M, Young S, et al. (1982) A case of Lassa fever: experience at St Thomas's Hospital. Br Med J Clin Res Ed 285:1003–1005

Cummins D, Bennett D, Fisher-Hoch SP, Farrar B, McCormick JB (1989a) Electrocardiographic abnormalities in patients with Lassa fever. J Trop Med Hyg 92:350–355

Cummins D, Fisher-Hoch SP, Walshe KJ, Mackie IJ, McCormick JB, Bennett D, et al. (1989b) A plasma inhibitor of platelet aggregation in patients with Lassa fever. Br J Haematol 72:543–548

Cummins D, McCormick JB, Bennett D, Samba JA, Farrar B, Machin SJ, et al. (1990a) Acute sensorineural deafness in Lassa fever [see comments]. JAMA 264:2093–2096

Cummins D, Molinas FC, Lerer G, Maiztegui JI, Faint R, Machin SJ (1990b) A plasma inhibitor of platelet aggregation in patients with Argentine hemorrhagic fever. Am J Trop Med Hyg 42:470–475

Cummins D, Bennett D, Fisher-Hoch SP, Farrar B, Machin SJ, McCormick JB (1992) Lassa fever encephalopathy: clinical and laboratory findings. J Trop Med Hyg 95:197–201

Di Simone C, Buchmeier MJ (1995) Protection of mice from lethal LCMV infection by a reconstituted glycoprotein vaccine. Cold Spring Harbor Laboratory Press, Cold Spring Harbor, pp 1–5

Elliott LH, McCormick JB, Johnson KM (1982) Inactivation of Lassa, Marburg, and Ebola viruses by gamma irradiation. J Clin Microbiol 16:704–708

Emond RT, Bannister B, Lloyd G, Southee TJ, Bowen ET (1982) A case of Lassa fever: clinical and virological findings. Br Med J (Clin Res Ed) 285:1001–1002

Fabiyi A, Tomori O, Pinneo P (1979) Lassa fever antibodies in hospital personnel in the Plateau State of Nigeria. Niger Med J 9:23–25

Feldmann H, Bugany H, Mahner F, Klenk HD, Drenckhahn D, Schnittler HJ (1996) Filovirus-induced endothelial leakage triggered by infected monocytes/macrophages. J Virol 70:2208–2214

Fisher-Hoch SP (1993) Stringent precautions are not advisable when caring for patients with viral haemorrhagic fevers. Rev Med Virol 3:7–13

Fisher-Hoch SP, McCormick JB (1987) Pathophysiology and treatment of Lassa fever. Curr Topics Microbiol Immunol 134:231–239

Fisher-Hoch SP, Price ME, Craven RB, Price FM, Forthall DN, Sasso DR, et al. (1985) Safe intensive-care management of a severe case of Lassa fever with simple barrier nursing techniques. Lancet 2:1227–1229

Fisher-Hoch SP, Mitchell SW, Sasso DR, Lange JV, Ramsey R, McCormick JB (1987) Physiological and immunologic disturbances associated with shock in a primate model of Lassa fever. J Infect Dis 155:465–474

Fisher-Hoch S, McCormick JB, Sasso D, Craven RB (1988) Hematologic dysfunction in Lassa fever. J Med Virol 26:127–135

Fisher-Hoch SP, McCormick JB, Auperin D, Brown BG, Castor M, Perez G, et al. (1989) Protection of rhesus monkeys from fatal Lassa fever by vaccination with a recombinant vaccinia virus containing the Lassa virus glycoprotein gene. Proc Natl Acad Sci USA 86:317–321

Fisher-Hoch SP, Tomori O, Nasidi A, Perez Oronoz GI, Fakile Y, Hutwagner L, et al. (1995) Review of cases of nosocomial Lassa fever in Nigeria: the high price of poor medical practice. BMJ 311:857–859

Fisher-Hoch SP, Hutwagner L, Brown B, McCormick JB (2000) Effective vaccine for lassa fever. J Virol 74:6777–6783

Frame JD, Baldwin JM Jr, Gocke DJ, Troup JM (1970) Lassa fever, a new virus disease of man from West Africa. I. Clinical description and pathological findings. Am J Trop Med Hyg 19:670–676

Frame JD, Casals J, Dennis EA (1979) Lassa virus antibodies in hospital personnel in western Liberia. Trans R Soc Trop Med Hyg 73:219–224

Frame JD, Jahrling PB, Yalley Ogunro JE, Monson MH (1984) Endemic Lassa fever in Liberia. II. Serological and virological findings in hospital patients. Trans R Soc Trop Med Hyg 78:656–660

Georges AJ, Gonzalez JP, Abdul Wahid S, Saluzzo JF, Meunier DM, McCormick JB (1985) Antibodies to Lassa and Lassa-like viruses in man and mammals in the Central African Republic. Trans R Soc Trop Med Hyg 79:78–79

Gonzalez JP, McCormick JB, Saluzzo JF, Herve JP, Georges AJ, Johnson KM (1983) An arenavirus isolated from wild-caught rodents (*Pramys* species) in the Central African Republic. Intervirology 19:105–112

Gonzalez JP, Josse R, Johnson ED, Merlin M, Georges AJ, Abandja J, et al. (1989) Antibody prevalence against haemorrhagic fever viruses in randomized representative Central African populations. Res Virol 140:319–331

Grundy DJ, Bowen ET, Lloyd G (1980) Isolated case of Lassa fever in Zaria, Northern Nigeria [letter]. Lancet 2:649–650

Helmick CG, Webb PA, Scribner CL, Krebs JW, McCormick JB (1986) No evidence for increased risk of Lassa fever infection in hospital staff. Lancet 2:1202–1205

Hirabayashi Y, Oka S, Goto H, Shimada K, Kurata T, Fisher-Hoch SP, et al. (1988) An imported case of Lassa fever with late appearance of polyserositis. J Infect Dis 158:872–875

Hirabayashi Y, Oka S, Goto H, Shimada K, Kurata T, Fisher-Hoch SP, et al. (1989) The first imported case of Lassa fever in Japan (in Japanese). Nippon Rinsho 47:71–75

Holmes GP, McCormick JB, Trock SC, Chase RA, Lewis SM, Mason CA, et al. (1990) Lassa fever in the United States. Investigation of a case and new guidelines for management [see comments]. N Engl J Med 323:1120–1123

Johnson KM, Webb PA, Kuns ML, Valverde L (1967) On the mode of transmission of Bolivian hemorrhagic fever. Jpn J Med Sci Biol 20:153–159

Johnson KM, Taylor P, Elliott LH, Tomori O (1981a) Recovery of a Lassa-related arenavirus in Zimbabwe. Am J Trop Med Hyg 30:1291–1293

Johnson KM, Elliott LH, Heymann DL (1981b) Preparation of polyvalent viral immunofluorescent intracellular antigens and use in human serosurveys. J Clin Microbiol 14:527–529

Johnson KM, McCormick JB, Webb PA, Smith ES, Elliott LH, King IJ (1987) Clinical virology of Lassa fever in hospitalized patients. J Infect Dis 155:456–464

Keenlyside RA, McCormick JB, Webb PA, Smith E, Elliott L, Johnson KM (1983) Case-control study of *Mastomys natalensis* and humans in Lassa virus-infected households in Sierra Leone. Am J Trop Med Hyg 32:829–837

Knobloch J, McCormick JB, Webb PA, Dietrich M, Schumacher HH, Dennis E (1980) Clinical observations in 42 patients with Lassa fever. Tropenmed Parasitol 31:389–398

Lukashevich IS (1992) Generation of reassortants between African arenaviruses. Virology 188:600–605

Lukashevich IS, Vasiuchkov AD, Stel'makh TA, Scheslenok EP, Shabanov AG (1991) The isolation and characteristics of reassortants between the Lassa and Mopeia arenaviruses. Vopr Virusol 36:146–150

Lukashevich IS, Maryankova R, Vladyko AS, Nashkevich N, Koleda S, Djavani M, et al. (1999) Lassa and Mopeia virus replication in human monocytes/macrophages and in endothelial cells: different effects on IL-8 and TNF-alpha gene expression. J Med Virol 59:552–560

Marta RF, Montero VS, Hack CE, Sturk A, Maiztegui JI, Molinas FC (1999) Proinflammatory cytokines and elastase-alpha-1-antitrypsin in Argentine hemorrhagic fever. Am J Trop Med Hyg 60:85–89

Martini GA, Schmidt HA (1968) Spermatogene Ubertragung des 'Virus Marburg'. (Erreger der 'Marburger Affenkrankheit'). Klin Wochenschr 46:398–400

McCormick JB (1986) Clinical, epidemiologic, and therapeutic aspects of Lassa fever. Med Microbiol Immunol Berl 175:153–155

McCormick JB (1987) Epidemiology and control of Lassa fever. Curr Topics Microbiol Immunol 134:69–78

McCormick JB (1988) Lassa fever: epidemiology, therapy and vaccine development. Kans-enshogaku.Zasshi 62 [Suppl]:353–366

McCormick JB (1990) Arenaviruses. In: Fields BN, Knipe DM (eds) Fields virology, 2nd edn. Raven Press, New York, pp 1245–1267

McCormick JB, Walker DH, King IJ, Webb PA, Elliott LH, Whitfield SG, et al. (1986) Lassa virus hepatitis: a study of fatal Lassa fever in humans. Am J Trop Med Hyg 35:401–407

McCormick JB, Webb PA, Krebs JW, Johnson KM, Smith ES (1987a) A prospective study of the epidemiology and ecology of Lassa fever. J Infect Dis 155:437–444

McCormick JB, King IJ, Webb PA, Johnson KM, O'Sullivan R, Smith ES, et al. (1987b) A case-control study of the clinical diagnosis and course of Lassa fever. J Infect Dis 155:445–455

McCormick JB, Mitchell SW, Kiley MP, Ruo S, Fisher-Hoch SP (1992) Inactivated Lassa virus elicits a non protective immune response in rhesus monkeys. J Med Virol 37:1–7

Mertens PE, Patton R, Baum JJ, Monath TP (1973) Clinical presentation of Lassa fever cases during the hospital epidemic at Zorzor, Liberia, March–April 1972. Am J Trop Med Hyg 22:780–784

Monath TP, Mertens PE, Patton R, Moser CR, Baum JJ, Pinneo L, et al. (1973) A hospital epidemic of Lassa fever in Zorzor, Liberia, March–April 1972. Am J Trop Med Hyg 22:773–779

Monath TP, Maher M, Casals J, Kissling RE, Cacciapuoti A (1974) Lassa fever in the Eastern Province of Sierra Leone, 1970–1972. II. Clinical observations and virological studies on selected hospital cases. Am J Trop Med Hyg 23:1140–1149

Monson MH, Cole AK, Frame JD, Serwint JR, Alexander S, Jahrling PB (1987) Pediatric Lassa fever: a review of 33 Liberian cases. Am J Trop Med Hyg 36:408–415

Morrison HG, Bauer SP, Lange JV, Esposito JJ, McCormick JB, Auperin DD (1989) Protection of guinea pigs from Lassa fever by vaccinia virus recombinants expressing the nucleoprotein or the envelope glycoproteins of Lassa virus. Virology 171:179–188

Morrison HG, Goldsmith CS, Regnery HL, Auperin DD (1991) Simultaneous expression of the Lassa virus N and GPC genes from a single recombinant vaccinia virus. Virus Res 18:231–241

Price ME, Fisher-Hoch SP, Craven RB, McCormick JB (1988) A prospective study of maternal and fetal outcome in acute Lassa fever infection during pregnancy. BMJ 297:584–587

Riviere Y, Ahmed R, Southern PJ, Buchmeier MJ, Oldstone MB (1985) Genetic mapping of lymphocytic choriomeningitis virus pathogenicity: virulence in guinea pigs is associated with the L RNA segment. J Virol 55:704–709

Robbins CB, Krebs JW Jr, Johnson KM (1983) *Mastomys* (Rodentia: Muridae) species distinguished by hemoglobin pattern differences. Am J Trop Med Hyg 32:624–630

Roberts PJ, Cummins D, Bainton AL, Walshe KJ, Fisher-Hoch SP, McCormick JB, Gribben JG, Machin SJ, Linch DC (1989) Plasma from patients with severe Lassa fever profoundly modulates f-met-leu-phe induced superoxide generation in neutrophils. Br J Haematol 73:152–157

Rowe AK, Bertolli J, Khan AS, Mukunu R, Muyembe-Tamfum JJ, Bressler D, et al. (1999) Clinical, virologic, and immunologic follow-up of convalescent Ebola hemorrhagic fever patients and their household contacts, Kikwit, Democratic Republic of the Congo. Commission de Lutte contre les Epidemies a Kikwit. J Infect Dis 179 [Suppl 1]:S28–S35

Saluzzo JF, Adam F, McCormick JB, Digoutte JP (1988) Lassa fever virus in Senegal [letter]. J Infect Dis 157:605

Schnittler HJ, Mahner F, Drenckhahn D, Klenk HD, Feldmann H (1993) Replication of Marburg virus in human endothelial cells. A possible mechanism for the development of viral hemorrhagic disease. J Clin Invest 91:1301–1309

Siegert R, Shu HL, Slenczka W (1968) Demonstration of the 'Marburg virus' in the patient (in German). Nachweis des "Marburg-Virus" beim Patienten. Dtsch Med Wochenschr 93:616–619

Swanepoel R, Leman PA, Shepherd AJ, Shepherd SP, Kiley MP, McCormick JB (1985) Identification of Ippy as a Lassa-fever-related virus [letter]. Lancet 1:639

Ter Meulen J, Lukashevich I, Sidibe K, Inapogui A, Marx M, Dorlemann A, et al. (1996) Hunting of peridomestic rodents and consumption of their meat as possible risk factors for rodent-to-human transmission of Lassa virus in the Republic of Guinea. Am J Trop Med Hyg 55:661–666

Ter Meulen J, Badusche M, Kuhnt K, Doetze A, Satoguina J, Marti T, et al. (2000) Characterization of human CD4(+) T-cell clones recognizing conserved and variable epitopes of the lassa virus nucleoprotein. J Virol 74:2186–2192

Tomori O, Fabiyi A, Sorungbe A, Smith A, McCormick JB (1988) Viral hemorrhagic fever antibodies in Nigerian populations. Am J Trop Med Hyg 38:407–410

Trappier SG, Conaty AL, Farrar BB, Auperin DD, McCormick JB, Fisher-Hoch SP (1993) Evaluation of the polymerase chain reaction for diagnosis of Lassa virus infection. Am J Trop Med Hyg 49:214–221

Troup JM, White HA, Fom AL, Carey DE (1970) An outbreak of Lassa fever on the Jos plateau, Nigeria, in January–February 1970. A preliminary report. Am J Trop Med Hyg 19:695–696

Walker DH, Johnson KM, Lange JV, Gardner JJ, Kiley MP, McCormick JB (1982) Experimental infection of rhesus monkeys with Lassa virus and a closely related arenavirus, Mozambique virus. J Infect Dis 146:360–368

Webb PA, McCormick JB, King IJ, Bosman I, Johnson KM, Elliott LH, et al. (1986) Lassa fever in children in Sierra Leone, West Africa. Trans R Soc Trop Med Hyg 80:577–582

White HA (1972) Lassa fever. A study of 23 hospital cases. Trans R Soc Trop Med Hyg 66:390–401

Winn WC Jr, Walker DH (1975) The pathology of human Lassa fever. Bull World Health Org 52:535–545

Wright KE, Salvato MS, Buchmeier MJ (1989) Neutralizing epitopes of lymphocytic choriomeningitis virus are conformational and require both glycosylation and disulfide bonds for expression. Virology 171:417–426

Wright KE, Spiro RC, Burns JW, Buchmeier MJ (1990) Post-translational processing of the glycoproteins of lymphocytic choriomeningitis virus. Virology 177:175–183

Wulff H, Fabiyi A, Monath TP (1975) Recent isolations of Lassa virus from Nigerian rodents. Bull World Health Org 52:609–613

Wulff H, McIntosh BM, Hamner DB, Johnson KM (1977) Isolation of an arenavirus closely related to Lassa virus from *Mastomys natalensis* in south-east Africa. Bull World Health Org 55:441–444

Yalley-Ogunro JE, Frame JD, Hanson AP (1984) Endemic Lassa fever in Liberia. VI. Village serological surveys for evidence of Lassa virus activity in Lofa County, Liberia. Trans R Soc Trop Med Hyg 78:764–770

Yang Z, Duckers HJ, Sullivan NJ, Sanchez A, Nabel EG, Nabel GJ (2000) Identification of the ebola virus glycoprotein as the main viral determinant of vascular cell cytotoxicity and injury. Nat Med 6:886–889

Receptor Structure, Binding, and Cell Entry of Arenaviruses

S. Kʌɴz[1], P. Bᴏʀʀᴏᴡ[2], and M.B.A. Oʟᴅsᴛᴏɴᴇ[1]

1 Virus-Receptor Binding and its Importance in Viral Tropism and Pathogenesis

In order for a virus to infect and replicate within the cells of its host, it must first gain entry into them. This is achieved by the attachment of virus particles to the host cell surface and subsequent transfer of viral nucleic acids and associated proteins into the cell cytoplasm. The latter may occur at the plasma membrane or following endocytosis of bound virions. In the case of enveloped viruses including the arenaviruses, the post-binding entry step is mediated by fusion of the virion and host cell membranes.

Virus attachment is achieved by the binding of virion component(s) to component(s) of the target cell membrane. This may sometimes involve a simple interaction between a virion attachment protein and a single host cell surface receptor; but in many cases when the process has been studied in detail, it has proved to entail a more complex series of stepwise interactions between distinct binding sites on the virion (which may be located on the same or different virion proteins) and a series of host cell receptors and co-receptors. A well-studied example

[1] Department of Neuropharmacology, Division of Virology, The Scripps Research Institute, 10550 North Torrey Pines Road, La Jolla, CA 92037, USA
[2] The Edward Jenner Institute for Vaccine Research, Compton, Newbury, Berkshire RG20 7NN, UK

is provided by the lentivirus human immunodeficiency virus type 1 (HIV-1). This is an enveloped virus with a single virus-encoded surface glycoprotein, gp160. The gp160 protein is composed of two subunits: gp41, a transmembrane protein that contains the fusion domain, and gp120, a more peripheral protein, which mediates virion attachment to host cells. Gp160 is thought to exist as trimers on the virion. Modeling suggests that the surface of the gp120 trimer which is oriented towards the host cell is very basic (KWONG et al. 2000), allowing electrostatic interactions between the approaching virion and polyanions such as heparan sulphate on the host cell surface that may mediate the initial binding of virions to some cell types (MONDOR et al. 1998). The primary receptor for HIV-1 is CD4 (DALGLEISH et al. 1984; KLATZMANN et al. 1984; MADDON et al. 1986). Gp120 binds to the N-terminal membrane-distal domain of CD4, an interaction that has been visualized at the atomic level (KWONG et al. 1998) CD4 binding induces conformation changes in gp120 that contribute to the formation or exposure of a binding site for members of the chemokine receptor family (primarily CCR5 or CXCR4), which act as host cell co-receptors for the virus (FENG et al. 1996; reviewed by MOORE 1997). Chemokine receptor binding to gp120 is in turn believed to trigger conformation changes in gp41, which ultimately mediates virus-cell membrane fusion. Likewise, the attachment of human herpesviruses such as herpes simplex viruses (HSV) and human cytomegalovirus (HCMV) to host cells is thought to involve initial electrostatic interactions with heparan sulphate (WUDUNN and SPEAR 1989; COMPTON et al. 1993) followed by binding of virion surface glycoproteins to specific host cell receptors/co-receptors (GERAGHTY et al. 1998; KRUMMENACHER et al. 1998; BOYLE and COMPTON 1998) and a subsequent fusion event.

As a critical first step in the infection process, virus-receptor interactions play a key role in determining the tropism of viruses; this was first emphasized by work carried out with polioviruses (HOLLAND et al. 1959; HOLLAND 1961). Receptor binding is not the only determinant of virus tropism: there can also be blocks to infection or productive replication of a virus within a cell after attachment has occurred. Conversely, viruses can also sometimes gain entry into cells that do not express the receptors to which they normally bind (e.g., via Fc receptor-mediated uptake of infectious virus-antibody complexes). Nonetheless, virus attachment is a critical determinant of viral tropism, and as such, of the in vivo pathogenicity of viruses. This was illustrated in the late 1970s by studies of reovirus infection of mice (WEINER et al. 1977, 1980; reviewed by FIELDS et al. 1980). Differences in the pathogenicity of reovirus types 1 and 3 in newborn mice were shown to relate to their tropism within the central nervous system (CNS), the more pathogenic type 3 virus infecting neurons and causing a fatal encephalitis, whilst the less pathogenic type 1 virus caused a non-fatal ependymal infection. Reassortant studies demonstrated that this difference mapped to the viral S1 gene, which encodes the reovirus attachment protein, the hemagglutinin (HA); the virulence pattern related to the specific interaction of the viral HA with (as yet unidentified) neuronal or ependymal surface receptors. A second, clinically important example of the importance of virus-receptor interactions in pathogenicity is provided by HIV-1. HIV-1 infection of humans is most commonly initiated by viral isolates that bind to CD4 and the co-receptor CCR5. Individuals homozygous for a deletion mutation in the CCR5 gene (CCR5Δ32) which renders the protein non-functional are relatively resistant to HIV-1 infection (Sampson et al. 1996; Liu et al. 1996), although they can become infected with HIV-1 isolates that utilize the alternative co-receptor CXCR4 (Michael et al. 1998). Further, heterozygotes who express CCR5 at reduced levels undergo a reduced rate of disease progression following infection (Dean et al. 1996; Huang et al. 1996; Michael et al. 1997). The role that receptor binding plays in determining the in vivo tropism and pathogenicity of different isolates of the arenavirus lymphocytic choriomeningitis virus (LCMV) in mice is discussed in detail later in this chapter.

The critical role that virus-receptor interactions play in viral tropism and pathogenicity is one of the reasons that so much attention is focused on characterizing this step in the infection process. However, in addition to increasing our understanding of viral pathogenesis, detailed analysis of the interaction between virion components and host cell surface receptors can also facilitate the design of antiviral agents that will inhibit this initial step in the infection process. This has provided additional impetus for the study of viral receptors, including those of arenaviruses.

2 A Wide Variety of Cellular Proteins can Function as Viral Receptors

Historically, the identification of virus receptors lagged behind knowledge about many other aspects of viral structure and replication. Before the late 1970s, only a few viral receptors had been unequivocally identified, for example sialic acid for influenza viruses (Paulson et al. 1979) and receptors for the third component of complement (C3) for Epstein-Barr virus (Jondal et al. 1976; Yefenof et al. 1976). However, the advent of monoclonal antibody technology and molecular cloning techniques in the following years resulted in a surge of discoveries of viral receptors (for reviews see Wimmer 1994; Norkin 1995; Weiss and Taylor 1995; Berger 1997; Evans and Almond 1998). A surprisingly wide variety of cellular molecules (proteins, glycoproteins, carbohydrates and lipids) can serve as viral receptors. Despite their pivotal importance for the biology and pathology of viruses, the endogenous functions of a large number of these receptor molecules are currently unknown.

A few common principles emerge from the staggering amount of new information which reveals a high degree of complexity in most viral-receptor relationships. Since one of the purposes of virus-receptor interaction can be to direct a virus to the cell populations in which it has evolved to replicate efficiently, the type and expression pattern of the receptor molecule may reflect the tropism of a virus. Thus, some viruses with restricted tropisms use cell surface molecules specifically expressed on their target cells for attachment, e.g., the use of CD4 as the principal receptor for HIV-1 targets it to $CD4^+$ T lymphocytes and macrophages (DALGLEISH et al. 1984; KLATZMANN et al. 1984; MADDON et al. 1986), and the binding of rabies virus to the acetylcholine receptor and/or N-CAM is thought to direct it to neurons (LENTZ et al. 1982; THOULOUZE et al. 1998). Likewise, viruses with a broad tissue tropism bind preferentially to widely expressed molecules that allow them to attach to many different cell types. Examples include the α_v integrins used as receptors by adenoviruses and certain picornaviruses, including foot and mouth disease virus and some coxsackieviruses (WICKHAM et al. 1993; ROIVAINEN et al. 1994; BERINSTEIN et al. 1995); the integrin VLA-2 used as a receptor by some echoviruses (BERGELSON et al. 1992); CD55 (decay accelerating factor), to which certain other coxsackieviruses and echoviruses bind (BERGELSON et al. 1995); and CD46 (membrane cofactor protein), the principal receptor for measles virus (NANICHE et al. 1993).

However, the sites of virus replication cannot always be predicted from the pattern of expression of the primary receptor, as, for example, there may be cell-type-specific modifications of the primary receptor which affect virus binding; the virus may also need to interact with co-receptor(s) that are not expressed on all cells bearing the major receptor; and/or virus replication may be restricted at a post-binding step in some receptor-expressing cells. Hence, although the poliovirus receptor (Pvr) is very broadly expressed (MENDELSOHN et al. 1989), poliovirus replication in infected primates is highly restricted; likewise, influenza viruses bind to sialic acid, a ubiquitously expressed cell-surface sugar (PAULSON et al. 1979; HIGA et al. 1985; WEIS et al. 1988), but in vivo replicate only within the lungs/respiratory tract.

In most cases, the specificity of the virus-receptor interaction is not a one-to-one relation. Many viruses are able to bind to host cells by more than one type of receptor, and some cellular molecules are used as receptors by a multitude of viruses from different families.

Among the cell surface proteins identified so far as virus receptors, cell surface proteins that are involved in cell adhesion and cell recognition processes in the host organism seem to be preferred candidates. A wide variety of viruses use cell adhesion molecules of the Ig superfamily or SCR family or ECM receptors like the integrins or dystroglycan (Table 1). Interestingly, the viral surface components that bind these cell recognition molecules frequently structurally mimic their host-derived ligands, for example the integrin-attachment sites of picornaviruses and adenoviruses (EVANS and ALMOND 1998) that contain a RGD-motif, similar to that recognized by integrins in their endogenous ligands. By this strategy, viruses make use of the previously existing cellular mechanisms for efficient attachment and subsequent entry. Since cell surface receptors like Ig superfamily molecules or integrins are also mediators of cellular signal transduction, the attachment of a virus to a cell by these molecules may elicit intracellular signals reminiscent of those triggered by their endogenous ligands. Activation of signal transduction pathways by virus binding to its receptor prior to viral entry may create a cellular environment optimal for subsequent viral gene expression, for example, by the activation of the cellular gene transcription machinery. On the other hand, signals elicited by

Table 1. Cell recognition molecules that function as virus receptors or co-receptors

Receptor	Virus	Virus family	Reference
Integrin			
$\alpha_v\beta_3$	Foot-and-mouth disease virus	Picornaviridae	BERINSTEIN et al. 1995
$\alpha_v\beta_5$	Coxackievirus A9	Picornaviridae	ROIVAINEN et al. 1994
$\alpha_2\beta_1$ (VLA-2)	Echoviruses 1 and 8	Picornaviridae	BERGELSON et al. 1992
$\alpha_v\beta_3$, $\alpha_v\beta_5$	Adenovirus	Adenoviridae	WICKHAM et al. 1993
Dystroglycan	Lymphocytic choriomeningitis virus	Arenaviridae	CAO et al. 1998
	Lassa fever virus	Arenaviridae	CAO et al. 1998
IgSF molecules			
CD4	Human immunodeficiency virus 1	Retroviridae	KLATZMANN et al. 1984
ICAM-1	Coxsackievirus A13, A18, A21	Picornaviridae	EVANS and ALMOND 1998
	Human rhinoviruses	Picornaviridae	GREVE et al. 1989
Pvr	Poliovirus	Picornaviridae	MENDELSOHN et al. 1989
HveB & C	Herpes simplex viruses 1 and 2	Herpesviridae	GERAGHTY et al. 1998
NCAM	Rabies virus	Rhabdoviridae	THOULOUZE et al. 1998
Biliary gps	MHV-A59	Coronaviridae	DVEKSLER et al. 1991
SCR-like molecules			
CD46	Measles virus	Paramyxoviridae	DORIG et al. 1993
CD55	Coxsackievirus A21 and B1, 3, 5	Picornaviridae	BERGELSON et al. 1995
	Echovirus 7 and others	Picornaviridae	BERGELSON et al. 1994

virus binding may interfere with normal host cell signal transduction and result in the perturbation of specific cellular functions, resulting in pathology.

3 The Identification of α-Dystroglycan as a Receptor for Arenaviruses Including Lymphocytic Choriomeningitis Virus and Lassa Fever Virus

At the beginning of the 1990s, very little was known about host cell receptor(s) for arenaviruses. The broad tissue and cell tropism of the prototypic arenavirus, Lymphocytic choriomeningitis virus (LCMV), in its natural murine host (for review see BORROW and OLDSTONE 1997) suggested that this virus may use a widely expressed cell surface component as its cellular receptor, but the nature of this receptor was not known.

At that time, the identity of the virion attachment protein (VAP) had also not been confirmed. LCMV (and by analogy, other arenaviruses) was known to encode a glycoprotein precursor that was post-translationally processed into two subunits, glycoproteins (GP) 1 and 2; these were generally accepted to be the only viral proteins exposed on the surface of intact virions. Of these candidate VAPs, GP-1 seemed the more likely one on the basis of structural evidence: GP-1 is a peripheral membrane protein non-covalently associated with GP-2, an integral membrane protein (BUCHMEIER and OLDSTONE 1979; BURNS and BUCHMEIER 1991). Further, of multiple monoclonal antibodies raised to epitopes on the LCMV glycoproteins,

116   S. Kunz et al.

those able to neutralize virus in vitro or mediate protection in vivo were all directed against GP-1, whereas antibodies to GP-2 were non-neutralizing (PAREKH and BUCHMEIER 1986; WRIGHT and BUCHMEIER 1991). The subsequent finding that GP-1-specific antibodies were able to block the binding of LCMV to murine cell lines, whereas antibodies against different epitopes on GP-2 failed to affect virus binding (BORROW and OLDSTONE 1992) provided further evidence that GP-1 likely did act as the VAP. With this premise, the interesting observation that a single amino acid change in GP-1 of LCMV was associated with marked differences in the in vivo pathogenesis of closely related LCMV variants (SALVATO et al. 1991) raised the intriguing possibility that the in vivo properties of different LCMV isolates may be affected by their in vivo tropism, which in turn was dictated by differences in their interaction with host cell receptors. This provided the impetus for investigation of arenavirus-receptor interactions.

Initial experiments aimed to determine the nature of the cell surface component(s) to which LCMV bound. The effect of selective removal of different host cell membrane components on the binding of LCMV to a murine fibroblast cell line was investigated (BORROW and OLDSTONE 1992). Phospholipase treatment did not reduce LCMV binding to cells, but a panel of proteases all ablated virus binding, indicating that the cellular receptor(s) for LCMV were either protein(s) or protein-bound entities. The membrane protein(s) on which LCMV binding was dependent were not attached to the host cell membrane by glycosyl-phosphatidylinositol linkage, as virus binding was not affected by phosphatidylinositol-specific phospholipase C. Further experiments addressed the role of carbohydrates in LCMV attachment to the cell surface. Treatment of cells with periodate, which oxidizes cell surface sialic acid, or neuraminidases, which remove sialic acid, had no effect on LCMV binding, nor did treatment with N- and O-glycanase, which remove N- and O-linked sugars, respectively, from proteins. In addition, LCMV was still able to bind to cells that had been grown overnight in the presence of tunicamycin, which inhibits N-linked glycosylation. Thus, although the cell surface protein(s) to which virus binding occurred might be glycoproteins, virus binding did not appear to be dependent on protein glycosylation.

The membrane protein(s) to which LCMV binds were then characterized using a virus overlay protein blot assay (VOPBA) (BORROW and OLDSTONE 1992). This is a modified form of the Western blot assay, in which test proteins (e.g., cell membrane proteins from different cell lines) are separated by SDS-PAGE and transferred onto a membrane which is incubated with virus, and virus binding to the test protein(s) is then visualized directly (if labelled virus was used) or indirectly (using antiviral antibodies and appropriate detection reagents). VOPBAs in which the binding of LCMV clone 13 to membrane proteins from different rodent cell lines was investigated revealed specific virus binding to a high-molecular-weight constituent of the membranes of those cells that were readily infected by LCMV (see Fig. 1, LCMV panel). By contrast, no viral binding was detected to membrane proteins of cell lines that were relatively resistant to LCMV clone 13 infection. Further experiments confirmed that the virus-binding entity was a heavily glycosylated protein, and that virus binding was not reduced by glycanase treatment.

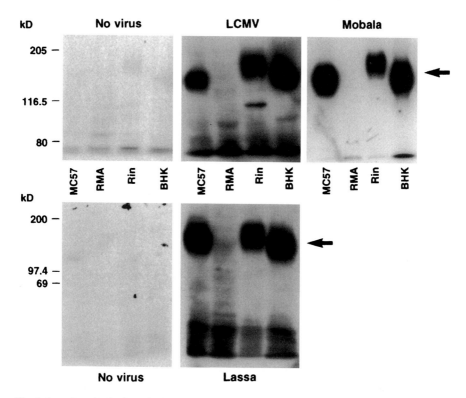

Fig. 1. Lymphocytic choriomeningitis virus (*LCMV*), Lassa and Mobala viruses show the same pattern of binding to cell membrane proteins in a virus overlay protein blot assay (VOPBA): membrane proteins from four different rodent cell lines (MC57, Rin and BHK, which are susceptible to arenavirus infection, and RMA, which is relatively resistant to infection) were separated by SDS-PAGE on replicate gels and transferred onto nitrocellulose. VOPBAs were performed on separate blots using LCMV, Mobala or Lassa virus as indicated: virus binding was detected using antiviral antibodies and ^{125}I-labelled protein A. Control VOPBAs were also performed in which the virus layer was omitted (*No virus*). The *arrows* indicate the position of the arenavirus-binding glycoprotein (subsequently identified as α-dystroglycan) in the membrane preparations from infection-susceptible cell lines: its apparent molecular weight varies slightly from one cell line to another

The apparent molecular mass of the protein was the same under both reducing and non-reducing conditions; it varied slightly from one cell line to another, but was generally in the 120–150kDa range (Fig. 1). This glycoprotein was a putative host cell receptor for LCMV (BORROW and OLDSTONE 1992).

VOPBAs were then carried out to determine whether other LCMV isolates also bound to the glycoprotein identified as a putative receptor for LCMV clone 13. Certain LCMV isolates, such as WE54 and Traub, exhibited an identical pattern of VOPBA binding to LCMV clone 13; interestingly, though, other LCMV isolates, including the Armstrong parental strain from which clone 13 was derived, WE2.2 and E350, exhibited no detectable VOPBA binding to total cell membrane preparations from rodent cell lines, indicating differences in receptor binding properties between LCMV isolates. This is discussed further below.

VOPBAs were also carried out with additional arenaviruses, including the highly pathogenic Lassa fever virus (LFV). As illustrated in Fig. 1, Old World arenaviruses LFV and Mobala exhibited a pattern of receptor binding in the VOPBA that was indistinguishable from that of LCMV clone 13, indicating that these diverse viruses may all share a common host cell receptor. Further VOPBAs performed with LCMV and LFV on membrane proteins from human cell lines also revealed parallel patterns of binding to ~120–150kDa proteins (P. Borrow, E. Ravkov, S. Nichol and M.B.A. Oldstone, unpublished data), suggesting that homologues of the same protein are likely utilized as receptors by these arenaviruses in both their natural rodent hosts and in humans.

Intensive efforts were then made to identify the putative LCMV/LFV host cell receptor. Membrane proteins from a murine fibroblast cell line were solubilized and separated by sequential column chromatography, the LCMV-binding fractions being tracked by VOPBA analysis. After enrichment for the LCMV-binding protein in this way, the remaining proteins were separated by SDS-PAGE, and the virus-binding band was excised, subjected to in-gel digestion with trypsin, and the resulting peptides sequenced. Three of the five peptide sequences obtained showed complete homology to dystroglycan (CAO et al. 1998). Dystroglycan is a protein involved in interactions between cells and the extracellular matrix (IBRAGHIMOV-BESKROVNAYA et al. 1992): it has a broad tissue and cellular expression pattern (DURBEEJ et al. 1998), as had been predicted for the arenavirus receptor. As discussed in more detail in Sect. 4 of this chapter, the dystroglycan gene encodes a precursor protein that is processed into two non-covalently associated subunits: α-dystroglycan, a peripheral membrane protein, and β-dystroglycan, an integral membrane protein (ERVASTI and CAMPBELL 1991; IBRAGHIMOV-BESKROVNAYA et al. 1992). All three tryptic peptide sequences were located near to the C-terminus of the α-dystroglycan subunit. This subunit is glycosylated and, depending on the tissue from which it is obtained, has an apparent molecular mass of between 110 and 156kDa, consistent with the putative LCMV/LFV receptor identified by VOPBA. LCMV and LFV were also shown to bind to purified α-dystroglycan on VOPBAs (CAO et al. 1998).

Further evidence that α-dystroglycan is probably used as the host cell receptor by LCMV was provided by experiments in which purified α-dystroglycan was shown to be able to block LCMV clone 13 infection of cells in a dose-dependent manner (CAO et al. 1998). However, the most unequivocal proof that dystroglycan does act as an arenavirus receptor came from experiments with dystroglycan knockout embryonic stem (ES) cell lines. A mouse ES cell line expressing dystroglycan was readily infected by LCMV clone 13, but dystroglycan-knockout ES cells were shown to be much more resistant to clone 13 infection. Further, infection susceptibility was conferred on the dystroglycan knockout cells when dystroglycan expression was restored by transduction with a rabbit dystroglycan cDNA (CAO et al. 1998).

It has thus now been clearly demonstrated that the α-subunit of dystroglycan is used as a host cell receptor by members of the arenavirus family (Table 2).

Table 2. α-dystroglycan is a receptor for LCMV, LFV and other arenaviruses

Arenaviruses bind to purified α-dystroglycan
Soluble α-dystroglycan blocks arenavirus binding
Removal of the dystroglycan gene converts a permissive cell to non-permissiveness
Restoration of dystroglycan expression to α-dystroglycan (−/−) cells restores virus permissivity

However, there are still many questions that remain unanswered, which current work is addressing. These include the following.

First, does arenavirus binding/entry into cells involve a stepwise series of interactions between virions and the host cell surface, as described earlier for HIV-1? If so, which of these steps does binding to α-dystroglycan represent, and what are the other interactions involved? It seems likely that there may be an initial electrostatic interaction between the incoming virion and the host cell surface (perhaps with, e.g., heparan sulphate, as has been reported for other viruses). Is binding to α-dystroglycan the next event? And is it in turn followed by interaction(s) with other cell surface receptors/co-receptors? Is the expression/accessibility of α-dystroglycan the major determinant of the susceptibility of different cell types to infection by α-dystroglycan-binding arenaviruses, or does the presence/absence of additional receptors also play a role?

Second, just how do arenaviruses bind to α-dystroglycan, and what are the consequences of virus-dystroglycan interaction? Which part of the virion surface glycoprotein binds to α-dystroglycan; is the tetrameric structure of the glycoprotein required; and can more than one GP-1 subunit within a tetramer contact α-dystroglycan simultaneously? Conversely which part of α-dystroglycan contacts the viral glycoprotein, and could this binding site be occluded by other components of the dystroglycan complex or natural ligands of α-dystroglycan? Does virus binding to dystroglycan trigger cell signalling and/or interfere with the normal functions of this protein, and what are the consequences of this? These issues are considered in more detail in Sect. 4 of this chapter.

Third, which arenaviruses bind to α-dystroglycan? Several different members of the arenavirus family have been shown to bind to purified α-dystroglycan on VOPBAs: these include both Old World arenaviruses (LCMV, LFV and Mobala viruses) and a New World arenavirus (Oliveros) (Cao et al. 1998). Although different members of a family of viruses frequently use very diverse host cell constituents as receptors, it is not unprecedented for different members of a family of viruses (or even unrelated viruses) to use common or homologous receptors on host cells – this is seen, for example, within the picornaviridae and retroviridae. It remains to be determined how many of the other arenaviruses utilize α-dystroglycan as a host cell receptor, and whether/how this relates to their relative pathogenicity in humans.

Finally, are all those arenaviruses that can bind to α-dystroglycan equally dependent on it for infection of host cells, and how does this relate to their in vivo tropism and pathogenesis? As mentioned above, there are differences between LCMV isolates in their binding to α-dystroglycan. Certain LCMV isolates (e.g., clone 13, WE54 and Traub) bind very strongly to purified α-dystroglycan in

VOPBAs, and display detectable binding to the levels of this protein in total membrane preparations from cell lines and tissues. In contrast, other LCMV isolates (e.g., Armstrong, WE2.2 and E350) bind much less well to α-dystroglycan. None of them show detectable binding to this protein in total membrane preparations from cells and tissues; WE2.2 does not even bind at detectable levels to purified α-dystroglycan on VOPBAs; and although binding of Armstrong and E350 to purified α-dystroglycan is seen on VOPBA, more than 100-fold more α-dystroglycan is required to detect this binding than that of, for example, clone 13 (SMELT et al. 2001; SEVILLA et al. 2000). Infection of cells by clone 13, Traub and WE54 is also much more readily inhibited by soluble α-dystroglycan than is infection by Armstrong, E350 and WE2.2 (SMELT et al. 2001; SEVILLA et al. 2000). Further, although α-dystroglycan knockout ES cells are relatively resistant to infection with clone 13, Traub and WE54 [only a low percentage of cells becoming infected even after incubation with these viruses at high multiplicity of infection (moi)], they can be infected with Armstrong, E350 and WE2.2. Armstrong and E350 do show some dependence on α-dystroglycan for infection, as they infect dystroglycan knockout ES cells less efficiently than dystroglycan-expressing ES cells, but WE2.2 infects dystroglycan-positive and -negative cells equally well even at low moi (SMELT et al. 2001; SEVILLA et al. 2000). Whether WE2.2 (and possibly also Armstrong and E350) binds to a unique receptor or is able to infect cells solely by means of co-receptor interactions [in the same way as macaque-derived SIV isolates are thought to infect simian cells by binding to chemokine receptors, with no requirement for binding to CD4 (reviewed by MARX and CHEN 1998)] has yet to be elucidated. The impact that these differences in interactions with host cell receptors have on the tropism and in vivo pathogenic properties of the different LCMV isolates is discussed in Sect. 5 of this chapter.

4 Dystroglycan: the Cellular Receptor for the Arenaviruses LCMV and LFV

Dystroglycan, the recently identified receptor for the arenaviruses Lymphocytic choriomeningitis virus (LCMV) and Lassa fever virus (LFV) (CAO et al. 1998; see Table 2) is a highly versatile cellular receptor for proteins of the extracellular matrix (ECM) that was originally isolated from skeletal muscle as a component of the dystrophin-glycoprotein complex (ERVASTI and CAMPBELL 1991b; IBRAGHIMOV-BESKROVNAYA et al. 1992). In muscle membrane, dystroglycan provides a molecular link between the extracellular matrix (ECM) and the actin-based cytoskeleton. In addition to its function in muscle, key findings in the past few years demonstrated that dystroglycan plays a fundamental role in the cell-mediated assembly and organization of basement membranes throughout the organism (for recent reviews see HEMLER 1999; HENRY and CAMPBELL 1999). Its broad tissue distribution, high evolutionary conservation, and ability to interact with extracellular proteins make α-dystroglycan an ideal candidate for a receptor for microbial pathogens. Not only arenaviruses make use of α-dystroglycan as a cellular receptor. Recent studies demonstrated that infection of Schwann cells of peripheral nerve tissue by *Mycobacterium leprae* is mediated by a complex of α-dystroglycan with laminin-2 (RAMBUKKANA et al. 1997, 1998; RAMBUKKANA 2000). A detailed understanding of the endogenous functions of dystroglycan is therefore of great importance for the study of the pathophysiology of these infectious diseases.

To date only a single, evolutionary highly conserved dystroglycan gene has been identified that is transcribed into a single mRNA species (IBRAGHIMOV-BESKROVNAYA et al. 1992). Initially encoded by a single polypeptide chain, dystroglycan undergoes proteolytic processing to form α-dystroglycan, a peripheral membrane protein, and the integral membrane protein β-dystroglycan (ERVASTI and CAMPBELL 1991; IBRAGHIMOV-BESKROVNAYA et al. 1992; HOLT et al. 2000). The apparent molecular masses of α-dystroglycan, as detected in gel electrophoresis, vary widely between different tissues, from 156kDa for α-dystroglycan isolated from skeletal muscle (ERVASTI and CAMPBELL 1991; IBRAGHIMOV-BESKROVNAYA et al. 1992) to 110kDa for α-dystroglycan from brain and peripheral nerve tissue (GEE et al. 1993; SMALHEISER and KIM 1995). Since the polypeptide core of α-dystroglycan is encoded by a single gene, these differences in apparent molecular mass between α-dystroglycans isolated from different tissues are presumably due to differential glycosylation. In contrast to α-dystroglycan, β-dystroglycan exhibits a constant molecular mass of 43kDa irrespective of the source. Only limited information is currently available regarding the structure of α-dystroglycan. Based on its amino acid sequence, a modular structure for dystroglycan is suggested (Fig. 2) that corresponds to the dumbbell-like appearance of the molecule in electron microscopic examinations (IBRAGHIMOV-BESKROVNAYA et al. 1992; BRANCACCIO et al. 1995). Analytical ultracentrifugation, electron microscopy and spectroscopic analysis revealed a globular structure for the N-terminal domain of α-dystroglycan that may represent an autonomous folding unit (BRANCACCIO et al. 1997). Recent studies suggest the existence of at least two subdomains within the globular N-terminal part of α-dystroglycan: a first subdomain may be formed by the sequence H30-S180, where amino acids 80–180 exhibit similarity to the Ig κ domain structure family. A second subdomain is formed by amino acids A181-A316 (BRANCACCIO et al. 1997; BOZIC et al. 1998). The sequence 160–180 is less conserved than the rest of the molecule, indicating a function as a spacer or linker between the two postulated subdomains. The central region of α-dystroglycan contains a high fraction of proline and threonine residues and is thought to represent a mucin-related structure (HILKENS et al. 1992; LI et al. 1996). Carbohydrate analysis revealed extensive O-glycosylation with a high abundance of terminally sialylated O-linked sugar chains which exhibit remarkable tissue-specific differences (CHIBA et al. 1997; ERVASTI et al. 1997). The polypeptide core of mucin-like proteins is thought to adopt an extended conformation with laterally protruding carbohydrate chains in a bottle brush-like manner. This model is in accordance with the extended central part of α-dystroglycan revealed by electron microscopic examination (BRANCACCIO et al. 1995). The same studies indicate a globular structure for the C-terminal

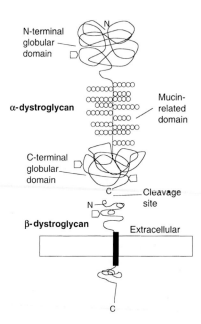

N-terminal globular domain

α-dystroglycan

Mucin-related domain

C-terminal globular domain

Cleavage site

β-dystroglycan

Extracellular

Fig. 2. Schematic representation of dystroglycan. The putative N-terminal and C-terminal globular domains are depicted as *coils* and the mucin-related central domain in an extended conformation with its O-linked carbohydrates (*chains of circles*) protruding in a perpendicular orientation. *N*-glycans are depicted as *pentagons*

domain of α-dystroglycan. The association of α- and β-dystroglycan is non-covalent in nature and appears to be of high stability, as harsh biochemical conditions are necessary to dissociate them (ERVASTI and CAMPBELL 1991). Which part of α-dystroglycan is involved in its attachment to β-dystroglycan is currently uncertain.

A striking feature of dystroglycan is its complex binding pattern with a wide variety of partners like ECM proteins, other membrane proteins like, for example, the sarcoglycans, as well as cystoskeletal components and effector molecules of signal transduction (Fig. 3). This complex binding pattern of dystroglycan result in the formation of tissue-specific α-dystroglycan-complexes at the cell surface. The structure and composition of the complex dystroglycan and its binding partners form at the cell surface is currently best characterized for skeletal muscle. In muscle fibers, α-dystroglycan binds to laminin-2 (merosin) at the extracellular face of the sarcolemma and β-dystroglycan interacts intracellularly with the cytoskeletal protein dystrophin. In this manner, dystroglycan provides a molecular link between the extracellular matrix and the actin-based cytoskeleton. The dystroglycan complex is further associated with four integral membrane proteins of 35–50kDa, α, β, γ and δ-sacroglycans (LIM and CAMPBELL 1998), as well as the 25-kDa tetraspan protein sarcospan (CROSBIE et al. 1997). Genetic mutations in many individual components of the dystrophin glycoprotein complex are manifested in muscular dystrophies (for review: STRAUB and CAMPBELL 1997; LIM and CAMPBELL 1998).

In order to bind to a cell, the virus has to recognize these tissue-specific complexes as they may represent the actual functional receptors for virus binding. At the extracellular face, α-dystroglycan undergoes high-affinity interactions with the ECM proteins laminin-1, laminin-2 (merosin) and the heparan sulphate

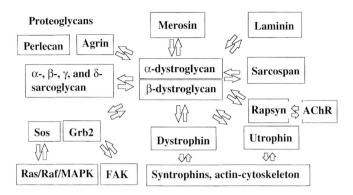

Fig. 3. The pattern of interactions of dystroglycan in skeletal muscle. The ECM proteins laminin-1, laminin-2 (merosin), and the heparan sulphate proteoglycans (HSPGs) agrin and perlecan bind to α-dystroglycan at the extracellular face. The sarcoglycans and sarcospan form a structurally discrete subcomplex within the muscle cell membrane that associates with α/β-dystroglycan. The intracellular domain of the transmembrane β-dystroglycan binds to the cytoskeletal protein dystrophin (replaced by utrophin in some non-muscle tissues) that provides a link to the actin-based cytoskeleton and other intracellular proteins like, for example, the syntrophins. β-dystroglycan binds further to the signal transduction molecule grb2 that is linked to the Ras/Raf/MEK/ERK MAP-kinase pathway and the focal adhesion kinase (*FAK*). At the neuromuscular synapse, β-dystroglycan interacts with rapsyn, a protein involved in acetylcholine receptor (*AchR*) clustering in the postsynaptic membrane

proteoglycans (HSPGs) agrin and perlecan (ERVASTI and CAMPBELL 1991, 1993; GEE et al. 1994; YAMADA et al. 1996b; TALTS et al. 1999). The binding sites of these ECM proteins overlap, raising the possibility of mutual competition between them in vivo (TALTS et al. 1999). The structural motifs within these large molecules recognized by α-dystroglycan are the laminin-type G domain (LG) modules. LG modules consist of ca 190 amino acids and have been identified in more than 60 variants. They occur in five-fold repeats at the C-termini of the laminin α1–α5 chains and in different arrangements in agrin and perlecan. LG modules are generally involved in binding to cellular receptors and sulphated ligands such as heparin or sulphatide glycolipids. The interactions between α-dystroglycan and the ECM molecules laminin1/2, agrin and perlecan share specific biochemical characteristics, such as the strict dependence on divalent cations (PALL et al. 1996; ANDAC et al. 1999), sensitivity towards ionic strength and, in some cases, inhibition by heparin (ERVASTI and CAMPBELL 1993; GEE et al. 1993; PALL et al. 1996; ANDAC et al. 1999). The recently solved crystal structure of the laminin-α2 chain LG5 module and previous analysis by point mutations revealed structural features of the α-dystroglycan binding site that reflect these biochemical characteristics (ANDAC et al. 1999; HOHENESTER et al. 1999). The binding site is formed by clusters of basic amino acid residues, contains a calcium ion as an integral structural component, and overlaps with the binding sites for heparin and sulphatide glycolipids.

The corresponding laminin binding site on α-dystroglycan is less well defined. Likely candidates for the α-dystroglycan structures recognized by the laminin LG modules are negatively charged carbohydrate moieties, although protein-protein interactions may also be involved. Treatment of α-dystroglycan with low concentrations of periodate eliminates laminin binding (ERVASTI and CAMPBELL 1993; SMALHEISER 1993). Further, removal of terminal sialic acid residues and competition with soluble sialic acid reduced laminin/α-dystroglycan binding in some studies (YAMADA et al. 1996a; CHIBA et al. 1997) but not others (ERVASTI et al. 1997), possibly reflecting tissue-specific differences in glycosylation of the α-dystroglycan used. These structural and biochemical data, together with the well described sensitivity of the LG/α-dystroglycan interaction in laminin and agrin towards heparin and high salt concentration (ERVASTI and CAMPBELL 1993; GEE et al. 1993), strongly supports an involvement of polyanionic carbohydrate structures of α-dystroglycan in this type of binding. Differential glycosylation of α-dystroglycan could therefore modulate its ligand binding properties. Indeed, a recent study demonstrated the developmental regulation of α-dystroglycan glycosylation in skeletal muscle and differential binding of laminin by distinct glycosylation variants (LESCHZINER et al. 2000).

Biochemical characterization of the LCMV/α-dystroglycan interaction revealed fundamental differences between virus binding and the interactions of α-dystroglycan with ECM proteins described above. In contrast to the ECM/α-dystroglycan interactions, the LCMV/α-dystroglycan binding is independent of cations and insensitive to chelating agents and heparin (KUNZ et al. 2000). Extensive neuraminidase treatment and oxidation by low concentrations of sodium periodate (< 1mM) that affects only terminal sialic acid residues have no effect on virus binding but abolish laminin-1/α-dystroglycan interaction (YAMADA et al. 1996a; RAMBUKKANA et al. 1998; KUNZ et al. 2001). The extensive deglycosylation of α-dystroglycan that is required to reduce virus binding (CAO et al. 1998; KUNZ et al. 2001) may reflect structural changes of the protein rather than a direct involvement of carbohydrates in the binding. Further, the dramatic changes in virus binding by the mutations F260L, F260I and S153F in the LCMV GP1 (SEVILLA et al. 2001; Fig. 4) suggest protein-protein interactions rather than a carbohydrate-mediated binding play a crucial role in the binding between viral GP1 and α-dystroglycan. However, a direct or indirect function of a specific post-translational modification of α-dystroglycan in virus binding cannot be ruled out currently.

As mentioned above, in muscle tissue, dystroglycan is found associated with two additional types of membrane proteins, the sarcoglycans and sarcospan. They are structurally organized into a distinct subcomplex, the sarcoglycan complex, which associates with the dystroglycan/dystrophin complex forming the dystrophin glycoprotein complex of the sarcolemma. Recent studies suggest a crucial role of the sarcoglycan complex in the stability of the dystroglycan complex. Specifically, the destabilization of the α/β-dystroglycan complex in sarcoglycan-deficient animals demonstrated a crucial function of the sarcoglycans for the structural integrity of the dystrophin glycoprotein complex in muscle tissue (ROBERDS et al. 1993; HOLT et al. 1998; HOLT and CAMPBELL 1998; DUCLOS et al. 1998; DURBEEJ et al. 2000). The association of sarcospan with the sarcoglycans is required for the correct targetting of sarcospan to the sarcolemma, where it contributes to the stabilization of α-dystroglycan in the muscle membrane (CROSBIE et al. 1999).

However, sarcospan-deficient mice show no overt abnormalities in their dystrophin glycoprotein complexes and have normal muscle function (LEBAKKEN et al. 2000), suggesting some redundancy in the components that contribute to the stability of the α/β-dystroglycan complex at the cell surface. The associations of dystroglycan with the sarcoglycans and sarcospan are cell-type specific. In smooth muscle, α-sarcoglycan is, for example, replaced by ε-sarcoglycan, resulting in an unique dystrophin glycoprotein complex (STRAUB et al. 1999). The dystroglycan complexes of epithelial cells and Schwann cells lack sarcoglycans and sarcospan completely (DURBEEJ and CAMPBELL 1999; SAITO et al. 1999). As expected from the studies discussed above, these dystroglycan complexes lacking the sarcoglycans appear to be less stable than those found in muscle that contain the sarcoglycan complex (SAITO et al. 1999).

α-dystroglycan is non-covalently associated with the membrane spanning β-dystroglycan. β-dystroglycan binds intracellularly to a variety of cytoskeletal proteins and signal transduction molecules. The best-described interaction is its binding to dystrophin and related molecules. Within the dystrophin glycoprotein complex of skeletal muscle, the C-terminal 15 amino acids of β-dystroglycan bind to dystrophin (JUNG et al. 1995). A WW motif and a calcium-binding site on dystrophin are essential for this interaction (RENTSCHLER et al. 1999). In tissues other than skeletal muscle and brain, full-length dystrophin is replaced by truncated dystrophin versions and the closely related molecule utrophin (SAITO et al. 1999). In all cases, dystrophin and utrophin provide a physical link to the actin-based cytoskeleton and are associated with further cytoskeletal components like, for example, the syntrophins. Other molecules that bind the cytoplasmatic tail of β-dystroglycan include the signal transduction molecule grb2 and the focal adhesion kinase (FAK) (YANG et al. 1995; CAVALDESI et al. 1999). The physiological relevance of these interactions is currently not known. However, since the adaptor protein grb2 is a crucial component in the activation of many signal transduction cascades, among them the MEK/ERK MAP kinase pathway, this opens the possibility that dystroglycan could be involved in cellular signal transduction.

Based on its highly complex binding pattern, α-dystroglycan at the cell surface might be virtually covered by ECM molecules and cellular proteins. Some of the α-dystroglycan-associated proteins may enhance virus binding and may be regarded as co-factors or co-receptors. Other binding partners may compete with the virus for overlapping binding sites on α-dystroglycan and therefore block its function as a viral receptor. Based on their large sizes, widespread co-expression with dystroglycan and their high binding affinities, the ECM molecules laminin-1/2, perlecan and agrin represent interesting candidates for competitors of virus binding. Indeed, recent studies revealed a competition between laminin-1 and LCMV for α-dystroglycan binding, suggesting a potential overlap in the binding sites of this ECM molecules with the α-dystroglycan structures required for virus attachment or simply a mutual steric hindrance based on the large size of both structures (KUNZ et al. 2001). The susceptibility of a specific cell for arenavirus infection in vivo may therefore depend not only on the expression of α-dystroglycan per se but also on α-dystroglycan's association with these host-derived proteins. In order to infect

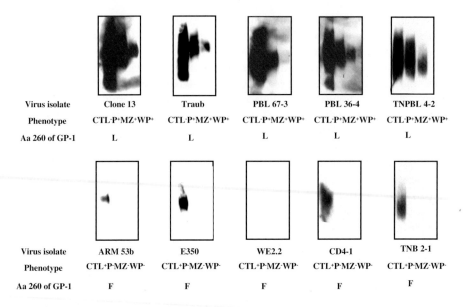

Fig. 4. VOPBA with purified α-DG and LCMV variants. Decreasing amounts (1, 0.1 and 0.01μg) of purified α-DG were incubated with 1×10^7 PFUs of each viral isolate and then detected with virus-specific antibody. The *upper panels* show the VOPBA of LCMV immunosuppressive isolates clone 13, Traub, PBL 67-3, PBL 36-4 and TNPBL4-2. The phenotype of these isolates is as follows: they induce immunosuppression (CTL⁻), cause persistent infection (P⁺) and show a tropism for the marginal zone (MZ⁺) and the white pulp (WP⁺) of the spleen. The *lower panel* shows the VOPBA of non-immunosuppressive LCMV isolates ARM53b, E350, We2.2, CD4-1 and TNB 2-1. These isolates are non-immunosuppressive (CTL⁺), are cleared by the host immune system (P⁻) and are unable to infect the marginal zone (MZ⁻) and the white pulp (WP⁻) of the spleen. Isolates in the *upper panel* have a L or I residue in position 260 of GP1, while isolates in the *lower panel* have F in position 260

specific cell populations, the virus would have to compete with these host-derived high-affinity ligands. It is conceivable that the binding affinity for α-dystroglycan represents a crucial property of a virus, determining its tissue tropism and therefore its pathological potential. Indeed, recent studies revealed a striking correlation between the pathological potential of different LCMV strains and variants and their binding affinity to α-dystroglycan (see Sect. 5). In line with that, recent in vitro studies demonstrated that only LCMV variants with a high binding affinity for α-dystroglycan can successfully compete with laminin-1 (KUNZ et al. 2001). Based on its competition with the α-dystroglycan/laminin binding, an arenavirus with sufficiently high binding affinity to α-dystroglycan may therefore interfere with the α-dystroglycan/ECM interactions. As a consequence, virus binding may perturb dystroglycan's function as an ECM receptor and contribute to viral pathology by disruption of cell/ECM contacts. Detailed knowledge of the endogenous function of α-dystroglycan is therefore mandatory for the understanding of the pathophysiology of arenaviruses.

What is the role of dystroglycan within the host organism? In the case of skeletal muscle, one hypothesis is that dystroglycan within the dystrophin glycoprotein complex protects muscle fibres against mechanical damage during contraction (MENKE and JOCKUSCH 1991; PASTERNAK et al. 1995). In this context, dystroglycan may act as a cell adhesion molecule to anchor cells to the extracellular matrix, as reflected by its reported role in clustering of laminin and agrin at the surface of muscle cells (CAMPANELLI et al. 1994; GEE et al. 1994; COHEN et al. 1997). However, recent studies have revealed more fundamental functions of dystroglycan's interactions with ECM proteins in non-muscle tissues. In addition to its prominent expression in skeletal and cardiac muscle, dystroglycan is expressed in many developing and adult tissues, typically in cell types that adjoin basement membranes, such as epithelial and neural tissue (TIAN et al. 1996; DURBEEJ et al. 1998). An elegant study by HENRY and CAMPBELL (1998) demonstrated that dystroglycan is required for the formation of basement membranes during early embryonic development and the formation of the sub-endodermal basement membrane in embryoid bodies. These results demonstrate a fundamental role for dystroglycan in the cell-mediated assembly of extracellular membrane proteins during the formation of basement membranes throughout the organism.

A specialized role for dystroglycan is described in the formation of the neuromuscular synapse, in particular in the clustering of postsynaptic acetylcholine receptors (GESEMANN et al. 1996; CARTAUD et al. 1998; RUEGG and BIXBY 1998). The localization of dystroglycan at the synapses in the central nervous system suggests a general role in synaptogenesis (MONTANARO et al. 1995; CAVALDESI et al. 1999). However, dystroglycan can mediate the formation of a receptor-cytoskeleton network over the entire surface of the muscle cell. This aggregation involves laminin polymerization, the cytoskeleton, as well as tyrosine phosphorylation and therefore resembles the formation of basal laminar structures (COLOGNATO et al. 1999). The function of α-dystroglycan in synaptogenesis may therefore turn out to be only a variation of the general function in basal membrane assembly, demonstrated by the study of HENRY and CAMPBELL (1998).

Based on these observations, it is conceivable that interference of virus binding to α-dystroglycan with its function as a receptor for ECM proteins may result in the perturbation of the assembly and structural integrity of basal laminae. Disruption of the cell-ECM interaction may in turn affect normal cell function and result in disease. Some aspects of arenavirus-mediated pathology may indeed be linked to such an interference of virus binding with the function of dystroglycan in the organization of basement membranes. A recent study demonstrated a crucial function of α-dystroglycan in the adhesion of vascular endothelial cells to the ECM (SHIMIZU et al. 1999). Perturbation of α-dystroglycan/ECM interactions in vascular endothelial cells by an arenavirus may therefore contribute to the hemorrhagic pathology observed in humans infected with Lassa fever virus, which binds α-dystroglycan with high affinity (CAO et al. 1998). In this context, it would be interesting to know to what extent the virus/α-dystroglycan binding interferes with the α-dystroglycan/ECM interactions. To this end, the study of a potential competition between virus and ECM proteins for α-dystroglycan binding as well as the determination of the relative affinities of arenaviruses and ECM proteins for α-dystroglycan are of great interest.

The link of dystroglycan to the cellular signal transduction network by grb2 and FAK (YANG et al. 1995; CAVALDESI et al. 1999) opens the possibility that binding of LCMV virions to dystroglycan on the cell surface activates signal transduction pathways in target cells prior to viral entry. Indeed, many virus receptors are proteins that are involved in cellular signal transduction processes of the host, like molecules of the immunoglobulin superfamily, integrins, and receptors for growth factors or cytokines (see Sect. 2). As the surface components of many viruses which interact with these receptors mimic their natural ligands, virus-receptor interaction frequently triggers similar intracellular signals like the host factors that normally bind the receptor proteins. Activation of specific cellular signal transduction cascades by the binding of LCMV to α-dystroglycan on the cell surface may be relevant for optimal viral replication and underlie some aspects of virus-induced pathology. The MAP kinase pathways are of particular interest in this context. The MEK/ERK MAP kinase pathway regulates the expression of many transcription factors and other components of the host cell gene expression machinery that may play a role in efficient viral replication. The p38 MAPK pathway and the SAPK/JNK pathway on the other hand are involved in cellular stress responses and regulate the expression of many immunoregulatory molecules such as chemokines and cytokines which may be linked to virus-induced pathology.

5 The Role of the Virus-Receptor Interaction in the Pathological Potential of LCMV Isolates

The investigation of virus-receptor interactions of variants of the same virus species may help to answer the important question of how different isolates of a particular virus can cause different diseases (OLDSTONE 1996). This aspect of viral pathogenesis is of particular interest in the case of arenaviruses, as long-term persistent infections will permit the generation of viral variants that have specific growth advantages in certain tissues. The selection of such viral variants is influenced in a critical way by the host tissue (AHMED et al. 1984; AHMED and OLDSTONE 1988; OLDSTONE et al. 1988). This host-influenced selection process may involve, among other factors, a different interaction of viral variants with their cellular receptor proteins.

In the course of persistent infection of mice with LCMV strain ARM53b, distinct viral variants can be isolated from the brain and lymphoid tissue (AHMED et al. 1984). Whereas the parental variant ARM53b predominated in brain tissue (neurotropic), the variant LCMV ARM53b clone 13 that was isolated from the spleen of persistently infected animals (lymphotropic) exhibits a remarkably changed pathogenic potential. Infection of immunocompetent mice with ARM53b elicits a vigorous immune response, and the virus is efficiently cleared by the host immune system. In contrast, infection with clone 13 results in a generalized immunosuppression and persistence of the virus (AHMED and OLDSTONE 1988). Clone 13 causes immunosuppression by infecting antigen-presenting cells (interdigitating dendritic cells) in the spleen and in lymph nodes. The subsequent destruction of these cells by CD8$^+$ anti-LCMV cytotoxic T lymphocytes (CTL) causes a generalized immunosuppression, which allows the virus to persist (ODERMATT et al. 1991; BORROW et al. 1995). Sequence analysis revealed only two amino acid changes in clone 13 compared with the parental Armstrong strain, F260L in GP1 (SALVATO et al. 1988) and K1079Q in the viral polymerase encoded by the L gene (SALVATO et al. 1991). The immunosuppressive potential of clone 13 was found to be associated with the single point mutation F260L in the viral glycoprotein (SALVATO et al. 1988, 1991), 200 to 500-fold enhanced binding to α-dystroglycan (SEVILLA et al. 2000) and a high dependence on α-dystroglycan for the infection of cells (SMELT et al. 2001). The recent study of a large number of LCMV variants generated in vivo demonstrated a consistent correlation between high receptor binding affinity and the immunosuppressive potential that is structurally reflected by a F260L or F260I mutation in LCMV-GP1 (SEVILLA et al. 2000). These viral variants causing immunosuppression consistently exhibit a remarkably altered tropism in spleen tissue. Like the prototypic immunosuppressive variant clone 13, they preferentially infect interdigitating dendritic cells (IDC), the major antigen-presenting cells in the T-cell area (white pulp) of the spleen. In contrast, the viruses that do not cause immunosuppression do not infect IDC and are restricted to the red pulp of the spleen (SEVILLA et al. 2000). These studies relate structural changes of the viral glycoprotein to receptor binding of a cell important in immune responses. The distinct binding affinities for α-dystroglycan observed with ARM53b and clone 13 most probably reflect structural differences in the complexes formed between the viral glycoprotein and α-dystroglycan. The differential tropism of high-affinity (immunosuppressive) and low-affinity (non-immunosuppressive) binding LCMV variants may relate to their ability to compete with host-derived ligands of α-dystroglycan. Variants with high-affinity receptor binding may out-compete host-derived ligands of α-dystroglycan, allowing them to infect cells co-expressing these factors and α-dystroglycan. In contrast, infection with variants with low affinity to α-dystroglycan, such as ARM 53b, may be blocked by host-derived ligands. Given the highly complex tissue-specific binding pattern of dystroglycan, the ability of a viral variant to compete for dystroglycan binding with host-derived ligands may be crucial for the infection of a particular cell type, like, for example, dendritic cells. Given further the potential role of dystroglycan in cell signal transduction, it is conceivable that the formation of structurally different complexes between viral glycoproteins of LCMV variants and the cellular receptor affects the host cell in a different way. LCMV variants with distinct receptor binding affinities may induce variant-specific intracellular signals in their target cells. A possible interference of these variant-specific signals with host cell signal transduction may be one mechanism by which these viral variants induce specific pathologies.

6 Post-Attachment Steps in the Arenavirus Entry Process

Following binding to cell surface receptors, enveloped viruses may enter host cells by direct fusion of the viral envelope with the plasma membrane, as occurs for example with certain paramyxoviruses (Sendai virus and Newcastle disease virus), retroviruses such as HIV-1 and some herpesviruses. More commonly, however, they are taken into the cell within vesicles (a process termed 'viropexis') and subsequently undergo a pH-dependent fusion event, as exemplified by influenza viruses, alphaviruses such as Semliki Forest virus and Sindbis virus and the rhabdoviruses rabies virus and vesicular stomatitis virus (reviewed by MARSH and HELENIUS 1989). Uptake most frequently occurs by receptor-mediated endocytosis in clathrin-coated vesicles, although virus uptake in large, smooth-walled vesicles has also been documented (e.g., NEMEROW and COOPER 1984; MILLER and HUTT-FLETCHER 1992).

Initial evidence that arenaviruses are taken up and undergo a pH-dependent fusion event within host cells was provided by experiments showing that infection of cells by both the Old World arenavirus LCMV and the New World arenavirus Junin could be inhibited at the entry stage by agents that raise the endosomal pH, e.g., the lysosomotropic weak bases chloroquine and ammonium chloride and the carboxylic ionophores monensin and nigericin (BORROW and OLDSTONE 1994; DI SIMONE et al. 1994; CASTILLA et al. 1994).

That LCMV entry occurs in vesicles rather than by direct fusion of virions with the plasma membrane was confirmed by immuno-electron microscopy (BORROW and OLDSTONE 1994). Following attachment, virions were observed to be taken up in large (150–300nm diameter), smooth-walled vesicles, which did not appear to be associated with clathrin. Although many viruses enter cells by classical endocytosis in clathrin-coated vesicles, it is perhaps not surprising that arenaviruses do not do so in view of their size. Arenavirus particles exhibit some pleomorphism, but an average LCMV virion is roughly spherical with a diameter of 90–120nm and is covered with 5–10nm glycoprotein spikes projecting from the envelope (VEZZA et al. 1977; PEDERSON et al. 1979). As the clathrin lattice restricts the size of coated vesicles to approximately 100nm in diameter, the majority of LCMV particles may be too large to enter via this route.

The large, smooth-walled vesicles in which LCMV entry occurs resemble phagocytic vesicles. Classical phagocytosis (e.g., as mediated by macrophages) is a microfilament-dependent process that is inhibited by cytochalasins. Cytochalasins bind to actin, preventing its proper polymerization into microfilaments and promoting microfilament disassembly (MACLEAN-FLETCHER and POLLARD 1980). Treatment of rodent fibroblast cell lines with cytochalasins B and D failed to inhibit the LCMV entry process (BORROW and OLDSTONE 1994), indicating that LCMV internalization involves a non-microfilament-dependent process distinct from classical phagocytosis. It is not known how this cytochalasin-resistant uptake process is mediated, and whether it is triggered by virion-receptor binding. The finding that LCMV uses the α-subunit of dystroglycan as its cellular receptor is of great interest in this regard. As discussed in Sect. 4 of this chapter, dystroglycan is a transmembrane protein, the cytoplasmic domain of which binds to a number of intracellular proteins including the signal transduction molecule grb2 and the cytoskeletal proteins dystrophin/utrophin. It is thus possible that LCMV binding to α-dystroglycan may initiate the internalization process either by directly triggering some form of signal through dystroglycan or by affecting the interaction of α-dystroglycan with its natural ligands and hence indirectly altering the pattern of signalling through dystroglycan. Recent evidence suggesting that LCMV may bind to α-dystroglycan in a manner distinct from that in which endogenous ligands such as laminin bind to this protein (KUNZ et al. 2001) would perhaps favour the latter hypothesis.

Following internalization of virions within vesicles, the vesicles enter the endocytic pathway and are acidified as they move through the cell. The intravesicular pH decreases from 6.2 in early endosomes to approximately 5.0 by the time the terminal compartments of the pathway (lysosomes) are reached. Fusion of the membrane of enveloped viruses with the vesicle membrane is triggered as the pH drops; the time and location of penetration of different viruses are determined by the pH dependence of the fusion activity. Thus, viruses such as Semliki Forest virus in which fusion is triggered at a pH close to neutral (pH 6.2) fuse in early endosomes, whereas viruses that fuse at lower pH (e.g., influenza virus, pH 5.3) fuse in late endosomes (reviewed by MARSH and HELENIUS 1989).

The pH at which the fusion activity of the LCMV glycoprotein is triggered has been investigated using fluorescence dequenching assays (DI SIMONE et al. 1994; DI SIMONE and BUCHMEIER 1995); fusion was found to be optimal at pH 5.3. Likewise, Junin virus was shown to induce fusion of infected cells, leading to polykaryocyte formation, at a similar pH (CASTILLA et al. 1994).

By analogy to the pH-triggered fusion events of other viruses such as influenza, it is likely that low pH triggers conformational changes in the arenavirus surface glycoprotein that result in exposure of a "fusion peptide" – a hydrophobic moiety which can mediate fusion of the virion and host cell membranes (reviewed by WEISSENHORN et al. 1999). In keeping with this hypothesis, the LCMV glycoprotein spike complex has been shown to undergo irreversible changes after exposure to acidic pH, in which GP-1 is dissociated from the virion, conformational epitopes on GP-1 are lost, and sequestered epitopes on GP-2 are exposed (DI SIMONE et al. 1994). Kinetic analysis of fusion and GP dissociation suggest a mechanism in which the viral glycoprotein is activated to a fusion-competent state where membrane lipid exchange occurs, and then undergoes an irreversible conformation change which includes loss of GP-1 from the spike complex (DI SIMONE and BUCHMEIER 1995). A "fusion peptide" has not been definitively identified within any of the arenavirus glycoproteins, although predictions as to putative sequences involved have been made (GLUSHAKOVA et al. 1990, 1992). Given the recent success of HIV-1 fusion inhibitors in clinical trials (KILBY et al. 1998), a more detailed analysis of the fusion process in arenaviruses is an important area for future investigation.

References

Ahmed R, Oldstone MB (1988) Organ-specific selection of viral variants during chronic infection. J Exp Med 167:1719–1724

Ahmed R, Salmi A, Butler LD, Chiller JM, Oldstone MB (1984) Selection of genetic variants of lymphocytic choriomeningitis virus in spleens of persistently infected mice. Role in suppression of cytotoxic T lymphocyte response and viral persistence. J Exp Med 160:521–540

Andac Z, Sasaki T, Mann K, Brancaccio A, Deutzmann R, Timpl R (1999) Analysis of heparin, alpha-dystroglycan and sulfatide binding to the G domain of the laminin alpha1 chain by site-directed mutagenesis. J Mol Biol 287:253–264

Bergelson JM, Shepley MP, Chan BMC, Hemler ME, Finberg RW (1992) Identification of the integrin VLA-2 as a receptor for echovirus 1. Science 255:1718–1720

Bergelson JM, Chan M, Solomon KR, St. John NF, Lin H, Finberg RW (1994) Decay-accelerating factor (CD55), a glycosylphosphatidylinositol-anchored complement regulatory protein, is a receptor for several echoviruses. Proc Natl Acad Sci USA 91:6245–6249

Bergelson JM, Mohanty JG, Crowell RL, St. John NF, Lublin DM, Finberg RW (1995) Coxsackievirus B3 adapted to growth in RD cells binds to decay-accelerating factor (CD55). J Virol 69:1903–1906

Berger EA (1997) HIV entry and tropism: the chemokine receptor connection. Aids 11:S3–16

Berinstein A, Roivainen M, Hovi T, Mason PW, Baxt B (1995) Antibodies to the vitronectin receptor (integrin alpha v beta 3) inhibit binding and infection of foot-and-mouth disease virus to cultured cells. J Virol 69:2664–2666

Borrow P, Oldstone MBA (1992) Characterization of lymphocytic choriomeningitis virus-binding protein(s): a candidate cellular receptor for the virus. J Virol 66:7270–7281

Borrow P, Oldstone MBA (1994) Mechanism of lymphocytic choriomeningitis virus entry into cells. Virology 198:1–9

Borrow P, Oldstone MBA (1997) Lymphocytic choriomeningitis virus. In: Nathanson N (ed) Viral pathogenesis. Lippincott-Raven, New York

Borrow P, Evans CF, Oldstone MB (1995) Virus-induced immunosuppression: immune system-mediated destruction of virus-infected dendritic cells results in generalized immune suppression. J Virol 69:1059–1070

Boyle KA, Compton T (1998) Receptor-binding properties of a soluble form of human cytomegalovirus glycoprotein B. J Virol 72:1826–1833

Bozic D, Engel J, Brancaccio A (1998) Sequence analysis suggests the presence of an IG-like domain in the N-terminal region of alpha-dystroglycan which was crystallized after mutation of a protease susceptible site (Arg168→His). Matrix Biol 17:495–500

Brancaccio A, Schulthess T, Gesemann M, Engel J (1995) Electron microscopic evidence for a mucin-like region in chick muscle alpha-dystroglycan. FEBS Lett 368:139–142

Brancaccio A, Schulthess T, Gesemann M, Engel J (1997) The N-terminal region of alpha-dystroglycan is an autonomous globular domain. Eur J Biochem 246:166–172

Buchmeier MJ, Oldstone MBA (1979) Protein structure of lymphocytic choriomeningitis virus: evidence for a cell-associated precursor of the virion glycopeptides. Virology 99:111–120

Burns JW, Buchmeier MJ (1991) Protein-protein interactions in lymphocytic choriomeningitis virus. Virology 183:620–629

Campanelli JT, Roberds SL, Campbell KP, Scheller RH (1994) A role for dystrophin-associated glycoproteins and utrophin in agrin-induced AChR clustering. Cell 77:663–674

Cao W, Henry MD, Borrow P, Yamada H, Elder JH, Ravkov EV, Nichol ST, Compans RW, Campbell KP, Oldstone MB (1998) Identification of alpha-dystroglycan as a receptor for lymphocytic chorio-meningitis virus and Lassa fever virus. Science 282:2079–2081

Cartaud A, Coutant S, Petrucci TC, Cartaud J (1998) Evidence for in situ and in vitro association between beta-dystroglycan and the subsynaptic 43K rapsyn protein. Consequence for acetylcholine receptor clustering at the synapse. J Biol Chem 273:11321–11326

Castilla V, Mersich SE, Candurra NA, Damonte EB (1994) The entry of Junin virus into Vero cells. Arch Virol 136:363–374

Cavaldesi M, Macchia G, Barca S, Defilippi P, Tarone G, Petrucci TC (1999) Association of the dystroglycan complex isolated from bovine brain synaptosomes with proteins involved in signal transduction. J Neurochem 72:1648–1655

Chiba A, Matsumura K, Yamada H, Inazu T, Shimizu T, Kusunoki S, Kanazawa I, Kobata A, Endo T (1997) Structures of sialylated O-linked oligosaccharides of bovine peripheral nerve alpha-dystroglycan. The role of a novel O-mannosyl-type oligosaccharide in the binding of alpha-dystroglycan with laminin. J Biol Chem 272:2156–2162

Cohen MW, Jacobson C, Yurchenco PD, Morris GE, Carbonetto S (1997) Laminin-induced clustering of dystroglycan on embryonic muscle cells: comparison with agrin-induced clustering. J Cell Biol 136:1047–1058

Colognato H, Winkelmann DA, Yurchenco PD (1999) Laminin polymerization induces a receptor-cytoskeleton network. J Cell Biol 145:619–631

Compton T, Nowlin DM, Cooper NR (1993) Initiation of human cytomegalovirus infection requires initial interaction with cell surface heparan sulfate. Virology 193:834–841

Crosbie RH, Heighway J, Venzke DP, Lee JC, Campbell KP (1997) Sarcospan, the 25-kDa transmembrane component of the dystrophin-glycoprotein complex. J Biol Chem 272:31221–31224

Crosbie RH, Lebakken CS, Holt KH, Venzke DP, Straub V, Lee JC, Grady RM, Chamberlain JS, Sanes JR, Campbell KP (1999) Membrane targeting and stabilization of sarcospan is mediated by the sarcoglycan subcomplex. J Cell Biol 145:153–165

Dalgleish AG, Beverley PCL, Clapham PR, Crawford DH, Greaves MF, Weiss RA (1984) The CD4 (T4) antigen is an essential component of the receptor for the AIDS retrovirus. Nature 312:763–767

Dean M, Carrington M, Winkler C, Huttley GA, Smith MW, Allikmets R, Goedert JJ, Buchbinder SP, Vittinghoff E, Gomperts E (1996) Genetic restriction of HIV-1 infection and progression to AIDS by a deletion allele of the CKR5 structural gene. Science 273:1856–1862

Di Simone C, Buchmeier MJ (1995) Kinetics and pH dependence of acid-induced structural changes in the lymphocytic choriomeningitis virus glycoprotein complex. Virology 209:3–9

Di Simone C, Zandonatti MA, Buchmeier MJ (1994) Acidic pH triggers LCMV membrane fusion activity and conformational change in the glycoprotein spike. Virology 198:455–465

Dockter J, Evans CF, Tishon A, Oldstone MB (1996) Competitive selection in vivo by a cell for one variant over another: implications for RNA virus quasispecies in vivo. J Virol 70:1799–1803

Dorig RE, Marcil A, Chopra A, Richardson CD (1993) The human CD46 molecule is a receptor for measles virus (Edmonston strain). Cell 75:295–305

Duclos F, Straub V, Moore SA, Venzke DP, Hrstka RF, Crosbie RH, Durbeej M, Lebakken CS, Ettinger AJ, Meulen J van der, Holt KH, Lim LE, Sanes JR, Davidson BL, Faulkner JA, Williamson R, Campbell KP (1998) Progressive muscular dystrophy in alpha-sarcoglycan-deficient mice. J Cell Biol 142:1461–1471

Durbeej M, Campbell KP (1999) Biochemical characterization of the epithelial dystroglycan complex. J Biol Chem 274:26609–26616

Durbeej M, Henry MD, Ferletta M, Campbell KP, Ekblom P (1998) Distribution of dystroglycan in normal adult mouse tissues. J Histochem Cytochem 46:449–457

Durbeej M, Cohn RD, Hrstka RF, Moore SA, Allamand V, Davidson BL, Williamson RA, Campbell KP (2000) Disruption of the beta-sarcoglycan gene reveals pathogenetic complexity of limb-girdle muscular dystrophy type 2 E. Mol Cell 5:141–151

Dveksler GS, Pensiero MN, Cardellichio CB, Williams RK, Jiang GS, Holmes KV, Dieffenbach CW (1991) J Virol 65:6881–6891

Ervasti JM, Campbell KP (1991) Membrane organization of the dystrophin-glycoprotein complex. Cell 66:1121–1131

Ervasti JM, Campbell KP (1993) A role for the dystrophin-glycoprotein complex as a transmembrane linker between laminin and actin. J Cell Biol 122:809–823

Ervasti JM, Kahl SD, Campbell KP (1991) Purification of dystrophin from skeletal muscle. J Biol Chem 266:9161–9165

Ervasti JM, Burwell AL, Geissler AL (1997) Tissue-specific heterogeneity in alpha-dystroglycan sialoglycosylation. Skeletal muscle alpha-dystroglycan is a latent receptor for *Vicia villosa* agglutinin b4 masked by sialic acid modification. J Biol Chem 272:22315–22321

Evans CF, Borrow P, Torre JC de la, Oldstone MB (1994) Virus-induced immunosuppression: kinetic analysis of the selection of a mutation associated with viral persistence. J Virol 68:7367–7373

Evans DJ, Almond JW (1998) Cell receptors for picornaviruses as determinants of cell tropism and pathogenesis. Trends Microbiol 6:198–202

Feng F, Broder CC, Kennedy PE, Berger EA (1996) HIV-1 entry cofactor: functional cDNA cloning of a seven-transmembrane, G protein-coupled receptor. Science 272:872–877

Fields BN, Weiner HL, Drayna DT, Sharpe AH (1980) The role of the reovirus hemagglutinin in viral virulence. Ann N Y Acad Sci 354:125–134

Gee SH, Blacher RW, Douville PJ, Provost PR, Yurchenco PD, Carbonetto S (1993) Laminin-binding protein 120 from brain is closely related to the dystrophin-associated glycoprotein, dystroglycan, and binds with high affinity to the major heparin binding domain of laminin. J Biol Chem 268: 14972–14980

Gee SH, Montanaro F, Lindenbaum MH, Carbonetto S (1994) Dystroglycan-alpha, a dystrophin-associated glycoprotein, is a functional agrin receptor. Cell 77:675–686

Geraghty RJ, Krummenacher C, Cohen GH, Eisenberg RJ, Spear PG (1998) Entry of alphaherperviruses mediated by poliovirus receptor-related protein 1 and poliovirus receptor. Science 280:1618–1620

Gesemann M, Cavalli V, Denzer AJ, Brancaccio A, Schumacher B, Ruegg MA (1996) Alternative splicing of agrin alters its binding to heparin, dystroglycan, and the putative agrin receptor. Neuron 16:755–767

Gesemann M, Brancaccio A, Schumacher B, Ruegg MA (1998) Agrin is a high-affinity binding protein of dystroglycan in non-muscle tissue. J Biol Chem 273:600–605

Glushakova SE, Lukashevich IS, Baratova LA (1990) Prediction of arenavirus fusion peptides on the basis of computer analysis of envelope protein sequences. FEBS Lett 269:145–147

Glushakova SE, Omelyanenko VG, Lukashevitch IS, Bogdanov AA, Moshnikova AB, Kozytch AT, Torchilin VP (1992) The fusion of artificial lipid membranes induced by the synthetic arenavirus "fusion peptide". Biochim Biophys Acta 1110:202–208

Greve JM, Davis G, Meyer AM, Forte CP, Yost SC, Marlor CW, Kamarck ME, McClelland A (1989) The major human rhinovirus receptor is ICAM-1. Cell 56:839–847

Hemler ME (1999) Dystroglycan versatility. Cell 97:543–546

Henry MD, Campbell KP (1998) A role for dystroglycan in basement membrane assembly. Cell 95: 859–870

Henry MD, Campbell KP (1999) Dystroglycan inside and out. Curr Opin Cell Biol 11:602–607

Henry MD, Williamson RA, Campbell KP (1998) Analysis of the role of dystroglycan in early postim-plantation mouse development. Ann N Y Acad Sci 857:256–9.

Higa HH, Rogers GN, Paulson JC (1985) Influenza virus haemagglutinins differentiate between receptor determinants bearing N-acetyl-N-glycollyl- and N-O-diacetylneuraminic acid groups. Virology 144:279–282

Hilkens J, Ligtenberg MJ, Vos HL, Litvinov SV (1992) Cell membrane-associated mucins and their adhesion-modulating property. Trends Biochem Sci 17:359–363

Hohenester E, Sasaki T, Timpl R (1999) Crystal structure of a scavenger receptor cysteine-rich domain sheds light on an ancient superfamily. Nat Struct Biol 6:228–232

Hohenester E, Tisi D, Talts JF, Timpl R (1999) The crystal structure of a laminin G-like module reveals the molecular basis of alpha-dystroglycan binding to laminins, perlecan, and agrin. Mol Cell 4: 783–792

Holland JJ (1961) Receptor affinities as major determinants of enterovirus tissue tropism in humans. Virology 15:312–326

Holland JJ, McLaren LC, Syverton JJ (1959) The mammalian cell-virus relationship. IV. Infection of naturally insusceptible cells with enterovirus nucleic acid. J Exp Med 110:65–80

Holt KH, Campbell KP (1998) Assembly of the sarcoglycan complex. Insights for muscular dystrophy. J Biol Chem 273:34667–34670

Holt KH, Lim LE, Straub V, Venzke DP, Duclos F, Anderson RD, Davidson BL, Campbell KP (1998) Functional rescue of the sarcoglycan complex in the BIO 14.6 hamster using delta-sarcoglycan gene transfer. Mol Cell 1:841–848

Holt KH, Crosbie RH, Venzke DP, Campbell KP (2000) Biosynthesis of dystroglycan: processing of a precursor propeptide. FEBS Lett 468:79–83

Huang Y, Paxton WA, Wolinsky SM, Neumann AU, Zhang L, He T, Kang S, Ceradini D, Jin Z, Yazdanbakhsh K (1996) The role of a mutant CCR5 allele in HIV-1 transmission and disease pro-gression. Nat Med 2:1240–1243

Ibraghimov-Beskrovnaya O, Ervasti JM, Leveille CJ, Slaughter CA, Sernett SW, Campbell KP (1992) Primary structure of dystrophin-associated glycoproteins linking dystrophin to the extracellular matrix. Nature 355:696–702

Jondal M, Klein G, Oldstone MB, Bokish V, Yefenof E (1976) Surface markers on human B and T lymphocytes. VIII. Association between complement and Epstein-Barr virus receptors on human lymphoid cells. Scand J Immunol 5:401–410

Jung D, Yang B, Meyer J, Chamberlain JS, Campbell KP (1995) Identification and characterization of the dystrophin anchoring site on beta-dystroglycan. J Biol Chem 270:27305–27310

Kilby JM, Hopkins S, Venetta TM, DiMassimo B, Cloud GA, Lee JY, Alldredg L, Hunter E, Lambert D, Bolognesi D, Matthews T, Johnson MR, Nowak MA, Shaw GM, Saag MS (1998) Potent suppression of HIV-1 replication in humans by T-20, a peptide inhibitor of gp41-mediated virus entry. Nat Med 4:1302–1307

Klatzmann D, Champagne E, Chamaret S, Gruest J, Guetard D, Hercend T, Gluckman JC, Montagnier L (1984) T-lymphocyte T4 molecule behaves as the receptor for human retrovirus LAV. Nature 312:767–768

Krummenacher C, Nicola AV, Whitbeck JC, Lou H, Hou W, Lambris JD, Geraghty RJ, Spear PG, Cohen GH, Eisenberg RJ (1998) J Virol 72:7064–7074

Kunz S, Sevilla N, Mc Gavern Campbell KP, Oldstone MB (2001) Molecular analysis of the interaction of LCMV with its cellular receptor α-dystroglycan. J Cell Biol (in press)

Kwong PD, Wyatt R, Robinson J, Sweet RW, Sodroski J, Hendrickson WA (1998) Structure of an HIV gp120 envelope glycoprotein in complex with the CD4 receptor and a neutralizing human antibody. Nature 393:648–659

Kwong PD, Wyatt R, Sattentau QJ, Sodroski J, Hendrickson WA (2000) Oligomeric modeling and electrostatic analysis of the gp120 envelope glycoprotein of human immunodeficiency virus. J Virol 74:1961–1972

Lebakken CS, Venzke DP, Hrstka RF, Consolino CM, Faulkner JA, Williamson RA, Campbell KP (2000) Sarcospan-deficient mice maintain normal muscle function. Mol Cell Biol 20:1669–1677

Lentz TL, Burrage TG, Smith AL, Crick J, Tignor GH (1982) Is the acetylcholine receptor a rabies virus receptor? Science 215:182–184

Leschziner A, Moukhles H, Lindenbaum M, Gee SH, Butterworth J, Campbell KP, Carbonetto S (2000) Neural regulation of alpha-dystroglycan biosynthesis and glycosylation in skeletal muscle. J Neurochem 74:70–80

Li F, Erickson HP, James JA, Moore KL, Cummings RD, McEver RP (1996) Visualization of P-selectin glycoprotein ligand-1 as a highly extended molecule and mapping of protein epitopes for monoclonal antibodies. J Biol Chem 271:6342–6348

Lim LE, Campbell KP (1998) The sarcoglycan complex in limb-girdle muscular dystrophy. Curr Opin Neurol 11:443–452

Liu R, Paxton WA, Choe S, Ceradini D, Martin SR, Horuk R, MacDonald ME, Stuhlmann H, Koup RA, Landau NR (1996) Homozygous defect in HIV-1 co-receptor accounts for resistance of some multiply-exposed individuals to HIV-1 infection. Cell 86:367–377

MacLean-Fletcher S, Pollard DT (1980) Mechanism of action of cytochalasin B on actin. Cell 20:329–341

Maddon PJ, Dalgleish AG, McDougal JS, Clapham PR, Weiss RA, Axel R (1986) The T4 gene encodes the AIDS virus receptor and is expressed in the immune system and the brain. Cell 47:333–348

Marsh M, Helenius A (1989) Virus entry into animal cells. Adv Virus Res 36:107–151

Marx PA, Chen Z (1998) The function of simian chemokine receptors in the replication of SIV. Semin Immunol 10:215–223

Mendelsohn CL, Wimmer E, Racaniello VR (1989) Cellular receptor for poliovirus: molecular cloning, nucleotide sequence, and expression of a new member of the immunoglobulin superfamily. Cell 56:855–865

Menke A, Jockusch H (1991) Decreased osmotic stability of dystrophin-less muscle cells from the mdx mouse. Nature 349:69–71

Michael NL, Chang G, Louie LG, Mascola JR, Dondero D, Birx DL, Sheppard HW (1997) The role of viral phenotype and CCR-5 gene defects in HIV-1 transmission and disease progression. Nat Med 3:338–340

Michael NL, Nelson JA, Kewal-Ramini VN, Chang G, O'Brien SJ, Mascola JR, Volsky B, Louder M, White GC II, Littman DR (1998) Exclusive and persistent use of the entry coreceptor CXCR4 by human immunodeficiency virus type 1 from a subject homozygous for CCR5 delta 32. J Virol 72:6040–6047

Miller N, Hutt-Fletcher LM (1992) Epstein-Barr virus enters B cells and epithelial cells by different routes. J Virol 66:3409–3414

Mondor I, Ugolini S, Sattentau QJ (1998) Human immunodeficiency virus type 1 attachment to HeLa cells is CD4 independent and gp120 dependent and requires cell surface heparans. J Virol 72:3623–3634

Montanaro F, Carbonetto S, Campbell KP, Lindenbaum M (1995) Dystroglycan expression in the wild type and mdx mouse neural retina: synaptic colocalization with dystrophin, dystrophin-related protein but not laminin. J Neurosci Res 42:528–538

Moore JP (1997) Co-receptors: implications for HIV pathogenesis and therapy. Science 276:51–52

Naniche D, Varior-Krishnan G, Cervoni F, Wild TF, Rossi B, Rabourdin-Combe C, Gerlier D (1993) Human membrane cofactor protein (CD46) acts as a cellular receptor for measles virus. J Virol 67:6025–6032

Nemerow GR, Cooper NR (1984) Early events in the infection of B lymphocytes by Epstein-Barr virus: the internalization process. Virology 132:186–198

Norkin LC (1995) Virus receptors: implications for pathogenesis and the design of antiviral agents. Clin Microbiol Rev 8:293–315

Odermatt B, Eppler M, Leist TP, Hengartner H, Zinkernagel RM (1991) Virus-triggered acquired immunodeficiency by cytotoxic T-cell-dependent destruction of antigen-presenting cells and lymph follicle structure. Proc Natl Acad Sci USA 88:8252–8256

Oldstone MB (1996) Principles of viral pathogenesis. Cell 87:799–801

Oldstone MB, Salvato M, Tishon A, Lewicki H (1988) Virus-lymphocyte interactions. III. Biologic parameters of a virus variant that fails to generate CTL and establishes persistent infection in immunocompetent hosts. Virology 164:507–516

Pall EA, Bolton KM, Ervasti JM (1996) Differential heparin inhibition of skeletal muscle alpha-dystroglycan binding to laminins. J Biol Chem 271:3817–3821

Parekh BS, Buchmeier MJ (1986) Proteins of LCMV: antigenic topography of the viral glycoproteins. Virology 153:168–178

Pasternak C, Wong S, Elson EL (1995) Mechanical function of dystrophin in muscle cells. J Cell Biol 128:355–361

Paulson JC, Sadler JE, Hill RL (1979). Restoration of specific myxovirus receptors to asialoerythrocytes by incorporation of sialic acid with pure sialyltransferases. J Biol Chem 254:2120–2124

Pederson IR (1979) Structural components and replication in arenaviruses. Adv Virus Res 24:277–330

Rambukkana A (2000) How does *Mycobacterium leprae* target the peripheral nervous system? Trends Microbiol 8:23–28

Rambukkana A, Salzer JL, Yurchenco PD, Tuomanen EI (1997) Neural targeting of *Mycobacterium leprae* mediated by the G domain of the laminin-alpha2 chain. Cell 88:811–821

Rambukkana A, Yamada H, Zanazzi G, Mathus T, Salzer JL, Yurchenco PD, Campbell KP, Fischetti VA (1998) Role of alpha-dystroglycan as a Schwann cell receptor for *Mycobacterium leprae*. Science 282:2076–2079

Rentschler S, Linn H, Deininger K, Bedford MT, Espanel X, Sudol M (1999) The WW domain of dystrophin requires EF-hands region to interact with beta-dystroglycan. Biol Chem 380:431–442

Roberds SL, Ervasti JM, Anderson RD, Ohlendieck K, Kahl SD, Zoloto D, Campbell KP (1993) Disruption of the dystrophin-glycoprotein complex in the cardiomyopathic hamster. J Biol Chem 268:11496–11499

Roivainen M, Piirainen L, Hovi T, Virtanen I, Riikonen T, Heino J, Hyypia T (1994) Entry of coxsackievirus A9 into host cells: specific interactions with alpha v beta 3 integrin, the vitronectin receptor. Virology 203:357–365

Ruegg MA, Bixby JL (1998) Agrin orchestrates synaptic differentiation at the vertebrate neuromuscular junction. Trends Neurosci 21:22–27

Saito F, Masaki T, Kamakura K, Anderson LV, Fujita S, Fukuta-Ohi H, Sunada Y, Shimizu T, Matsumura K (1999) Characterization of the transmembrane molecular architecture of the dystroglycan complex in Schwann cells. J Biol Chem 274:8240–8246

Salvato M, Shimomaye E, Southern P, Oldstone MB (1988) Virus-lymphocyte interactions. IV. Molecular characterization of LCMV Armstrong (CTL+) small genomic segment and that of its variant, Clone 13 (CTL−). Virology 164:517–522

Salvato M, Borrow P, Shimomaye E, Oldstone MB (1991) Molecular basis of viral persistence: a single amino acid change in the glycoprotein of lymphocytic choriomeningitis virus is associated with suppression of the antiviral cytotoxic T-lymphocyte response and establishment of persistence. J Virol 65:1863–1839

Sampson M, Libert F, Doranz BL, Rucker J, Liesnard C, Farber C-M, Saragosti S, Lapoumeroulie C, Cognaux J, Forceille C (1996) Resistance to HIV-1 infection in caucasian individuals bearing mutant alleles of the CCR-5 chemokine receptor gene. Nature 382:722–725

Sevilla NS, Kunz S, Holz A, Lewicki H, Homann D, Yamada H, Campbell KP, de La Torre JC, Oldstone MB (2000) Immunosuppression and resultant viral persistence by specific viral targeting of dendritic cells. J Exp Med 192:1249–1260

Shafren DR, Bates RC, Agrez MV, Herd RL, Burns GF, Barry RD (1995) Coxsackieviruses B1, B3, and B5 use decay accelerating factor as a receptor for cell attachment. J Virol 69:3873–3877

Shimizu H, Hosokawa H, Ninomiya H, Miner JH, Masaki T (1999) Adhesion of cultured bovine aortic endothelial cells to laminin-1 mediated by dystroglycan. J Biol Chem 274:11995–12000

Smalheiser NR (1993) Cranin interacts specifically with the sulfatide-binding domain of laminin. J Neurosci Res 36:528–538

Smalheiser NR, Kim E (1995) Purification of cranin, a laminin binding membrane protein. Identity with dystroglycan and reassessment of its carbohydrate moieties. J Biol Chem 270:15425–15433

Smelt SC, Borrow P, Kunz S, Cao W, Tishon A, Lewicki H, Campbell KP, Oldstone MB (2001) Differences in affinity of binding of lymphocytic choriomeningitis virus strains to the cellular receptor alpha-dystroglycan correlate with viral tropism and disease kinetics. J Virol 75:448–457

Staub V, Campbell KP (1997) Muscular dystrophies and the dystrophin-glycoprotein complex. Curr Opin Neurol 10:168–175

Straub V, Ettinger AJ, Durbeej M, Venzke DP, Cutshall S, Sanes JR, Campbell KP (1999) Epsilon-sarcoglycan replaces alpha-sarcoglycan in smooth muscle to form a unique dystrophin-glycoprotein complex. J Biol Chem 274:27989–27996

Talts JF, Andac Z, Gohring W, Brancaccio A, Timpl R (1999) Binding of the G domains of laminin alpha1 and alpha2 chains and perlecan to heparin, sulfatides, alpha-dystroglycan and several extra-cellular matrix proteins. EMBO J 18:863–870

Thoulouze MI, Lafage M, Schachner M, Hartmann U, Cremer H, Lafon M (1998) The neural cell adhesion molecule is a receptor for rabies virus. J Virol 72:7181–7190

Tian M, Jacobson C, Gee SH, Campbell KP, Carbonetto S, Jucker M (1996) Dystroglycan in the cerebellum is a laminin alpha 2-chain binding protein at the glial-vascular interface and is expressed in Purkinje cells. Eur J Neurosci 8:2739–2747

Vezza AC, Gard GP, Compans RW, Bishop DHL (1977) Structural components of the arenavirus Pichinde. J Virol 23:776–786

Weiner HL, Drayna D, Averill DR Jr, Field BN (1977) Molecular basis of reovirus virulence: role of the S1 gene. Proc Natl Acad Sci USA 74:5744–5748

Weiner HL, Powers ML, Fields BN (1980) Absolute linkage of virulence and central nervous system cell tropism of reoviruses to viral hemagglutinin. J Infect Dis 141:609–616

Weis W, Brown JH, Cusack S, Paulson JC, Skehel JJ, Wiley DC (1988) Structure of the influenza virus haemagglutinin complexed with its receptor, sialic acid. Nature 333:426–431

Weiss RA, Tailor CS (1995) Retrovirus receptors. Cell 82:531–533

Weissenhorn W, Dessen A, Calder LJ, Harrison SC, Skehel JJ, Wiley DC (1999) Structural basis for membrane fusion by enveloped viruses. Mol Membr Biol 16:3–9

Wickham TJ, Mathias P, Cheresh DA, Nemerow GR (1993) Integrins alpha v beta 3 and alpha v beta 5 promote adenovirus internalization but not virus attachment. Cell 73:309–319

Wimmer E (1994) Cellular receptors for animal viruses. Cold Spring Harbor Press, New York

Wright KE, Buchmeier MJ (1991) Antiviral antibodies attenuate T-cell-mediated immunopathology following acute lymphocytic choriomeningitis virus infection. J Virol 65:3001–3006

WuDunn D, Spear PG (1989) Initial interaction of herpes simplex virus with cells is binding to heparan sulfate. J Virol 63:52–58

Yamada H, Chiba A, Endo T, Kobata A, Anderson LV, Hori H, Fukuta-Ohi H, Kanazawa I, Campbell KP, Shimizu T, Matsumura K (1996a) Characterization of dystroglycan-laminin interaction in peripheral nerve. J Neurochem 66:1518–1524

Yamada H, Denzer AJ, Hori H, Tanaka T, Anderson LV, Fujita S, Fukuta-Ohi H, Shimizu T, Ruegg MA, Matsumura K (1996b) Dystroglycan is a dual receptor for agrin and laminin-2 in Schwann cell membrane. J Biol Chem 271:23418–23423

Yang B, Jung D, Motto D, Meyer J, Koretzky G, Campbell KP (1995) SH3 domain-mediated interaction of dystroglycan and Grb2. J Biol Chem 270:11711–11714

Yefenof E, Klein G, Jondal M, Oldstone MB (1976) Surface markers on human B and T-lymphocytes. IX. Two-color immunofluorescence studies on the association between ebv receptors and complement receptors on the surface of lymphoid cell lines. Int J Cancer 17:693–700

Arenaviruses: Genomic RNAs, Transcription, and Replication

B.J. Meyer[1], J.C. de la Torre[2], and P.J. Southern[3]

1 Genome Organization

The arenavirus genome comprises two single-stranded RNA molecules of negative polarity, designated L and S, that contain essentially nonoverlapping sequence information (for extensively referenced reviews see BUCHMEIER et al. 1980; LEHMANN-GRUBE 1984; HOWARD 1986; SALVATO 1993a; SOUTHERN 1996). There is some variability in the lengths of the genomic RNA segments for individual arenaviruses (L approximately 7,200 bases, S approximately 3,400 bases), but the general organization of the L and S genomic RNA species appears to be well conserved across the virus family. An extensive compilation of arenavirus genomic RNA sequence is now available, and this information has been used to derive

[1] Air Force Technical Applications Center, Patrick Air Force Base, FL 32925, USA
[2] Division of Virology, Department of Neuropharmacology, The Scripps Research Institute, La Jolla, CA 92037, USA
[3] Department of Microbiology, University of Minnesota, Mayo Mail Code 196, 420 Delaware Street, SE, Minneapolis, MN 55455, USA

phylogenetic relationships amongst the known arenaviruses (BOWEN et al. 1997; ALBARINO et al. 1998). Sequence alignments have also facilitated the development of a generalized scheme to amplify arenavirus genomic RNAs by RT-PCR (LOZANO et al. 1997) This innovative diagnostic resource, together with a specific RT-PCR assay for LCMV (PARK et al. 1997), should have a significant positive impact on the rapid recognition and characterization of new arenavirus infections.

Arenaviruses have been grouped with other single-stranded, negative-polarity RNA viruses by standard criteria that include the lack of direct infectivity for purified virion RNAs and the presence of a virion-associated RNA-dependent-RNA polymerase. However, the actual coding organization of the L and S are-navirus genomic RNA segments does not conform with the coding arrangements for prototypical negative-polarity viruses, like paramyxoviruses and rhabdoviruses. The term "ambisense" has been widely accepted to designate a sub-group of neg-ative-polarity viruses that includes arenaviruses and bunyaviruses (BISHOP 1986). Ambisense viruses are recognized by a distinctive transcription pattern in infected cells such that one region of genomic RNA is transcribed into a genomic com-plementary mRNA, while genetic information in a nonoverlapping region of the same genomic RNA can only be expressed as a genomic sense mRNA (AUPERIN et al. 1984) (Fig. 1). Genomic sense mRNAs are not transcribed until viral RNA replication has been initiated because the full-length genomic complementary replication intermediate serves two roles – as the template for the synthesis of full-length genomic sense RNAs (replication) and as the template for the synthesis of a genomic sense mRNA (transcription). The ambisense coding arrangement, there-fore, provides and imposes a mechanism for the regulation of arenavirus gene expression within infected cells.

2 Virion RNAs

The arenavirus L and S genomic RNAs are present within virions as helical nucleocapsid structures that are organized into circular configurations, with lengths ranging from 400 to 1300nm (YOUNG and HOWARD 1983). Highly purified virion preparations routinely contain electron-dense granules that have been identified as host ribosomes (FARBER and RAWLS 1975; MURPHY and WHITFIELD 1975). This physical characteristic accounts for the term "arena" which was taken from *arenosus*, the Latin for "sandy". Further evidence in support of encapsidation of ribosomes is provided by denaturing gel electrophoresis of virion RNA preparations that consistently shows abundant RNAs co-migrating with markers representing host 28S and 18S RNA species (CARTER et al. 1973; PEDERSEN 1979; SOUTHERN et al. 1987). These virion 28S- and 18S-sized RNAs have identical RNA finger-prints to host ribosomal RNAs (DUTKO and OLDSTONE 1983). There is no evidence to support the contention that host ribosomes should be considered an integral component of the arenavirus infectious virion because virions harvested at an early

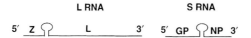

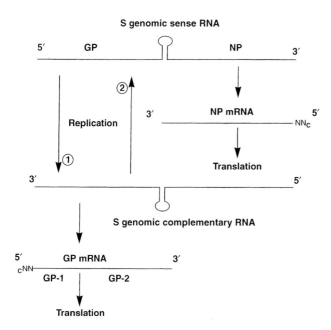

Fig. 1. Arenavirus gene organization and expression. The stem-loop structures represent the intergenic noncoding regions. The *lower part* of the figure outlines transcription, translation, and replication events for the S genomic RNA. A similar pattern of events supports L and Z gene expression and RNA replication for the genomic L RNA segment. Note that GP mRNA (and Z mRNA) transcription does not occur prior to the onset of RNA replication. The 5′ ends of the subgenomic mRNAs contain nontemplated extensions (NN) and a 7-methyl G cap structure (C). (Modified from MEYER and SOUTHERN 1993)

stage of acute infection display normal infectivity and a significantly diminished ribosome content. In addition, the infectivity of Pichinde virus was not affected by propagation at the nonpermissive temperature in host cells with a *ts* lesion in a ribosomal protein (LEUNG and RAWLS 1977). The process of arenavirus virion assembly, at least with respect to the internal components of the virion, appears to be imprecise, and ribosomes may be fortuitously encapsidated into budding virions. Similarly, a serine threonine kinase of presumptive cellular origin has been detected in preparations of highly purified LCMV virions (HOWARD and BUCHMEIER 1983). Although clear connections have now been established between negative-strand virus replication and cellular kinase activity (DE and BANERJEE 1997), there is little current insight into the role that a virion-associated cellular kinase might play in the arenavirus lifecycle.

Purified arenavirus virions routinely contain an abundant, heterogeneous, low-molecular-weight RNA component of about 4–7S that consists of a mixture of host- and viral-encoded species. The host RNAs, comprising 5/5.8S ribosomal RNAs and tRNAs, are probably not essential for virion infectivity, while one viral-encoded, low-molecular-weight RNA species, Z mRNA, may participate in the initiation of arenavirus infection (SALVATO et al. 1992). Currently, it is not possible to determine if Z mRNA should be regarded as an essential virion RNA component – this would mean that Z protein could be immediately translated in the newly infected cell and/or that Z mRNA has a key structural role in the newly infected cell – or whether the detection of Z mRNA within virions can simply be explained by an imprecise encapsidation process. Support for the argument that any and all virus-encoded RNAs may be encapsidated randomly is provided by the finding that low levels of genomic complementary L and genomic complementary S RNAs could be detected by PCR amplification of LCMV virion RNAs (MEYER and SOUTHERN 1994). However, because of the relatively high molar equivalence of Z mRNA in virions (SALVATO and SHIMOMAYE 1989), it is extremely unlikely that encapsidated Z mRNA is devoid of function. Additional support for the general concept of the selective incorporation of cytoplasmic viral mRNAs into infectious virions has been obtained from recent experiments with human cytomegalovirus (BRESNAHAN and SHENK 2000).

The L and S genomic arenavirus RNAs are not present in equimolar amounts, either within virions or within infected cells, and the S RNA has always been found to be more abundant (ROMANOWSKI and BISHOP 1983; SOUTHERN et al. 1987; IAPALUCCI et al. 1994). Estimates of L:S stoichiometry can vary widely according to the precise conditions of infection but, under optimal conditions with low multiplicity of infection and a low-passage virus stock, the L:S ratio does not exceed 2:5. Furthermore, the progression from acute to persistent arenavirus infection may be associated with a significant shift, in favor of S accumulation, in the relative content of intracellular viral RNAs (FRANCIS and SOUTHERN 1988; IAPALUCCI et al. 1994; MEYER and SOUTHERN 1997). The S genomic RNA segment encodes the major virion structural components: the internal nucleoprotein, NP, and the two external glycoproteins, GP-1 and GP-2 (AUPERIN et al. 1984; RIVIERE et al. 1985; BUCHMEIER et al. 1987; FRANZE-FERNANDEZ et al. 1987; SOUTHERN et al. 1987). The L genomic RNA segment encodes the viral RNA-dependent RNA polymerase, L, and an 11-kDa protein, Z, that has been assigned both structural and regulatory roles in the infectious cycle (IAPALUCCI et al. 1989a,b; SALVATO and SHIMOMAYE 1989; SALVATO et al. 1989; DJAVANI et al. 1997; LUKASHEVICH et al. 1997). Z contains a RING finger (zinc-binding) domain and may therefore be directly involved with the regulation of gene expression within infected cells (SALVATO 1993b, see below). Both Z mRNA and Z protein are encapsidated into virions, suggesting an important role for Z in the newly infected cell (SALVATO et al. 1992). Z has been shown to be associated with NP, and it is probable that Z and NP, together with L, comprise the viral protein components of virion nucleocapsids (SALVATO 1993b). The arenavirus coding capacity is therefore limited to four defined, nonoverlapping open reading frames that are individually transcribed into subgenomic mRNAs. The NP, L, and Z mRNAs are translated into single mature protein products, whereas the primary translation product from the GP mRNA,

GP-C, is cleaved post-translationally to yield the mature glycoproteins GP-1 and GP-2 (BUCHMEIER et al. 1987).

3 Terminal Nucleotide Sequences

The nucleotide sequences at the 3′ termini of the arenavirus genomic L and S RNAs are conserved (17 of the first 19 nucleotides are identical between the L and S RNAs) (AUPERIN et al. 1982a,b), and the inverted complement of this sequence is positioned at the 5′ termini of the genomic RNAs. The conserved terminal sequence element is retained in all arenavirus genomes examined to date. A minor modification has been reported in the 5′ S sequence for Junin (GHIRINGHELLI et al. 1991), but the arrangement of 3′/5′ complementarity is still preserved. It has been suggested that this conserved terminal sequence may represent part or all of a binding site for the viral RNA-dependent RNA polymerase. Models that have been proposed to account for the initiation of replication suggest that intramolecular duplexes may form as a consequence of the sequence complementarity at the termini of individual L or S RNA molecules and/or that intermolecular duplexes are generated by annealing between the termini of L and S RNA molecules (SALVATO and SHIMOMAYE 1989; SALVATO et al. 1989; HARNISH et al. 1993; SALVATO 1993b). Physical evidence for the formation of intramolecular and intermolecular RNA complexes has been derived from electron microscopic spreads of arenavirus nucleocapsids (YOUNG and HOWARD 1983), but there is currently only limited mechanistic insight into events regulating the initiation of arenavirus replication and transcription.

4 Open Reading Frames

Extensive nucleic acid mapping, cloning, sequencing, analyses, and protein analyses are all fully consistent with a genome organization for arenaviruses that encompasses four distinct open reading frames and four distinct primary translation products. Additional open reading frames have been identified by computer analysis of arenavirus genomic RNA sequences, most notably the X region at the 5′ end of the L RNA (SALVATO and SHIMOMAYE 1989), but there is no current evidence to suggest either the presence of appropriate subgenomic mRNAs or the actual synthesis of these hypothetical proteins in arenavirus-infected cells. The 5′ nontranslated region of most mRNAs is relatively short (about 30–80 nucleotides) and, apart from the conserved terminal sequences, no function has yet been ascribed to these regions that, in total, constitute 2%–4% of the arenavirus genetic information.

Lassa L mRNA has an extended 5′ noncoding region (157 nucleotides), but the functional significance, if any, has yet to be recognized (LUKASHEVICH et al. 1997).

5 Intergenic Regions

The open reading frames in the 3′ and 5′ regions of the genomic RNAs do not overlap, and therefore both the L and S RNA segments contain an intergenic, noncoding region. These intergenic regions have the potential to form relatively stable stem-loop structures which appear to be involved in regulating transcriptional termination. For the S RNA, transcription termination occurs at multiple sites in the stem (FRANZE-FERNANDEZ et al. 1993; MEYER and SOUTHERN 1993), suggesting that arenavirus polymerase molecules may dissociate from template RNAs in response to an RNA structure rather than by recognition of a precise termination site or sequence. There is a single stem-loop in the S RNA for Pichinde (AUPERIN et al. 1984), LCMV (ROMANOWSKI et al. 1985; SALVATO et al. 1988) and Lassa (AUPERIN and McCORMICK 1988; CLEGG et al. 1990), but the S sequence for Tacaribe (FRANZE-FERNANDEZ et al. 1987, 1993), Junin (GHIRINGHELLI et al. 1991), and Mopeia (WILSON and CLEGG 1991) can be folded to produce two distinct stem-loops that are positioned just beyond the translation termination codons for NP and GP-C.

With Tacaribe virus, the L intergenic region can be folded into a single hairpin structure, and the 3′ termini of the L and Z mRNAs map to the base of the distal sides of this hairpin. As a consequence of this arrangement, the 3′ termini of Tacaribe L-derived mRNAs overlap by approximately 24–34 nucleotides (FRANZE-FERNANDEZ et al. 1993). These RNA 3′ terminus mapping studies with Tacaribe have provided the first direct evidence for an arenavirus subgenomic L mRNA (FRANZE-FERNANDEZ et al. 1993).

6 Arenavirus Lifecycle: Acute Infections

The arenavirus lifecycle occurs exclusively within the cytoplasm of acutely infected cells, and progeny virions are released by budding from the plasma membrane within 16–24h of the initiation of infection (Fig. 2). Many acute arenavirus infections are noncytolytic, and there is a ready progression into long-term persistent infection. The overall outcome of any infection, however, is profoundly influenced by the combination of host species, the infected cell type, the strain of virus, and the precise conditions of infection. Thus, despite their generally noncytolytic properties, arenaviruses will form plaques under defined laboratory conditions. Plaque

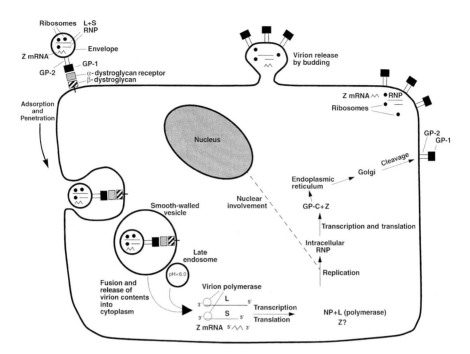

Fig. 2. Arenavirus lifecycle. The arenavirus genome organization and the intracellular patterns of transcription, translation and replication are summarized in Fig. 1. (Modified from Southern 1996)

assays have provided an extremely valuable experimental tool both for virus titrations and for plaque purifications in the derivation of homogeneous virus stocks. The absence of direct virus-induced cytolysis does not necessarily imply an absence of clinical symptoms in an infected host because there are numerous examples of acute immunopathological sequelae that are induced by arenavirus infections.

The arenaviruses are known to display a broad host range and cell type tropism. Consistent with these properties, a widely conserved cell surface protein, α-dystroglycan, has recently been identified as an arenavirus receptor (Cao et al. 1998). Several arenaviruses including LCMV, Lassa fever virus, Oliveros, and Mobala all bind to α-dystroglycan, but, curiously, no binding was observed for Guanarito. This suggests that other cell surface proteins may also be recognized as receptors by different arenaviruses. The identification of a major cell surface receptor should now permit molecular investigations into the mechanism of relative resistance of some cell types to arenavirus infections. For example, can the impaired replicative capacity of LCMV in mouse lymphocytes and terminally differentiated neurons be explained by restricted surface expression of the essential virus receptor molecule, α-dystroglycan? Most arenavirus tissue culture infections have been performed in the experimentally robust BHK-21 cells or other well-characterized rodent cell lines, but there has been some expansion into human target cells. Pichinde virus replicates in normal human peripheral blood monocytes (POLYAK et al. 1991). Lassa fever virus and Mopeia replicate in human macrophages and endothelial cells (LUKASHEVICH et al. 1999), and LCMV can replicate in a variety of primary human cell lines (P.J. Southern, unpublished data). These primary human cell systems appear to represent a very fertile experimental area for further study of the interactions between human cells and the pathogenic arenaviruses.

7 Transcription

Three prominent subgenomic mRNAs, transcribed from the NP, GP-C, and Z coding regions, are readily detectable in acute arenavirus infections. The presence of a fourth subgenomic mRNA, transcribed from the L coding region, is inferred, but the L mRNA is not easily visualized on denaturing gels because of close similarity in size to the genomic sense and genomic complementary L RNA segments. A complete molecular description of the events underlying arenavirus transcription initiation and termination is not currently available, but considerable insight has been derived from transcription mapping studies. The 5′ ends of the S-derived subgenomic mRNAs have been shown to extend beyond the ends of the genomic RNA templates (GARCIN and KOLAKOFSKY 1990; RAJU et al. 1990; MEYER and SOUTHERN 1993). These nontemplated extensions are variable in length (1–7 nucleotides) and terminate with 5′ cap structures. The derivation of these nontemplated nucleotides and the 5′ cap has yet to be explained. The process of "cap-stealing" has been well documented for influenza virus and bunyaviruses, but a similar mechanism for cap acquisition by arenaviruses has not been confirmed. There are various experimental indicators that the cell nucleus is important for completion of the arenavirus lifecycle (BANERJEE et al. 1976); for example, the nucleus may be required to provide capped cellular mRNAs for priming of arenavirus transcripts. This possibility is consistent with the observed inhibition of Junin virus replication in cells that have been treated with α-amanitin (MERSICH et al. 1981). Additionally, the nuclear membrane may be required to provide structural support for arenavirus transcription and replication. Productive arenavirus infections can be completed in cells treated with actinomycin D, but yields of infectious progeny virions are reduced relative to untreated cells (RAWLS et al. 1976; LOPEZ et al. 1986). Conversely, productive Pichinde infection of the human monocytic cell line THP-1 requires PMA treatment to induce the target cell population to differentiate into monocytes, and this positive host cell influence on virus replication can be blocked by actinomycin D treatment (POLYAK et al. 1991, 1995). Arenavirus transcription and replication can be inhibited by ribavirin (GESSNER and LOTHER 1989; DE LA TORRE and OLDSTONE 1992), which has a beneficial therapeutic effect if administered sufficiently early in the course of patient infections with pathogenic arenaviruses. However, there is still considerable uncertainty over the molecular mechanism(s) of action for ribavirin, and it is unclear whether ribavirin disrupts arenavirus mRNA capping and/or the extension of newly initiated RNA chains. In extrapolating from other viral systems (DE and BANERJEE 1997; LAI 1998), it would now seem timely to reevaluate and clarify the contribution of host cell factors to the productive arenavirus life cycle.

The arenavirus subgenomic mRNAs terminate within the intergenic noncoding region, and they are not polyadenylated (SINGH et al. 1987; SOUTHERN et al. 1987). In many cases, it appears that transcription termination occurs on the distal side of the intergenic stem-loop structure so that the 3' termini of the mRNAs could be stabilized by the formation of terminal hairpin structures (FRANZE-FERNANDEZ et al. 1987, 1993; MEYER and SOUTHERN 1993). NP mRNA synthesis can occur within infected cells that have been treated with protein synthesis inhibitors, but further progression through the arenavirus lifecycle is blocked (FRANZE-FERNANDEZ et al. 1987). This has led to the suggestion that NP may be involved in regulating transcription termination in the intergenic region. At the onset of infection, when the intracellular levels of NP are low, polymerase progression would be arrested within the intergenic region, and NP mRNA would be released. As NP accumulates within the cytoplasm of infected cells, NP binding to the intergenic regions of some template molecules would allow polymerase to progress to the 5' end of the template and complete an RNA replication cycle. GP-C mRNA is not transcribed until RNA replication has commenced because the full length genomic complementary S RNA is utilized both as a replication intermediate and as the template for GP mRNA transcription. This temporal separation of NP and GP-C gene expression has been validated in kinetic studies of acute arenavirus infections. Similar temporal studies with expression of the genomic L RNA segment have not yet been reported, but this experimental approach could be valuable in establishing the importance of virion-encapsidated Z mRNA. Based strictly on the ambisense coding arrangement, newly synthesized L protein would be expected to appear in the cytoplasm before newly synthesized Z protein. Conversely, if Z mRNA from virions is immediately translated at the initiation of infection, then newly synthesized Z protein should be present before newly synthesized L protein.

By analogy with other RNA viruses, it is highly probable that the intracellular content and distribution of NP are critical in regulating the relative levels of transcription and replication within arenavirus-infected cells. There have been various suggestions that NP may be subject to post-translational modification, but the primary NP translation product is the single most abundant species in acutely infected cells. A phosphorylated derivative of NP may be involved with the attenuation of viral gene expression that marks the progression from acute to persistent infection (BRUNS et al. 1988), and NP cleavage products have frequently been detected in infected cells and in purified virions. Given the limited coding capacity of the arenavirus genome, it is conceivable that fragments of NP could function as minor structural proteins. A 28-kDa NP cleavage product has been shown to accumulate in the nucleus of Pichinde-infected cells (YOUNG et al. 1987).

8 Replication

On one level of analysis, replication of single-stranded RNAs can be considered a straightforward process involving the synthesis of genomic complementary RNA intermediates which, in turn, are copied repeatedly to produce newly synthesized genomic sense strands. RNA replication requires a viral-encoded RNA-dependent RNA polymerase that binds at the 3' end of the templates and traverses the template RNA from end to end, synthesizing a full-length complementary RNA. Unfortunately, this simplistic scheme overlooks major mechanistic problems that arise from constraints regarding the initiation of RNA synthesis and the requirement to copy the RNA terminal sequences precisely. Several aspects of arenavirus RNA replication have not been fully resolved, but as is the case with arenavirus transcriptional regulation, much has been learnt from detailed molecular analysis of the RNA molecules involved. The precise 5' terminus of arenavirus genomic S RNA segments has one nontemplated nucleotide (RAJU et al. 1990; GARCIN and KOLAKOFSKY 1990). A model has been proposed that incorporates this nontemplated nucleotide into a novel mechanism for the initiation of arenavirus RNA replication (GARCIN and KOLAKOFSKY 1992; KOLAKOFSKY and GARCIN 1993). The model suggests that after the initiation of RNA synthesis at the 3' terminus of the template and formation of the first phosphodiester bond, the newly synthesized dinucleotide product then slips backwards on the template (movement in the direction 5 → 3' with respect to the template RNA) to create the appearance of a "nontemplated" nucleotide. Alternatively, a pre-existing dinucleotide or a newly synthesized dinucleotide, formed by either a cellular RNA polymerase or the viral RNA polymerase, could anneal to the template as part of an initiation complex and then slip backwards. The precise composition of the arenavirus replication initiation complex remains unknown, but extensive biochemical studies with Tacaribe polymerase have shown that exogenous primers, complementary to varying positions at the terminus of the RNA template, stimulate the synthesis of RNA products and have a predictable impact on the presence or absence of 5' extensions for the newly synthesized products. Results from this Tacaribe system have also established a requirement for Z protein in both mRNA synthesis and genomic RNA replication (GARCIN et al. 1993). More recently, however, the role of Z has been called into question by the finding that the transcription and replication of an LCMV minigenome could be supported with the provision of only NP and L as essential *trans*-acting factors (LEE et al. 2000). It is to be expected that the continued combination of biochemical assays for polymerase function and reverse genetics with experimentally modified viral genomic segments will provide further insight into the regulation of arenavirus transcription and replication under different conditions of infection.

There have been several attempts to identify the protein and enzymatic constituents of the viral RNA-dependent RNA polymerase. By analogy with other negative-strand viruses, it has been assumed that L protein constitutes part or all of the viral polymerase. Inspection of the predicted amino acid sequences for arenavirus L proteins has identified conserved residues that are found in other RNA-dependent RNA polymerases (LUKASHEVICH et al. 1997). L protein is detectable in virions at low levels, as would be expected for a virion-associated RNA polymerase (SINGH et al. 1987). Specific RNA-dependent RNA polymerase activity has been detected in purified Pichinde virions (LEUNG et al. 1979) and in extracts of cells acutely infected with LCMV (FULLER-PACE and SOUTHERN 1989), but the most extensive study of polymerase activity has been conducted with Tacaribe (GARCIN and KOLAKOFSKY 1990, 1992; GARCIN et al. 1993).

The intracellular concentration of L protein has been found to increase dramatically over the time course of acute infection, but results derived from LCMV polymerase assays suggest that an inverse correlation may exist between the amount of L protein and the level of detectable polymerase activity (FULLER-PACE and SOUTHERN 1989). This finding could explain the observed downregulation of viral transcription and replication that occurs at late times in acute infections (SOUTHERN et al. 1987) and may signal the transition from acute to persistent infection. A similar correlation between elevated polymerase protein levels and diminished polymerase activity has also been reported in the readout from a VSV transfection system (MEIER et al. 1987). Conversely, in the context of transcription and replication of an LCMV minigenome template, there is no obvious effect on RNA synthesis that can be correlated with changes in the levels of L protein (LEE et al. 2000).

9 Persistent Arenavirus Infections

The noncytolytic acute arenavirus infection in tissue culture cells can frequently progress to a long-term persistent or chronic infection (LEHMANN-GRUBE et al. 1969). Additionally, there are notable examples where persistent arenavirus infection has been detected in well-studied cell lines that had never been deliberately exposed to virus infection (VAN DER ZEIJST et al. 1983a,b; REISEROVA et al. 1999). The transition from acute to persistent infection is marked by a reduction in the release of infectious progeny virions and downregulation of the expression of GP-1 and GP-2 at the cell surface (OLDSTONE and BUCHMEIER 1982). Viral RNP remain in the cytoplasm of infected cells and partition randomly to daughter cells at cell division. The dynamic state of persistently infected cell populations is well illustrated by the periodic release of infectious virus particles and also by a novel analysis of intracellular viral RNA species (Fig. 3). Persistent arenavirus infections are associated with the formation and release of noninfectious particles that have been variously called interfering particles and/or defective interfering particles. These noninfectious particles can block the infectivity of standard virus preparations, but for arenaviruses, it is not clear how interference occurs at the molecular level or why the interfering particles are defective (WELSH and OLDSTONE 1977; DUTKO and PFAU 1978; WELSH and BUCHMEIER 1979; D'AIUTOLO and COTO 1986;

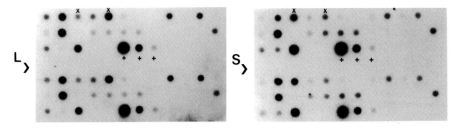

Fig. 3. Variability in LCMV RNA content in single cell clones from a persistently infected cell population. Single cell clones were established from a population of persistently-infected BHK-21 cells, and total
cell nucleic acid was extracted when the clones had expanded up to the 50–100 cell stage. Nucleic acid
samples were applied in duplicate to a nitrocellulose membrane. (*Arrowheads* indicate the boundary
between one set of samples and the duplicate set) The membrane was hybridized sequentially with
LCMV L-specific and S-specific probes that were matched for length of target sequence and specific
activity of radiolabeling. Serial dilutions of a positive control sample, BHK cells acutely infected with
LCMV, are indicated with (+). In this experimental format, each *spot* represents an independent clone,
and comparison of the hybridization signals with the L and S probes provides a direct indication of the
relative levels of L and S RNA in that clone. One pair of designated spots (x) shows the anticipated result
with RNA levels S > L; however, the other pair of designated spots shows the opposite result, with RNA
levels L > S. This novel experiment reveals a previously unrecognized and unexpected complexity in the
total intracellular LCMV RNA content of persistently infected cells

IAPULUCCI et al. 1994). In sharp contrast to persistent infections with other RNA
viruses, where extensively deleted viral genomes (DI RNAs) rapidly accumulate,
the persistent arenavirus infection is usually associated with prominent retention of
apparently full-length genomic-sized RNAs. During persistent LCMV infection,
RNAs with subtle alterations in their terminal sequences have been found to
accumulate, and there is indirect evidence suggesting active replication of genomic
RNAs with modified termini (MEYER and SOUTHERN 1997). Extensively deleted
RNA species can be formed and maintained in persistent arenavirus infections, but
it is presently unclear if such deleted RNAs are causal, consequential, or even
coincidental to the state of persistent infection. No systematic molecular analysis of
deleted RNAs has been performed to identify the minimal *cis*-acting sequences for
an arenavirus replicon. Such studies are now highly feasible with the ready availability of cloned genomic sequences and the newly developed reverse genetics
system to assess RNA synthesis from defined templates (LEE et al. 2000).

New insight into the molecular basis of arenavirus persistence has come from
RNA terminal mapping studies with LCMV. By using a procedure to create
intramolecular RNA circles, it is possible to derive both the 5′ and 3′ terminal
sequence from the same set of RNA molecules (MEYER and SOUTHERN 1993, 1994,
1997). These studies revealed unexpected sequence microheterogeneity (predominantly short deletions) at the termini of genomic sense and genomic complementary
RNAs that would not have been recognized by standard denaturing gel electrophoretic methods. The identification of similar types of deletions in both the
genomic sense and genomic complementary RNAs raises the possibility that RNA
molecules with terminal alterations may be capable of replicating and thereby
interfering with the replication of standard virus genomes. It is very significant that

no deleted RNA species were observed when the circularization procedure was used to analyze LCMV mRNAs. Because the 5′ termini of the mRNAs extend up to and beyond the termini of the template RNAs, this suggests that transcription is not supported by genomic templates with terminal deletions. By this reasoning, LCMV genomic RNAs with short 5′ and 3′ terminal deletions could represent a novel class of DI RNA (MEYER and SOUTHERN 1997). Similar patterns of terminal sequence heterogeneity have also been observed in RNA mapping studies with a distinctly different negative-polarity virus, Seoul virus (MEYER and SCHMALJOHN 2000). The finding of microheterogeneity at the termini of LCMV genomic RNAs raises a question over the precise function of the conserved terminal sequences that characterize the arenavirus genomic RNAs. There is some evidence from positive-polarity RNA viruses that viral polymerases can initiate RNA synthesis by recognizing internal sequences within templates that lack the prototypical 3′ terminal sequence, generally considered to represent the polymerase initiation site (YOSHINARI et al. 2000). Additional complexity in the parameters affecting template recognition by viral polymerases has been revealed by deletion mapping studies of an MHV DI RNA: successful replication of the DI RNA required extensive regions from both the 5′ and 3′ termini and an internal, noncontiguous sequence (LIN and LAI 1993). Further clarification of the importance of signals and sequences at the termini of arenavirus genomic RNA segments, and the possible involvement of essential internal sequences, should emerge from the continued development and analysis of arenavirus reverse genetics systems (LEE et al. 2000).

10 Disruption of Host Cell Gene Expression

Infection with noncytolytic arenaviruses that replicate exclusively in the cytoplasm of infected cells is known to cause distinct alterations in the host cell's gene expression (OLDSTONE et al. 1982, 1984; DE LA TORRE and OLDSTONE 1996). The most dramatic examples occur in experimental infections of newborn mice where virus infection can induce profound alterations in the normal course of development. In a number of cases, additional molecular investigation has been done with virus infections of appropriately specialized cell lines in vitro. LCMV-induced disruption of growth hormone transcription in anterior pituitary cells (VALSAMAKIS et al. 1987; KLAVINSKIS and OLDSTONE 1989; DE LA TORRE and OLDSTONE 1992) and of GAP43 expression in neuronal cells (CAO et al. 1997) can both be explained by disturbances in the signalling pathways that connect the cytoplasm to the nucleus. The effect on growth hormone expression is caused by a reduction in the intracellular content of functional Pit1, a *trans*-activation factor that is essential for efficient growth hormone transcription. The reduction in GAP43 transcription is apparently caused by alterations in the NGF signalling pathway. The evolutionary significance of these highly specialized virus/host molecular interactions has not yet been appreciated, but as was pointed out many years ago (ROWE 1954; HOTCHIN

1962), there are multiple layers and a multitude of subtleties to the virus/host interaction.

An intriguing new concept, relating directly to changes that are induced in the intracellular environment in arenavirus-infected cells, has emerged from continuing investigations into the role(s) for Z protein. In a series of elegant studies with both transfected cells and virus-infected cells, Z has been shown to associated with the promyelocytic leukemia protein PML and the ribosomal P proteins and to cause redistribution of PML from the nucleus to the cytoplasm (BORDEN et al. 1998a,b). Parenthetically, this interaction between Z and ribosomal P proteins may be connected with the encapsidation of ribosomes into arenavirus virions. Recently, specific interactions between Z and the eukaryotic initiation factor 4 E (eIF-4 E) have been shown to cause down-modulation of the host cell translation in an eIF-4E-dependent manner (CAMPBELL DWYER et al. 2000). However, in virus-infected cells, the availability of Z to interact with specific cellular target proteins appears to be influenced by levels of NP, as NP/Z complexes have been readily visualized by protein cross-linking methods. Collectively, it appears that Z may be highly significant in regulating translation in infected cells and that the interplay between Z and NP may impact directly on the level of viral gene expression, in determining a state of acute or persistent infection. In this respect, it is interesting to note that Z expression has been found to be elevated in human Ma Tu cells persistently infected with the MX strain of LCMV (GIBADULINOVA et al. 1998).

11 Indications for the Future

There has been tremendous progress over the last 30 years in gaining an understanding of the genetic organization of arenaviruses and in developing a molecular profile for productive arenavirus infections. However, several major questions remain unresolved that, both individually and collectively, impact profoundly on the interaction between arenaviruses and their hosts and the molecular mechanisms for arenavirus-induced diseases. Additional insight into the regulation of both transcription and replication may facilitate the development of therapeutic agents for rapid and highly selective inhibition of arenavirus replication in infected patients. It is also conceivable that a more complete understanding of the progression from acute to persistent infection will contribute to the development of safe and effective arenavirus vaccines that can be administered under conditions of restricted virus replication. There is clearly much still to be learnt regarding the dependence on host cellular factors for completion of the arenavirus lifecycle. In addition, although the contribution of host factors to the induction of pathogenic processes and overall outcome of infection has now been recognized, many details may still be missing from the cascades of virus-induced change that occur within infected hosts. The importance of Z in the arenavirus lifecycle is now established beyond question, but Z remains enigmatic. It is probable that Z has key regulatory and/or structural roles in both acute and persistent arenavirus infections; it is distinctive because of a clear propensity to interact with both viral and cellular proteins. The newly developed reverse genetics system offers considerable promise for the delineation of essential regulatory sequences located within viral RNA templates and clarification of the roles played by viral proteins and host cell proteins in acute and persistent arenavirus infections. However, because the course of infection within a host is determined by the cumulative effects of arenavirus infection in multiple cell types, it may be informative as the reverse genetics procedures become more facile to extend these experiments into a range of host cell types. Finally, it is hoped that the collective efforts of the many talented and dedicated investigators who have contributed to the current molecular store of arenavirus knowledge will be matched and then exceeded in the coming years.

References

Albarino CG, Posik DM, Ghiringhelli PD, Lozano ME, Romanowski V (1998) Arenavirus phylogeny: a new insight. Virus Genes 16:39–46

Auperin DD, McCormick JB (1988) Nucleotide sequence of the Lassa virus (Josiah strain) S genome RNA and amino acid sequence comparison of the N and GPC proteins to other arenaviruses. Virology 168:421–425

Auperin DD, Compans RW, Bishop DHL (1982a) Nucleotide sequence conservation at the 3' termini of the virion RNA species of New World and Old World arenaviruses. Virology 121:200–203

Auperin D, Dimock K, Cash P, Rawls WE, Leung W-C, Bishop DHL (1982b) Analyses of the genome of prototype Pichinde arenavirus and a virulent derivative of Pichinde Munchique: evidence for sequence conservation at the 3' termini of their viral RNA species. Virology 116:363–367

Auperin DD, Romanowski V, Galinski M, Bishop DHL (1984) Sequencing studies of Pichinde arenavirus S RNA indicate a novel coding strategy, an ambisense viral S RNA. J Virol 52:897–904

Banerjee SN, Buchmeier M, Rawls WE (1976) Requirement of a cell nucleus for the replication of an arenavirus. Intervirology 6:190–196

Bishop DHL (1986) Ambisense RNA genomes of arenaviruses and phleboviruses. Adv Virus Res 31:1–51

Borden KLB, Campbell Dwyer EJ, Carlile GW, Djavani M, Salvato MS (1998a) Two RING finger proteins, the oncoprotein PML and the arenavirus Z protein, colocalize with the nuclear fraction of the ribosomal P proteins. J Virol 72:3819–3826

Borden KLB, Campbell Dwyer EJ, Salvato MS (1998b) An arenavirus RING (zinc-binding) protein binds the oncoprotein promyelocyte leukemia protein (PML) and relocates PML nuclear bodies to the cytoplasm. J Virol 72:758–766

Bowen MD, Peters CJ, Nichol SJ (1997) Phylogenetic analysis of the Arenaviridae: patterns of virus evolution and evidence for cospeciation between arenaviruses and their rodent hosts. Mol Phylog Evol 8:301–316

Bresnahan WA, Shenk T (2000) A subset of viral transcripts packaged within human cytomegalovirus particles. Science 288:2373–2376

Bruns M, Gessner A, Lother H, Lehmann-Grube F (1988) Host cell-dependent homologous interference in lymphocytic choriomeningitis virus infection. Virology 166:133–139

Buchmeier MJ, Welsh RM, Dutko FJ, Oldstone MBA (1980) The virology and immunobiology of lymphocytic choriomeningitis virus infection. Adv Immunol 30:275–331

Buchmeier MJ, Southern PJ, Parekh BS, Wooddell MK, Oldstone MBA (1987) Site-specific antibodies define a cleavage site conserved among arenavirus GP-C glycoproteins. J Virol 61:982–985

Campbell Dwyer EJ, Lai H, MacDonald RC, Salvato MS, Borden KLB (2000) The lymphocytic choriomeningitis virus RING protein Z associates with eukaryotic initiation factor 4 E and selectively represses translation in a RING-dependent manner. J Virol 74:3293–3300

Cao W, Oldstone MBA, De la Torre JC (1997) Viral persistent infection affects both transcriptional and posttranslational regulation of neuron-specific molecule GAP43. Virology 230:147–154

Cao W, Henry MD, Borrrow P, Yamada H, Elder JH, Ravkov EV, Nichol ST, Compans RW, Campbell KP, Oldstone MBA (1998) Identification of alpha-dystroglycan as a receptor for lymphocytic choriomeningitis virus and Lassa fever virus. Science 282:279–281

Carter MF, Biswal N, Rawls WE (1973) Characterization of the nucleic acid of Pichinde virus. J Virol 11:61–68

Clegg JCS, Wilson SM, Oram JD (1990) Nucleotide sequence of the S RNA of Lassa virus (Nigerian strain) and comparative analysis of arenavirus gene products. Virus Res 18:151–164

D'Aiutolo AC, Coto CE (1986) Vero cells persistently infected with Tacaribe virus: role of interfering particles in the establishment of the infection. Virus Res 6:235–244

De BP, Banerjee AK (1997) Role of host proteins in gene expression of nonsegmented negative strand RNA viruses. Adv Virus Res 48:169–204

De la Torre JC, Oldstone MBA (1992) Selective disruption of growth hormone transcription machinery by viral infection. Proc Natl Acad Sci USA 89:9939–9943

De la Torre JC, Oldstone MBA (1996) Anatomy of viral persistence: mechanisms of virus persistence and associated disease. Adv Virus Res 46:311–343

Djavani M, Lukashevich IS, Sanchez A, Nichol ST, Salvato MS (1997) Completion of the Lassa fever virus sequence and identification of a RING finger open reading frame at the 5' end. Virology 235:414–418

Dutko FJ, Oldstone MBA (1983) Genomic and biological variation among commonly used lymphocytic choriomeningitis virus strains. J Gen Virol 64:1689–1698

Dutko FJ, Pfau CJ (1978) Arenavirus defective interfering particles mask the cell-killing potential of standard virus. J Gen Virol 38:195–208

Farber FE, Rawls WE (1975) Isolation of ribosome-like structures from Pichinde virus. J Gen Virol 26:21–31

Francis SJ, Southern PJ (1988) Deleted viral RNAs and lymphocytic choriomeningitis virus persistence in vitro. J Gen Virol 69:1893–1902

Franze-Fernandez M-T, Zetina C, Iapalucci S, Lucero MA, Bouissou C, Lopez R, Rey O, Deheli M, Cohen GN, Zakin MM (1987) Molecular structure and early events in the replication of Tacaribe arenavirus S RNA. Virus Res 7:309–324

Franze-Fernandez M-T, Iapalucci S, Lopez N, Rossi C (1993) Subgenomic RNAs of Tacaribe virus. In: Salvato MS (ed) The Arenaviridae. Plenum Press, New York, pp 113–132

Fuller-Pace FV, Southern PJ (1989) Detection of virus-specific RNA-dependent RNA polymerase activity in extracts from cells infected with lymphocytic choriomeningitis virus: in vitro synthesis of full-length viral RNA species. J Virol 63:1938–1944

Garcin D, Kolakofsky D (1990) A novel mechanism for the initiation of Tacaribe arenavirus genome replication. J Virol 64:6196–6203

Garcin D, Kolakofsky D (1992) Tacaribe arenavirus RNA synthesis in vitro is primer dependent and suggests an unusual model for the initiation of genome replication. J Virol 66:1370–1376

Garcin D, Rochat S, Kolakofsky D (1993) The Tacaribe arenavirus small zinc finger protein is required for both mRNA synthesis and genome replication. J Virol 67:807–812

Gessner A, Lother H (1989) Homologous interference of lymphocytic choriomeningitis virus involves a ribavirin-susceptible block in virus replication. J Virol 63:1827–1832

Ghiringhelli PD, Rivera-Pomar RV, Lozano ME, Grau O, Romanowski V (1991) Molecular organization of Junin virus S RNA: complete nucleotide sequence, relationship with other members of the Arenaviridae and unusual secondary structures. J Gen Virol 72:2129–2141

Gibadulinova A, Zelnik V, Reiserova L, Zavodska E, Zatovicova M, Ciampor F, Pastorekova S, Pastorek J (1998) Sequence and characterisation of the Z gene encoding ring finger protein of the lymphocytic choriomeningitis virus MX strain. Acta Virol 42:369–374

Harnish DG, Polyak SJ, Rawls WE (1993) Arenavirus replication: molecular dissection of the role of protein and RNA. In: Salvato MS (ed) The Arenaviridae. Plenum Press, New York, pp 157–174

Hotchin J (1962) The biology of lymphocytic choriomeningitis infection: virus-induced immune disease. Cold Spring Harbor Symp Quant Biol 27:479–499

Howard CR (1986) Arenaviruses. Perspectives in Medical Virology, Vol 2. Elsevier, Amsterdam

Howard CR, Buchmeier MJ (1983) A protein kinase activity in lymphocytic choriomeningitis virus and identification of the phosphorylated product using a monoclonal antibody. Virology 126:538–547

Iapalucci S, Chernavsky A, Rossi C, Burgin MJ, Franze-Fernandez M-T (1994) Tacaribe virus gene expression in cytopathic and non-cytopathic infections. Virology 200:613–622

Iapalucci S, Lopez R, Rey O, Lopez N, Franze-Fernandez M-T, Cohen GN, Lucero M, Ochoa A, Zakin MM (1989a) Tacaribe virus L gene encodes a protein of 2210 amino acid residues. Virology 170:40–47

Iapalucci S, Lopez N, Rey O, Zakin MM, Cohen GN, Franze-Fernandez M-T (1989b) The 5' region of Tacaribe virus L RNA encodes a protein with a potential metal binding domain. Virology 173: 357–361

Klavinskis LS, Oldstone MBA (1989) Lymphocytic choriomeningitis virus selectively alters differentiated but not housekeeping functions: block in expression of growth hormone gene is at the level of transcriptional initiation. Virology 168:232–235

Kolakofsky D, Garcin D (1993) The unusual mechanism of arenavirus RNA synthesis. In: Salvato MS (ed) The Arenaviridae. Plenum Press, New York, pp 103–112

Lai MMC (1998) Cellular factors in the transcription and replication of viral genomes: a parallel to DNA-dependent RNA transcription. Virology 244:1–12

Lee KJ, Novella IS, Teng MN, Oldstone MBA, De la Torre JC (2000) NP and L proteins of lymphocytic choriomeningitis virus (LCMV) are sufficient for efficient transcription and replication of LCMV genomic analogs. J Virol 74:3470–3477

Lehmann-Grube F (1984) Portraits of viruses: arenaviruses. Intervirology 22:121–145

Lehmann-Grube F, Slenczka W, Tees R (1969) A persistent and inapparent infection of L cells with the virus of lymphocytic choriomeningitis. J Gen Virol 5:63–81

Leung W-C, Rawls WE (1977) Virion-associated ribosomes are not required for the replication of Pichinde virus. Virology 81:174–176

Leung W-C, Leung MFKL, Rawls WE (1979) Distinctive RNA transcriptase, polyadenylic acid polymerase and polyuridylic acid polymerase activities associated with Pichinde virus. J Virol 30:98–107

Lin Y-J, Lai MMC (1993) Deletion mapping of a mouse hepatitis virus defective interfering RNA reveals the requirement of an internal and discontiguous sequence for replication. J Virol 67:6110–6118

Lopez R, Franze-Fernandez MT (1985) Effect of Tacaribe virus infection on host cell protein and nucleic acid synthesis. J Gen Virol 66:1753–1761

Lopez R, Grau O, Franze-Fernandez MT (1986) Effect of actinomycin D on arenavirus growth and estimation of the generation time for a virus particle. Virus Research 5:123–220

Lozano ME, Posik DM, Albarino CG, Schujman G, Ghiringhelli PD, Calderon G, Sabattini M, Romanowski V (1997) Characterization of arenaviruses using a family-specific primer set for RT-PCR amplification and RFLP analysis. Its potential use for detection of uncharacterized arenaviruses. Virus Res 49:79–89

Lukashevich IS, Djavani M, Shapiro K, Sanchez A, Ravkov E, Nichol ST, Salvato MS (1997) The Lassa fever virus L gene: nucleotide sequence, comparison, and precipitation of a predicted 250kDa protein with monospecific antiserum. J Gen Virol 78:547–551

Lukashevich IS, Maryankova R, Vladyko AS, Nashkevich N, Koleda S, Djavani M, Horejsh D, Voitenok NN, Salvato MS (1999) Lassa and Mopeia virus replication in human monocytes/macrophages and in epithelial cells: different effects on IL-8 and TNF-alpha gene expression. J Med Virol 59: 552–560

Meier E, Hermison GG, Schubert M (1987) Homotypic and heterotypic exclusion of vesicular stomatitis virus replication by high levels of recombinant polymerase protein L. J Virol 61:3133–3142

Mersich SE, Damonte EB, Coto CE (1981) Induction of RNA polymerase II activity in Junin virus-infected cells. Intervirology 16:123–127

Meyer BJ, Schmaljohn C (2000) Accumulation of terminally deleted RNAs may play a role in Seoul virus persistence. J Virol 74:1321–1331

Meyer BJ, Southern PJ (1993) Concurrent sequence analysis of 5' and 3' RNA termini by intramolecular circularization reveals 5' nontemplated bases and 3' terminal heterogeneity for lymphocytic choriomeningitis virus mRNAs. J Virol 67:2621–2627

Meyer BJ, Southern PJ (1994) Sequence heterogeneity in the termini of lymphocytic choriomeningitis virus genomic and antigenomic RNAs. J Virol 68:7659–7664

Meyer BJ, Southern PJ (1997) A novel type of defective viral genome suggests a unique strategy to establish and maintain persistent lymphocytic choriomeningitis virus infections. J Virol 71:6757–6764

Murphy FA, Whitfield SG (1975) Morphology and morphogenesis of arenaviruses. Bull WHO 52: 409–419

Oldstone MBA, Buchmeier MJ (1982) Restricted expression of viral glycoprotein in cells of persistently infected mice. Nature 300:360–362

Oldstone MBA, Sinha YN, Blount P, Tishon A, Rodriguez M, Wedel R von, Lampert PW (1982) Virus-induced alterations in homeostasis: alterations in differentiated functions of infected cells in vivo. Science 218:1125–1127

156   B.J. Meyer et al.

Oldstone MBA, Rodriguez M, Daughaday WH, Lampert PW (1984) Viral perturbation of endocrine function: disordered cell function leads to disturbed homeostasis and disease. Nature 307:278–281

Park JY, Peters CJ, Rollin PE, Ksiazek TG, Gray B, Waites KB, Stephensen CB (1997) Development of a reverse transcription-polymerase chain reaction assay for the diagnosis of lymphocytic choriomeningitis virus infection and its use in a prospective surveillance study. J Med Virol 51:107–114

Pedersen IR (1979) Structural components and replication of arenaviruses. Adv Virus Res 24:277–330

Polyak SJ, Rawls WE, Harnish DG (1991) Characterization of Pichinde virus infection of cells of the monocytic lineage. J Virol 65:3575–3582

Polyak SJ, Zheng S, Harnish DG (1995) Analysis of Pichinde arenavirus transcription and replication in human THP-1 monocytic cells. Virus Res 36:37–48

Raju R, Raju L, Hacker D, Garcin D, Compans RW, Kolakofsky D (1990) Nontemplated bases at the 5′ ends of Tacaribe virus mRNAs. Virology 174:53–59

Rawls WE, Banerjee SN, McMillan CA, Buchmeier MJ (1976) Inhibition of Pichinde virus replication by actinomycin D. J Gen Virol 33:421–434

Reiserova L, Kaluzova M, Kaluz S, Willis AC, Zavada J, Zavodska E, Zavadova Z, Ciampor F, Pastorek J, Pastorekova S (1999) Identification of MaTu-MX agent as a new strain of lymphocytic choriomeningitis virus (LCMV) and serological indication of horizontal spread of LCMV in population. Virology 257:73–83

Riviere Y, Ahmed R, Southern PJ, Buchmeier MJ, Dutko FJ, Oldstone MBA (1985) The S RNA segment of lymphocytic choriomeningitis virus codes for the nucleoprotein and glycoproteins 1 and 2. J Virol 53:966–968

Romanowski V, Bishop DHL (1983) The formation of arenaviruses that are genetically diploid. Virology 126:87–95

Romanowski V, Matsuura Y, Bishop DHL (1985) Complete sequence of the S RNA of lymphocytic choriomeningitis virus (WE strain) compared to that of Pichinde arenavirus. Virus Res 3:101–114

Rowe WP (1954) Studies on pathogenesis and immunity in lymphocytic choriomeningitis infection of the mouse. Res Rept Naval Med Res Inst 12:167–220

Salvato MS (ed) (1993a) The Arenaviridae. Plenum Press, New York

Salvato MS (1993b) Molecular biology of the prototype arenavirus, lymphocytic choriomeningitis virus. In: Salvato MS (ed) The Arenaviridae. Plenum Press, New York, pp 133–156

Salvato MS, Shimomaye EM (1989) The completed sequence of lymphocytic choriomeningitis virus reveals a unique RNA structure and a gene for a zinc finger protein. Virology 173:1–10

Salvato M, Shimomaye E, Southern P, Oldstone MBA (1988) Virus-lymphocyte interactions: IV. Molecular characterization of LCMV Armstrong (CTL+) small genomic segment and that of its variant, clone 13 (CTL−). Virology 164:517–522

Salvato M, Shimomaye EM, Oldstone MBA (1989) The primary structure of the lymphocytic choriomeningitis virus L gene encodes a putative RNA polymerase. Virology 169:377–384

Salvato MS, Schweighofer KJ, Burns J, Shimomaye EM (1992) Biochemical and immunological evidence that the 11kDa zinc-binding protein of lymphocytic choriomeningitis virus is a structural component of the virus. Virus Res 22:185–198

Singh MK, Fuller-Pace FV, Buchmeier MJ, Southern PJ (1987) Analysis of the genomic L RNA segment of lymphocytic choriomeningitis virus. Virology 161:448–456

Southern PJ (1996) Arenaviridae: the viruses and their replication. In: Fields BN, Knipe DM, Howley PM, et al. (eds) Fields virology. Lippincott-Raven, Philadelphia, pp 1505–1519

Southern PJ, Singh MK, Riviere Y, Jacoby DR, Buchmeier MJ, Oldstone MBA (1987) Molecular characterization of the genomic S RNA segment from lymphocytic choriomeningitis virus. Virology 157:145–155

Valsamakis A, Riviere Y, Oldstone MBA (1987) Perturbation of differentiated functions in vivo during persistent viral infection. III. Decreased growth hormone mRNA. Virology 156:214–220

Welsh RM, Buchmeier MJ (1979) Protein analysis of defective interfering lymphocytic choriomeningitis virus and persistently infected cells. Virology 96:503–515

Welsh RM, Oldstone MBA (1977) Inhibition of immunologic injury of cultured cells infected with lymphocytic choriomeningitis virus: role of defective interfering virus in regulating viral antigen expression. J Exp Med 145:1449–1468

Wilson SM, Clegg JCS (1991) Sequence analysis of the S RNA of the African arenavirus Mopeia: an unusual secondary structure feature in the intergenic region. Virology 180:543–552

Yoshinari S, Nagy PD, Simon AE, Dreher TW (2000) CCA initiation boxes without unique promoter elements support in vitro transcription by three viral RNA-dependent RNA polymerases. RNA 6:698–707

Young PR, Howard CR (1983) Fine structure of Pichinde virus nucleocapsids. J Gen Virol 64:833–842
Young PR, Chanas AC, Lee SR, Gould EA, Howard CR (1987) Localization of an arenavirus protein in the nuclei of infected cells. J Gen Virol 68:2465–2470
Zeijst BAM van der, Bleumink N, Crawford LV, Swyryd EA, Stark GR (1983a) Viral proteins and RNAs in BHK cells persistently infected by lymphocytic choriomeningitis virus. J Virol 48:262–270
Zeijst BAM van der, Noyes BE, Mirault M-E, Parker B, Osterhaus ADME, Swyryd EA, Bleumink N, Horzinek MC, Stark GR (1983b) Persistent infection of some standard cell lines by lymphocytic choriomeningitis virus: transmission of infection by an intracellular agent. J Virol 48:249–261

Arenaviruses: Protein Structure and Function

M.J. BUCHMEIER

1 Introduction

The Arenaviruses are structurally quite simple, consisting of only four primary gene products encoded on two RNA strands. Despite this very simple genetic plan, these viruses are capable of interacting with the host in a bewildering variety of permutations that result in a range of infections from a lifelong persistent carrier state, as is evident in the neonatally or congenitally infected carrier mouse, to the lethal acute diseases typical of Lassa, Machupo, Junin, and other arenavirus hemorrhagic fevers. These differing disease courses are, in part, determined by the clash of two factors: the cellular and tissue site(s) of virus replication in vivo, defined as tropism, and the genetically determined host response to the infecting virus. When the virus replicates in critical tissues like the meninges and choroid plexi of the mouse brain, as is the case in acute LCMV infection, and the host is capable of mounting a strong T-cell response, the end result is a fatal choriomeningitis (Fig. 1). However, replication of the virus in these same tissues results in little tissue injury or disease in a mouse that has been immunosuppressed, or in a neonate prior to maturation of

Division of Virology, Mailcode CVN-8, The Scripps Research Institute, 10550 N. Torrey Pines Road, La Jolla, CA 92037, USA

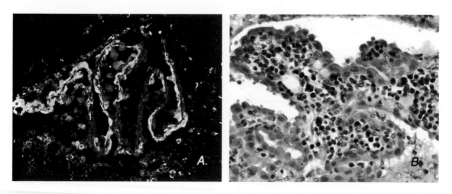

Fig. 1A,B. Expression of lymphocytic choriomeningitis virus (LCMV) antigen in critical membranes of the brain leads to the fatal choriomeningitis syndrome in mice. In this example, GP1, expressed at 7 days after infection in cells of the choroid plexus of the third ventricle (**A**) provides the target against which highly activated mononuclear infiltrates are directed (**B**)

the T-cell response. This immunopathological paradox is at the core of understanding the pathogenesis of LCM disease and has provided a singularly important biological model for probing cellular immunology for more than six decades (BUCHMEIER and ZAJAC 1999). In this brief chapter, the nature of the arenavirus proteins and their functions will be discussed with particular emphasis on their role in infection and disease.

The proteins of arenaviruses were first studied by Smadel and his colleagues (SMADEL et al. 1942), with reference to their antigenicity. These investigators described the presence of a virus-specific soluble (S) antigen detectable by complement fixation (CF) in homogenates of spleen and lung from LCMV-infected guinea pigs. Soluble antigen could be separated from infectious virus by ultracentrifugation. Repeatedly washed virions reacted poorly in CF tests, while the S antigen lost none of its immunoreactivity after ultracentrifugation. These studies were not extended until nearly three decades later when BROWN and KIRK (1969), CHASTEL (1970), SIMON (1970), and BRO-JORGENSEN (1971) described antigens detectable by CF and immunodiffusion in tissues or cell cultures infected with LCMV. BRO-JORGENSEN (1971) found two antigenic species by immunodiffusion using infected BHK-21 cells as the antigen source. One antigen was heat stable and resistant to proteolysis, while the second was degraded by both heating and pronase digestion. Both antigens sedimented at a rate of 3.5 S in rate zonal sucrose gradient centrifugation, and based on this S value, the molecular weight of the thermolabile S antigen was estimated to be 48,000.

Studies by GESCHWENDER et al. (1976) with LCMV established that the extractable complement-fixing antigen (ECFA) was an internal component of the virion. Antiserum directed against ECFA did not neutralize infectious LCMV, and it did not mediate complement-dependent lysis of LCMV-infected cells. Purified LCMV, disrupted by detergents, liberated an antigen, which reacted with anti-ECFA in a CF test and produced a band of identity with ECFA by immunodiffusion.

Rawls and colleagues (RAWLS and BUCHMEIER 1975) arrived at similar conclusions, working with the S antigens of Pichinde virus. Antisera directed against partially purified CF antigen from cells infected by Pichinde virus were shown to react against the internal nucleocapsid protein of the virus but not with surface antigens of infected cells. Subsequent studies (BUCHMEIER et al. 1977) demonstrated that the S antigen was a degradation product of the viral nucleocapsid protein (NP). Moreover, the antigenic cross-reactivity observed by CF among the New World Tacaribe complex arenaviruses (RAWLS and LEUNG 1979) was shown to be due to conservation of NP-related antigens (BUCHMEIER and OLDSTONE 1977).

Persistent arenavirus infections, whether in vitro (LEHMANN-GRUBE et al. 1969; WELSH et al. 1977; WELSH and BUCHMEIER 1979; VAN DER ZEIJST et al. 1983a,b) or in vivo (TRAUB 1936a,b; WILSNACK and ROWE 1964; OLDSTONE and BUCHMEIER 1982; RODRIGUEZ et al. 1983), are characterized by the persistence of nucleoprotein, often in the absence of viral glycoprotein antigens and infectious virus production. This phenomenon, which we now recognize may be a consequence of the ambisense genomic arrangement of the S RNA segment, led to a great deal of confusion and ambiguity in early attempts to grow and purify arenaviruses (RAWLS and LEUNG 1979). Only when factors, such as multiplicity of infection, rigorous plaque purification of the infecting virus, and time of harvest, were carefully controlled did a consistent picture of the structural features of these viruses begin to emerge.

All of the arenaviruses share a common strategy of gene organization in which the single-stranded RNA genome is divided between two segments of approximately 3.4 (S) and 7.2kb (L). Each of these RNAs is further partitioned by a unique ambisense coding strategy with the 5' end reading in the positive or message sense and the 3' end reading in the negative or anti-message sense. Coding assignments and the corresponding viral polypeptides are shown in (Fig. 2). Implicit in the ambisense-replication strategy is the ability of the virus to exert control over negatively and positively encoded genes independently of one another. This feature translates into the ability of a virus to modulate expression of glycoprotein mRNA transcription and translation independently of NP expression in vitro and in vivo (OLDSTONE and BUCHMEIER 1982; BLOUNT et al. 1986).

2 Specific Arenavirus Proteins and their Functions

2.1 Nucleocapsid Protein

The Nucleocapsid protein, NP, is the most abundant structural protein of arenaviruses and has a molecular mass of 60–68kDa. In the Pichinde virus, the NP represents 70% of the labeled virion proteins, and 1,530 molecules of NP are present in each virion. The NP is the major protein component of nucleocapsids and associates with virion RNA to form the string of bead-like structures observed by electron microscopy (YOUNG and HOWARD 1983). NP can become phosphory-

A Coding assignments

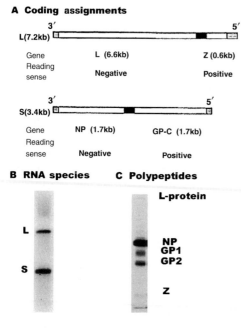

Fig. 2A–C. Coding assignments and polypeptides of arenaviruses. **A** RNA segments and the identification of each of the four open reading frames. **B** 28 S L and 18 S S RNA segments as separated on an agarose gel. **C** Virion polypeptides *L*, 180kDa, *NP*, 63kDa, *GP1*, 44kDa, *GP2*, 35kDa, and *Z*, 10–14kDa

lated in the latter stages of acute infection, and this form increases in abundance during persistent infections in vitro (HOWARD and BUCHMEIER 1983). In infected cells, full-length NP is normally localized exclusively in the cell cytoplasm but a 28-kDa degradation fragment of NP has been reported to accumulate in the nucleus of Pichinde-infected cells (YOUNG et al. 1987).

Various arenaviruses encode NPs ranging from 558 to 570 residues in length. MAXHOM alignment of the nine available NP sequences reveals a high degree of conservation of sequence and structural motifs among these. Notable among them are frequent arginine and lysine residues, appearing singly, in pairs, and in clusters of three or more, which may serve to neutralize the nucleic acid. One stretch located near the carboxyl terminus of NP contains a conserved segment of 4 or 5 consecutive basic residues and may be an RNA-binding domain. Although NP has several potential N-linked glycosylation sites, it is not known to be glycosylated. Overall, the structure of NP is consistent with a globular, basic protein with the primary function of protecting the viral RNA within the cell. Immune precipitation with anti-NP antibodies has been used in the author's laboratory to recover viral nucleocapsids containing vRNA.

2.2 Glycoproteins

The cell-associated glycoprotein precursor, GPC, is a 70–80-kDa polyprotein that is post-translationally cleaved within the cell to release the virion glycoproteins GP1 and GP2. A predictive computer algorithm suggested that the N-terminal 58 amino acids of GP-C constituted a cleavable signal sequence. This was confirmed by amino acid sequencing of isolated LCMV glycoproteins, which established the N-terminal residues of GP-1 and GP-2 as met$_{59}$ and gly$_{266}$, respectively. Similar N-termini were demonstrated in the glycoproteins of the related arenaviruses Pichinde and Tacaribe. The signal sequence is exceptionally long and contains two hydrophobic domains, raising the possibility that the signal may serve an additional functional role in viral glycoprotein transport or particle assembly. Cleavage of GPC to GP1 and GP2 occurs late in the secretory pathway at the medial Golgi or trans-Golgi network and requires prior glycosylation and trimming. GP1 derives from the amino terminal portion of GPC, and cleavage occurs at a unique motif that is conserved in all arenaviruses except Tacaribe virus (BURNS and BUCHMEIER 1993; LENZ et al. 2000) (Fig. 3). Equimolar amounts of the two glycoproteins are found in virions. GP1 (40–46kDa) is the peripheral membrane glycoprotein with 4 to 11 potential N-linked glycosylation sites (AUPERIN et al. 1984; WRIGHT et al. 1990; CLEGG 1993). Because GP1 runs as a heterogeneous species on SDS-PAGE, it has been speculated that not all potential glycosylation sites are always used; however, WRIGHT et al. (1990) were able to demonstrate utilization of all six potential glycosylation sites on LCMV GP1 and two of the three sites on GP2.

GP1 molecules assemble into homotetrameric complexes, which are held together by disulfide bonds. GP2 (MW 35kDa) is the integral membrane glycoprotein, which contains one to four potential N-linked glycosylation sites and a membrane-spanning domain. The carboxy terminus of GP2 contains charged residues and is thought to interact with NP in the cytosol and within the interior of the virion, as evidenced by cross-linking studies. GP2 molecules, which are predicted to assume a coiled-coil conformation due to the presence of two heptad-repeat sequences in the amino-terminal half of the molecule, also assemble into homotetramers and form the stalk portion of the glycoprotein spike. GP2 homo-

	SP	GP1	GP2
LCMV [1]		59	265
		ASCG *MYGLK*	FTRRLA *GTFTWT*
Pichinde		59	273
		SCDS *MMIDR*	VSRKLL *GFFTW*
Tacaribe		58	261
		RSCS *EETFTK*	VGRTLK *AFFSWT*
Lassa		58	259
		RSCT *TSLYK*	ISRRLL *GTFTWT* [2]

1 N-terminal sequences of LCMV, Pichinde and Tacaribe determined by Burns and Buchmeier1993
2 N-terminal sequence of the Lassa GP2 determined by Lenz et al. 2000

Fig. 3. Signal peptide (*SP*) and glycoprotein (*GP1:GP2*) cleavage sites of several arenaviruses. Sequences of the N termini of GP1 and GP2 have been determined by BURNS and BUCHMEIER (1993) for lymphocytic choriomeningitis virus (*LCMV*), Pichinde, and Tacaribe viruses, and the N terminal sequence of Lassa GP2 and the protease cleavage motif have been determined by LENZ et al. (2000) for Lassa Virus

tetramers bind through ionic interactions with GP1 homotetramers, which comprise the globular head of glycoprotein spikes. GP2 is the viral fusion protein. Structural modelling of GP2 has shown that it contains two αhelical coiled-coil regions in the ectodomain.

The ultrastructure and composition of the lymphocytic choriomeningitis virus (LCMV) glycoprotein spike has been examined by cryo-electron microscopic, immunochemical and biophysical techniques in the author's laboratory. We used cryo-electron microscopy to examine LCM virions frozen under physiological pH and salt conditions. With this method, the virions were imaged in positive contrast (Fig. 4), and a number of features were apparent. The virions were spherical particles of variable diameter consisting of a poorly resolved electron-dense core enclosed by a lipid bilayer. The outer surface of the bilayer was studded with spike projections composed of the glycoproteins. A series of exposures was made at different levels of defocus to visualize these features more clearly. At a focus of −1.5μm, where 50Å spacings were emphasized in the images, the bilayer was clearly visible (Fig. 4A). The high electron-scattering density of the phosphate head groups of the lipids gives rise to the characteristic trilamellar appearance of the bilayer. The spikes, while apparent in these images, are more clearly visualized in more strongly defocussed images (−3.0μm, Fig. 4B,C). Details in the images (Fig. 4C) suggest that the spikes are T-shaped, with the stalk anchored in the lipid bilayer and major axis of the head structures lying parallel to the bilayer approximately 80–100Å from the surface.

Viral particles were observed to be decidedly variable in size and in morphology. To obtain an estimate of this variability and to assess the range of size variation in the preparations, measurement of the mean particle diameter for the virions resolved by cryo-electron microscopy was performed. To correct for

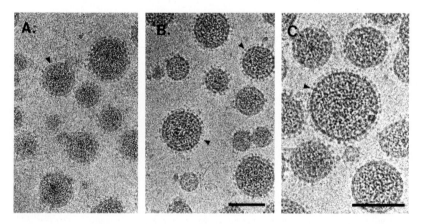

Fig. 4A–C. Cryo-electron micrographs of purified lymphocytic choriomeningitis (LCM) virions. Purified lymphocytic choriomeningitis virus (LCMV) preparations were analyzed by cryoelectron microscopy using underfocus values of –1.5μm (**A**) or –3.0μm (**B,C**). In **A** the lipid bilayer of the virion envelope is emphasized (*arrow head*). **B,C** The surface topography and t-shaped glycoprotein spikes are emphasized (*arrow heads*). Magnification **A,B** 167,100× and **C** is 232,750×. *Bar scales* = 1000Å

aspherical particles, two measurements were made at 90°, and the mean of these two measurements taken as the diameter of the individual particle. Analysis of the distribution of diameters of 100 particles revealed a range of virion diameters from 62 to 150nm, with a modal distribution at 92nm. There were prominant populations of particles at 62, 79, 92, and 113nm, which may represent virions encapsidating variable numbers of genomic RNA segments. It has been shown that virions can be genetically diploid, suggesting the incorporation of multiple copies of L or S RNA (ROMANOWSKI and BISHOP 1983), and nonstoichiometric ratios of L and S RNA are regularly observed in highly purified virion preparations, lending support to this concept.

By immunoblotting virions digested with proteinase K using an anti-peptide antibody to the carboxy-terminal sequence of GP-C, it was established that GP-2 was anchored in the membrane by its carboxy-terminus. A region of heptad repeats was located near the amino-terminus of GP-2, suggesting an extended alpha-helical coiled-coil structure, consistent with a "stalk-like" structural domain. Incubation of virions in 1M LiCl or NaCl resulted in the quantitative release of GP-1 from otherwise intact virions, demonstrating a role for ionic interactions in the association of GP-1 with the virion. These findings support a model of the Arenavirus glycoprotein spike consisting of a globular tetrameric GP-1 head bound by ionic interactions to a membrane anchored GP-2 stalk with a 15–18 amino acid transmembrane domain and a 42 residue cytoplasmic tail.

2.3 Polymerase Protein

The arenavirus L (large) protein is the viral RNA-dependent RNA polymerase, and is encoded in the 3' open reading frame of the L RNA segment. The L protein has a reported molecular mass of 180–250kDa (SALVATO et al. 1989; LUKASHEVICH et al. 1997). Motifs that are common to all RNA-dependent RNA polymerases and the polymerases of segmented negative strand RNA viruses, as well as two regions found only in the polymerases of arenaviruses and Bunyaviruses, are conserved in arenavirus L proteins. The L protein is a component of nucleocapsids, since polymerase activity has been associated with these structures.

2.4 Zinc-Binding Protein

The smallest protein encoded by the arenaviral genome is the Z (also called p11) protein, which has a molecular size of 11kDa. The Z protein contains a RING-finger motif and binds zinc. It has been suggested that the Z protein is both a structural component of viral nucleocapsids (SALVATO et al. 1992) and that it acts as a cofactor in viral replication and/or transcription (GARCIN et al. 1993). Immunodepletion of Z protein in Tacaribe virus-infected cell extracts strongly inhibited synthesis of genomic RNA and NP mRNA, but a requirement of Z protein for transcription was seen only during the early stages of infection. However, recent studies (LEE et al. 2000), using an artificially constructed LCMV

RNA analog, show clearly that L and NP are the minimal viral trans-acting factors required for efficient RNA synthesis mediated by the LCMV polymerase.

Z protein has been detected in the cytoplasm and nucleus of LCMV-infected cells. Recent work by Salvato and colleagues (BORDEN et al. 1997; BORDEN et al. 1998a,b; CAMPBELL DWYER et al. 2000; DJAVANI et al. 2001) revealed a possible interaction with the nuclear oncoprotein, PML. These investigators have suggested that the Z-protein-PML interaction may act to modulate the interferon response in infected cells (DJAVANI et al. 2001).

3 Viral Binding and Entry into Cells

The GP1 portion of the glycoprotein spike is responsible for initial binding to cellular receptors, and antibodies directed to epitopes on GP1 can block viral binding and neutralize viral infectivity (BORROW and OLDSTONE 1992). Virus binds to a 120–140-kDa cellular glycoprotein identified as alpha-dystroglycan (CAO et al. 1998). Variations in binding affinity to alpha-dystroglycan have been observed among the LCMV strains, with LCMV Cl-13 and -WE strains being typical of high-affinity binders, while LCMV-ARM binds at low affinity. Other arenaviruses (i.e. Lassa, Mobala, Oliveros) also bind to this glycoprotein, but Guanarito virus does not, suggesting that more than one cellular protein may serve as a receptor for arenaviruses.

After attachment to cellular receptors, virions are internalized into in large, smooth-walled endocytic vesicles that do not appear to be clathrin-coated. Viral nucleocapsids are delivered into the cell cytoplasm by pH-dependent fusion of virion and endosomal membranes in response to acidification of the endosome (BORROW and OLDSTONE 1994; DI SIMONE et al. 1994). At acidic pH, GP1 dissociates from GP2 exposing the putative GP2 fusion peptide (DI SIMONE et al. 1994). Evidence from several laboratories showed that LCMV infection was blocked by inhibitors of lysosomal acidification, including chloroquine, ammonium chloride and monensin. DI SIMONE et al. (DI SIMONE et al. 1994; DI SIMONE and BUCHMEIER 1995) extended these findings by demonstrating that exposure of LCMV to acidic pH (pH 5.3) similar to that expected in the endocytic vesicle resulted in elution of GP-1 from virions and activation of a fusion function mediated by GP-2. Fusion activity was shown to be accompanied by exposure of core epitopes on the GP-2 stalk domain, suggesting that significant conformational changes in the spike structure had occurred. The pH optimum for fusion activation was 5.3–5.5, as determined in a fluorescence-dequenching system. LCMV differs from other acid pH-dependent enveloped RNA viruses in that it does not induce synctium formation in cell culture. LCMV GP-2 lacks a long hydrophobic amino acid sequence characteristic of other fusion-inducing viruses and possesses relatively weak membrane-fusing activity. Once nucleocapsids have been delivered into the cyto-plasm, replication is initiated by transcription of subgenomic, genome-complementary NP and L mRNAs by the viral L-protein, an RNA-dependent RNA polymerase (Fig. 5).

NP mRNAs can be detected as early as 2h post-infection, and NP protein can be detected after 6–12h, depending upon the multiplicity of infection and sensitivity of the assay. New L protein synthesis protein cannot be detected until 12–24h post infection, and its concentration increases dramatically during acute infection. NP mRNA and protein accumulate earlier than GPC mRNA and the glycoproteins. NP protein accumulation either precedes replication, or the two processes are contemporary, suggesting that the first transcript produced by the incoming nucleoprotein complex is NP and that this early message is transcribed by the incoming viral RNA polymerase. These data illustrate how the ambisense coding arrangement of the arenavirus genome temporally separates initial expression of NP and L proteins from expression of the glycoproteins and Z protein. In the presence of the protein synthesis inhibitor pactamycin, NP mRNA accumulates, but replication and GPC mRNA transcription do not occur, thus demonstrating the need for de novo protein synthesis for replication to take place. To obtain expression of the GPC and Z proteins, a round of replication must take place in which S and L antigenomes, full-length complements to the genomic RNAs, are produced. The GPC is cleaved 75–90min post-translation after conversion of high-mannose oligosaccharides precursors to complex carbohydrates (glucosamine, fucose, galactose) and transport to the Golgi (BURNS and BUCHMEIER 1993). There is little information available describing Z protein expression, largely due to the lack of widely available reagents for study.

The assembly process of arenavirus particles is poorly characterized. Newly synthesized genomic RNAs, NP protein, and L protein are assembled into nucle-ocapsids intracellularly. Arenaviruses also package host-cell ribosomes into virion particles; however, the numbers of ribosomes encapsidated is highly variable. Within arenavirus-infected cells, the intracytoplasmic distribution of ribosomes is altered, and inclusion bodies can be found that consist of ribosomes embedded in a matrix of virus-specific proteins (RODRIGUEZ et al. 1983). Aggregates of electron-dense granules are found free in the cytoplasm of infected cells, as well as in close apposition to the cytoplasmic face of the plasma membrane near patches of glycoprotein spikes. NP can be cross-linked to the carboxy terminus of GP2 (BURNS and BUCHMEIER 1991), suggesting that interaction of these two proteins is essential for the assembly of virions at the cell membrane. After association of electron-dense structures with the plasma membrane, budding takes place by "pinching off" of the lipid bilayer and subsequent separation of the virion and plasma membranes.

4 Arenavirus Protein Expression in Persistent Infections

Arenaviruses establish persistent infections in their rodent host, and persistent infections are easily established in cell culture in vitro. The two systems differ, however, in the fact that persistence in vitro is due solely to alterations in viral gene expression and replication, whereas in vivo persistence is likely to be a combination of molecular biological mechanisms and a failure of the host immune response to clear infection (BUCHMEIER et al. 2001) The molecular mechanisms of arenaviral persistence have been investigated both in cell culture as well as in infected rodents. In vitro, most arenavirus infections progress over time from the acute phase to a persistent phase, characterized by a reduction in the amount of infectious virus produced. During the acute phase of arenavirus infection in vitro, there is active viral replication and virus production and usually little, if any, cytopathic effect. In persistent infection, cells remain infected for life with alterations in transcription, replication and expression of viral proteins, though is it is possible that some cells may spontaneously clear arenavirus infections. There is an increase in the number of S genomic RNAs relative to the number of L genomic RNAs in cells persistently infected with LCMV (ROMANOWSKI and BISHOP 1983). In both cultured cells (WELSH and BUCHMEIER 1979) and mice persistently infected with LCMV (OLDSTONE and BUCHMEIER 1982), there is a down-regulation of viral glycoprotein expression. In persistently infected L cells, GPC, GP1, and GP2 expression are reduced, but a truncated GPC protein can be detected in abundance along with increased levels of NP (BRUNS et al. 1990). In persistent infections, full-length genomic segments and mRNAs can be detected along with populations of heterogeneously sized, truncated RNAs that accumulate over time. The truncated RNAs detected in persistently infected cells in vitro tend to be less heterogeneous in size than those detected in vivo. Defective-interfering (DI) RNAs of arenaviruses are poorly characterized. DI RNAs from the brain tissue of mice persistently infected with LCMV have short deletions (three to 41 bases) at the termini of both the S and L RNA genomes and antigenomes. These DI RNAs are thought to be competent for replication but not transcription and, therefore, are able to compete with genomes and antigenomes for viral proteins (MEYER and SOUTHERN 1994).

Defective interfering particles (DI), which are able to interfere with the infectivity of standard virus, are produced during both acute and persistent arenavirus infections. Infection of L cells with LCMV at a high multiplicity of infection results in lower titers of standard virus and a higher ratio of DI to standard virus compared to an infection at a low multiplicity (LEHMANN-GRUBE et al. 1983). When LCMV stocks were passed at a high multiplicity of infection in cell culture, the titer of infectious virus and DIs alternatively rises and falls synchronously with each passage. This cycling effect is presumably due to increased production of DIs during high titer infection, which interferes with standard virus production. DIs are smaller than infectious virions (mean diameter 55–56nm) and probably lack one or both genomic RNAs. In DIs, GP1 and GP2 can be absent or non-glycosylated, and the GPC and NP often display alterations in molecular size (GIMENEZ and COMPANS 1980; MARTINEZ PERALTA et al. 1981; LEHMANN-GRUBE et al. 1983). Treatment of cultured cells with DIs prior to or up to 8h post-infection with standard LCMV dramatically inhibits replication of the standard virus (PEDERSEN 1979; LEHMANN-GRUBE et al. 1983). Concurrent intracranial injection of DIs with standard LCMV inhibits cerebellar disease in a suckling rat model. The mechanism of DI interference and its potential role in the development and maintenance of persistent infections has yet to be determined.

A DNA form of the LCMV S RNA has been detected in the spleen tissues of persistently infected mice and in persistently infected murine cell lines (KLENERMAN et al. 1997). Production of the DNA form of the LCMV S RNA was inhibited by the reverse transcriptase inhibitor AZT, suggesting that endogenous reverse transcriptases are responsible for this activity. The exact relevance of genomic reverse transcription to the biology of arenaviruses and its potential roles in the maintenance of persistent infection and the immune response remains to be elucidated.

5 Prospects for Future Research

Progress in understanding the basic structure and function of the arenavirus proteins has lagged behind that of other negative stranded RNA viruses for several reasons. First among these has been the lack of both reliable and efficient expression systems for producing suitable a substrate for experiments. Two of the most widely utilized systems, the vaccinia and baculovirus expression vectors perform rather badly when called upon to express Arenavirus proteins, particularly GPC. Vaccinia has been found by the author to produce large quantities of uncleaved and unprocessed GPC, which while acceptable for CTL targeting protocols, is not satisfactory for structural and functional studies. Similarly, the baculovirus-expression system (MATSUURA et al. 1986) yields excellent expression of NP in *Spodoptera* cells but performs poorly with respect to GPC. Baculovirus-expressed glycoprotein has been shown to accumulate in the ER in an unprocessed form, leading to cell death. This failure has been attributed to differences in glycosylation between insect and mammalian cells, although in view of the findings of LENZ et al. (2000), the failure to cleave and transport GPC may also be due to the lack of an appropriate protease in the insect cells. Proper folding of GPC is critical to achieve the fidelity of structure necessary for meaningful structural and functional analysis. WRIGHT et al. (1989, 1990) have demonstrated that tunicamycin, which blocks glycosylation of GPC with high mannose core sugars, effectively blocks transport and cleavage to GP1 and GP2 and virus production. Restoration of just the high mannose core sugars in the absence of further trimming also restored posttranslational processing and viral maturation of GPC. In other studies (WRIGHT et al. 1989), we found that both the native conformation and recognition by neutralizing antibody to GP1 was disrupted by reduction of sulfhydryl bonds, while under the same conditions, reactivity against a linear epitope on GP2 (WEBER and BUCHMEIER 1988) was unaffected.

Current studies in the author's laboratory utilize the cytomegalovirus immediate early promoter to drive the expression of the GPC gene in a variety of mammalian cell types. This combination yields high-level expression of GPC with stoichiometric processing to GP1 and GP2; moreover, the products react well with conformation-dependent virus neutralizing antibodies – the best criterion we currently have to judge preservation of native structure. Taking this further, to perform functional analyses on GP, we have employed the three-vector transduction system described by Soneoka and co-workers (SONEOKA et al. 1995) to produce retroviral pseudotypes with the glycoproteins of Lassa and LCMV. These pseudotype viruses have been shown to exhibit receptor-binding and neutralization properties identical to their respective parental arenaviruses. The availability of such reagents allows us to entertain studies of the Lassa virus glycoprotein function outside of BSL4 containment for the first time.

Exciting progress has also been made toward the establishment of a recombinant system for recovery of genetically engineered arenaviruses. LEE et al. (2000) have described the establishment of a minigenome system to test the requirements for efficient transcription and replication of artificial LCMV genome analogs. In this system, it was observed that expression of L and NP proteins was sufficient to drive both transcription and replication. The establishment of this system and exploration of requirements for packaging the RNA genome are important steps in developing a "reverse genetic" approach to probe arenavirus pathogenesis and may make development of safe vaccines for highly pathogenic arenaviruses a reality.

6 Conclusion

Arenaviruses have provided one of the best experimental models for understanding the complex relationship between virus and host that constitutes pathogenesis. Studies in particular of the LCMV infection have yielded and continue to yield primary observations of the immune response including the first descriptions of virus-induced immune complex disease (OLDSTONE and DIXON 1969), the first observation of MHC restriction in the CD8 response (ZINKERNAGEL and DOHERTY 1974), and virus-induced NK cells (WELSH 1978), and the system remains fertile ground for studies of immunobiology of infection. Full appreciation of the nature of persistent infection and the ultimate goal of vaccination against pathogenic arenavirus infections will require a deeper understanding of how these viruses function. Fortunately, tools are now becoming available that will provide these answers, and it is hoped, also new data that will allow investigators to interpret the complex host-virus interactions that are unique to arenavirus biology and replication.

References

Auperin DD, Romanowski V, et al. (1984) Sequencing studies of pichinde arenavirus S RNA indicate a novel coding strategy, an ambisense viral S RNA. J Virol 52(3):897–904
Blount P, Elder J, et al. (1986) Dissecting the molecular anatomy of the nervous system: analysis of RNA and protein expression in whole body sections of laboratory animals. Brain Res 382(2):257–265

Borden KL, Campbell Dwyer EJ, et al. (1997) The promyelocytic leukemia protein PML has a pro-apoptotic activity mediated through its RING domain. FEBS Lett 418(1–2):30–34

Borden KL, Campbell Dwyer EJ, et al. (1998a) An arenavirus RING (zinc-binding) protein binds the oncoprotein promyelocyte leukemia protein (PML) and relocates PML nuclear bodies to the cytoplasm. J Virol 72(1):758–766

Borden KL, Campbell Dwyer EJ, et al. (1998b) Two RING finger proteins, the oncoprotein PML and the arenavirus Z protein, colocalize with the nuclear fraction of the ribosomal P proteins. J Virol 72(5):3819–3826

Borrow P, Oldstone MB (1992) Characterization of lymphocytic choriomeningitis virus-binding protein(s): a candidate cellular receptor for the virus. J Virol 66(12):7270–7281

Borrow P, Oldstone MB (1994) Mechanism of lymphocytic choriomeningitis virus entry into cells. Virology 198(1):1–9

Bro-Jorgensen K (1971) Characterization of virus-specific antigen in cell culture infected with lymphocytic choriomeningitis virus. Acta Pathol Microbiol Scand [B] Microbiol Immunol 79(4):466–474

Brown WJ, Kirk BE (1969) Complement-fixing antigen from BHK-21 cell cultures infected with lymphocytic choriomeningitis virus. Appl Microbiol 18(3):496–499

Bruns M, Kratzberg T, et al. (1990) Mode of replication of lymphocytic choriomeningitis virus in persistently infected cultivated mouse L cells. Virology 177(2):615–624

Buchmeier MJ, Bowen MD, et al. (2001) Chapter 50: Arenaviridae: the viruses and their replication. In: Knipe DM, Howley PM (eds) Fields Virology. Lippincott Williams and Wilkins, Philadelphia 2: 1635–1668

Buchmeier MJ, Gee SR, et al. (1977) Antigens of Pichinde virus I. Relationship of soluble antigens derived from infected BHK-21 cells to the structural components of the virion. J Virol 22(1):175–186

Buchmeier MJ, Oldstone MBA (1977) Identity of the viral protein responsible for serologic cross reactivity among the Tacaribe complex arenaviruses. Proc of Conf on Negative Strand Virus and the Host Cell. B. W. J. a. B. Mahy, R.D. London, Academic, pp 91–96

Buchmeier MJ, Zajac AJ (1999) Lymphocytic Choriomeningitis Virus. John Wiley & Sons Ltd, Chichester, Sussex, UK

Burns JW, Buchmeier MJ (1991) Protein-protein interactions in lymphocytic choriomeningitis virus. Virology 183(2):620–629

Burns JW, Buchmeier MJ (1993) Glycoproteins of the arenaviruses. In: Salvato MS (ed) The Arenaviridae. Plenum Press, New York, pp 17–35

Campbell Dwyer EJ, Lai H, et al. (2000) The lymphocytic choriomeningitis virus RING protein Z associates with eukaryotic initiation factor 4 E and selectively represses translation in a RING-dependent manner. J Virol 74(7):3293–3300

Cao W, Henry MD, et al. (1998) Identification of alpha-dystroglycan as a receptor for lymphocytic choriomeningitis virus and Lassa fever virus. Science 282(5396):2079–2081

Chastel C (1970) Immunodiffusion studies on a fluorocarbon-extracted antigen of lymphocytic choriomeningitis virus. Acta Virol (Praha) 14:507–509

Clegg JCS (1993) Molecular phylogeny of the arenaviruses and guide to published sequence data. In: Salvato MS (ed) The Arenaviridae. Plenum Press, New York, pp 175–185

Di Simone C, Buchmeier MJ (1995) Kinetics and pH dependence of acid-induced structural changes in the lymphocytic choriomeningitis virus glycoprotein complex. Virology 209(1):3–9

Di Simone C, Zandonatti MA, et al. (1994) Acidic pH triggers LCMV membrane fusion activity and conformational change in the glycoprotein spike. Virology 198(2):455–465

Djavani M, Rodas J, et al. (2001) Role of the promyelocytic leukemia protein PML in the interferon sensitivity of lymphocytic choriomeningitis virus. J Virol 75(13):6204–6208

Garcin D, Rochat S, et al. (1993) The Tacaribe arenavirus small zinc finger protein is required for both mRNA synthesis and genome replication. J Virol 67(2):807–812

Geschwender HH, Rutter G, et al. (1976) Lymphocytic choriomeningitis virus. II. Characterization of extractable complement-fixing activity. Med Microbiol Immunol (Berl) 162(2):119–131

Gimenez HB, Compans RW (1980) Defective interfering Tacaribe virus and persistently infected cells. Virology 107(1):229–239

Howard CR, Buchmeier MJ (1983) A protein kinase activity in lymphocytic choriomeningitis virus and identification of the phosphorylated product using monoclonal antibody. Virology 126(2):538–547

Klenerman P, Hengartner H, et al. (1997) A non-retroviral RNA virus persists in DNA form [see comments]. Nature 390(6657):298–301

Lee KJ, Novella IS, et al. (2000) NP and L proteins of lymphocytic choriomeningitis virus (LCMV) are sufficient for efficient transcription and replication of LCMV genomic RNA analogs. J Virol 74(8):3470–3477

Lehmann-Grube F, Slenczka W, et al. (1969) A persistent and inapparent infection of L cells with the virus of lymphocytic choriomeningitis. J Gen Virol 5(1):63–81

Lehmann-Grube F, Martinez Peralta LM, et al. (1983) Persistent infection of mice with the lymphocytic choriomeningitis virus. In: Fraenkel-Conrat H, Wagner RR (eds) Comprehensive Virology. Plenum Press, New York, pp 43–103

Lenz O, ter Meulen J, et al. (2000) Identification of a novel consensus sequence at the cleavage site of the Lassa Virus glycoprotein. J Virol 74:11418–11421

Lukashevich IS, Djavani M, et al. (1997) The Lassa fever virus L gene: nucleotide sequence, comparison, and precipitation of a predicted 250-kDa protein with monospecific antiserum. J Gen Virol 78(Pt 3):547–551

Martinez Peralta L, Bruns M, et al. (1981) Biochemical composition of lymphocytic choriomeningitis virus interfering particles. J Gen Virol 55:475–479

Matsuura Y, Possee RD, et al. (1986) Expression of the S-coded genes of lymphocytic choriomeningitis arenavirus using a baculovirus vector. J Gen Virol 67(8):1515–1529

Meyer BJ, Southern PJ (1994) Sequence heterogeneity in the termini of lymphocytic choriomeningitis virus genomic and antigenomic RNAs. J Virol 68(11):7659–7664

Oldstone MB, Buchmeier MJ (1982) Restricted expression of viral glycoprotein in cells of persistently infected mice. Nature 300(5890):360–362

Oldstone MB, Dixon FJ (1969) Pathogenesis of chronic disease associated with persistent lymphocytic choriomeningitis viral infection. I. Relationship of antibody production to disease in neonatally infected mice. J Exp Med 129(3):483–505

Pedersen IR (1979) Structural components and replication of arenaviruses. Adv Virus Res 24:277–330

Rawls WE, Buchmeier M (1975) Arenaviruses: purification and physicochemical nature. Bull World Health Organ 52(4–6):393–401

Rawls WE, Leung WC (1979) Arenaviruses. Compr Virol 14:157–192

Rodriguez M, Buchmeier MJ, et al. (1983) Ultrastructural localization of viral antigens in the CNS of mice persistently infected with lymphocytic choriomeningitis virus (LCMV) Am J Pathol 110(1): 95–100

Romanowski V, Bishop DH (1983) The formation of arenaviruses that are genetically diploid. Virology 126(1):87–95

Salvato M, Shimomaye E, et al. (1989) The primary structure of the lymphocytic choriomeningitis virus L gene encodes a putative RNA polymerase. Virology 169(2):377–384

Salvato MS, Schweighofer KJ, et al. (1992) Biochemical and immunological evidence that the 11kDa zinc-binding protein of lymphocytic choriomeningitis virus is a structural component of the virus. Virus Res 22(3):185–198

Simon M (1970) Multiplication of lymphocytic choriomeningitis virus in various systems. Acta Virol 14(5):369–376

Smadel JE, Green RM, et al. (1942) Lymphocytic choriomeningitis: two human fatalities following an unusual febrile illness. Proc Soc Exp Biol Med 49:683

Soneoka Y, Cannon PM, et al. (1995) A transient three-plasmid expression system for the production of high titer retroviral vectors. Nucleic Acids Res 23(4):628–633

Traub E (1936a) The epidemiology of lymphocytic choriomeningitis in white mice. J Exp Med 64:183–200

Traub E (1936b) Persistence of lymphocytic choriomeningitis virus in immune animals and its relation to immunity. J Exp Med 63:847–852

van der Zeijst BA, Bleumink N, et al. (1983a) Viral proteins and RNAs in BHK cells persistently infected by lymphocytic choriomeningitis virus. J Virol 48(1):262–270

van der Zeijst BAM, Noyes BE, et al. (1983b) Persistent infection of some standard cell lines by lymphocytic choriomeningitis virus: transmission of infection by an intracellar agent. J Virol 48: 249–264

Weber EL, Buchmeier MJ (1988) Fine mapping of an antigenic site conserved among arenaviruses. Virology 164:30–38

Welsh RM (1978) Cytotoxic cells induced during lymphocytic choriomeningitis virus infection of mice. I. Characterization of natural killer cell induction. J Exp Med 148:163–181

Welsh RM Jr., Buchmeier MJ (1979) Protein analysis of defective interfering lymphocytic choriomeningitis virus and persistently infected cells. Virology 96(2):503–515

Welsh RM, Lampert PW, et al. (1977) Prevention of virus-induced cerebellar diseases by defective-interfering lymphocytic choriomeningitis virus. J Infect Dis 136(3):391–399

Wilsnack RE, Rowe WP (1964) Immunofluorescent studies of the histopathogenesis of lymphocytic choriomeningitis virus infection. J Exp Med 120:829–841

Wright KE, Salvato MS, et al. (1989) Neutralizing epitopes of lymphocytic choriomeningitis virus are conformational and require both glycosylation and disulfide bonds for expression. Virology 171(2):417–426

Wright KE, Spiro RC, et al. (1990) Post-translational processing of the glycoproteins of lymphocytic choriomeningitis virus. Virology 177(1):175–183

Young PR, Chanas AC, et al. (1987) Localization of an arenavirus protein in the nuclei of infected cells. J Gen Virol 68(Pt 9):2465–2470

Young PR, Howard CR (1983) Fine structure analysis of Pichinde virus nucleocapsids. J Gen Virol 64(Pt 4):833–842

Zinkernagel RM, Doherty PC (1974) Restriction of in vitro T cell-mediated cytotoxicity in lymphocytic choriomeningitis within a syngeneic or semiallogeneic system. Nature 248(450):701–702

Reverse Genetics of Arenaviruses

K.J. Lee and J.C. de la Torre

1 Introduction

Arenaviruses merit significant attention both as experimental models to study acute and persistent infections and as clinically important human pathogens, including hemorrhagic fever agents such as Lassa virus.

Lymphocytic choriomeningitis virus (LCMV), the prototypic member of the family Arenaviridae, provides one of the most valuable model systems in the field of viral pathogenesis. Investigations using the LCMV model have been central to defining several basic virologic and immunologic concepts including major histocompatibility complex (MHC) restriction of T-cell recognition (Zinkernagel and Doherty 1974a,b, 1979), tolerance, immunological memory, immune-mediated pathology, mechanisms of viral clearance, as well as the strategies by which viruses evade the host immune responses (Rowe 1954; Oldstone and Dixon 1967,

Department of Neuropharmacology, The Scripps Research Institute, 10550 North Torrey Pines Road, IMM-6, La Jolla, CA 92037, USA

1969; COLE et al. 1972; GLIDEN et al. 1972a,b; OLDSTONE 1975, 1998). Studies of LCMV virus-host interaction have also uncovered the ability of noncytolytic persistent viruses to induce disease by interfering with specialized functions of infected cells, revealing a new way by which viruses do harm in the absence of the classic hallmarks of cytolysis and inflammation (OLDSTONE et al. 1982; DE LA TORRE and OLDSTONE 1996). Despite a wealth of knowledge about the immunobiology and pathogenesis of LCMV infection, there is only a limited understanding of the molecular mechanisms involved in the control of LCMV genome replication and expression, and how these processes relate to viral persistence and associated disease. As with other negative-strand RNA viruses, progress in these areas will benefit greatly from the establishment of a reverse genetic system to dissect the molecular biology of LCMV.

2 Molecular Biology of LCMV: Brief Overview

LCMV is an enveloped virus with a bisegmented, negative, single-stranded RNA genome. Virions are somewhat pleomorphic but typically spherical, with an average diameter of 90–110nm, and are covered with surface glycoprotein spikes (BURNS and BUCHMEIER 1993). Virions enclose the genomic RNAs as helical ribonucleo-protein structures in circular configurations (YOUNG and HOWARD 1983). Host-cell-derived ribosomes are also frequently included within virions, which give the virus particles the "sandy" appearance from which the family name is derived (FARBER and RAWLS 1975; PEDERSEN 1979).

The genomic L (ca. 7.3kb) and S (ca. 3.5kb) RNA segments contain nonoverlapping coding information. Each RNA segment has an ambisense coding strategy, encoding two polypeptides in opposite orientation, separated by an intergenic region with a predicted folding of a stable hairpin structure (Fig. 1). The S RNA encodes the viral glycoprotein precursor, GPC (ca. 75kDa), and the nucleoprotein, NP (ca. 63kDa) (AUPERIN et al. 1984; BUCHMEIER et al. 1987; FRANZE-FERNANDEZ et al. 1987; SOUTHERN et al. 1987), while the L RNA encodes the putative viral L polymerase (ca. 200kDa) and a small polypeptide Z (ca. 11kDa) that contains a RING finger-domain (SINGH et al. 1987; IAPALUCCI et al. 1989a,b; SALVATO et al. 1989; SALVATO and SHIMOMAYE 1989). The roles of Z during the LCMV life cycle are only barely understood. However, it has been postulated that Z participates in transcriptional regulation and virion morphogenesis (GARCIN and KOLAKOFSKY 1992; SALVATO et al. 1992; SALVATO 1993), as well as contributing to the noncytolytic nature of LCMV (BORDEN et al. 1998). The NP and L coding regions are transcribed into a genomic complementary mRNA, whereas the GPC and Z coding regions are transcribed into genomic sense mRNA (AUPERIN et al. 1984; ROMANOWSKI et al. 1985; FRANZE-FERNANDEZ et al. 1987; SOUTHERN et al. 1987; IAPALUCCI et al. 1989a; SALVATO and SHIMOMAYE 1989). The term *ambisense* refers to this situation in which in one region the S and L RNA are

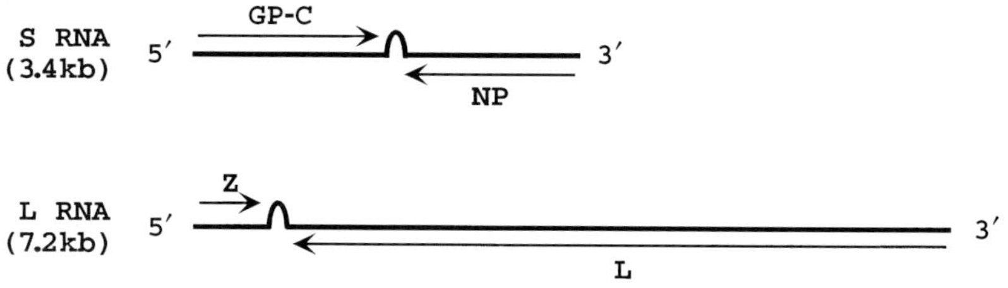

Fig. 1. Scheme of the lymphocytic choriomeningitis virus (LCMV) genome organization

negative sense and in a second, nonoverlapping region they are pseudo-positive sense. The qualifier *pseudo* is used because there is not yet any evidence that the genomic S and L RNAs can function as mRNAs and be directly translated into GPC and Z proteins, respectively.

The viral glycoprotein precursor GPC is posttranslationally cleaved to yield the two mature virion glycoproteins GP-1 (40–46kDa) and GP-2 (35kDa) (WRIGHT et al. 1990). GP-1 is located at the top of the spike, away from the membrane, and is held in place by ionic interactions with the N-terminus of the transmembrane GP-2 that forms the stalk of the spike (BURNS and BUCHMEIER 1991, 1993). Neutralizing antibodies predominantly recognize conformational epitopes within GP-1, which is the virion attachment protein that mediates virus interaction with host cell surface receptors. Alpha-dystroglycan (α-DG) has been recently identified as the receptor for LCMV (CAO et al. 1998). A detailed description of the interactions between α-DG and GP-1 is presented in the chapter by Kunz et al. LCMV assembly and release processes are currently very poorly understood (MANNWEILER and LEHMANN-GRUBE 1973; COMPANS 1993). For most enveloped viruses, a matrix (M) protein is involved in organizing the virion components prior to assembly. Interestingly, arenaviruses do not have an obvious counterpart of M. This could contribute to the apparently nonprecise packaging of arenaviruses. However, cross-linking studies have shown complex formation between NP and Z, suggesting a possible role of Z in virion morphogenesis (SALVATO et al. 1992; SALVATO 1993).

LCMV replication and transcription are confined to the cytoplasm of infected cells, although whether a nuclear component may be involved is still controversial. The LCMV mRNAs have extra nontemplated nucleotides (nt) and a cap structure at their 5′-ends, but it is still unclear how both the cap and 5′-nontemplated nt extensions are synthesized (GARCIN and KOLAKOFSKY 1990; RAJU et al. 1990; MEYER and SOUTHERN 1993). Transcription termination of subgenomic mRNAs does not appear to be precise, with their 3′-ends having been mapped to multiple sites within the distal side of the intergenic hairpin region (MEYER and SOUTHERN 1994). Subgenomic mRNAs are not polyadenylated (SINGH et al. 1987; SOUTHERN et al. 1987), but stabilization of the mRNA 3′-termini could result from the formation of a terminal hairpin following transcription termination (FRANZE-FERNANDEZ et al. 1987, 1993; MEYER and SOUTHERN 1993). The relationship between LCMV RNA replication and transcription and the regulatory mechanisms of the two processes remains to be defined. Intracellular levels of NP could influence the relative levels of transcription and replication, but the molecular bases are unknown. The polymerase could operate in a transcriptional mode until intracellular levels of NP become sufficient to begin co-synthetic encapsidation of the nascent RNA, which together with NP coating and unfolding of the intergenic hairpin would switch the polymerase into a read-through replicative mode. It is also possible that different LCMV polymerase complexes are involved in replication versus transcription. The capability to manipulate *cis*-acting RNA sequences and *trans*-acting proteins should provide new insights into the molecular mechanisms of LCMV transcription, RNA replication, and virion morphogenesis.

3 Genetic Manipulation of Negative-Strand RNA Virus Genomes

Direct manipulation of RNA virus genomes depends on the ability to produce recombinant RNAs that are accepted as template by the particular viral RNA-dependent polymerase. The template of the polymerases of negative-strand (NS) RNA viruses, such as LCMV, is exclusively a nucleocapsid consisting of the genomic RNA tightly encapsidated by the virus nucleoprotein (NP) and associated with the virus polymerase proteins to form a ribonucleoprotein (RNP) complex. This RNP is active in transcription and replication and is the minimum unit of infectivity (Tordo et al. 1992; Garcia-Sastre and Palese 1993). In contrast to positive-stranded RNA viruses, deproteinized genomic and antigenomic RNAs of NS RNA viruses cannot function as mRNAs and are not infectious. Thus, generation of biologically active synthetic virus from cDNA will require *trans* complementation by all viral proteins involved in virus replication and transcription. These considerations have severely hindered the application of recombinant DNA technology to the genetic analysis of these viruses. However, during the past few years, following the pioneer work of Palese's group (Luytjes et al. 1989), significant progress has been made in this area, and for several NS RNA viruses, short model genomes could be encapsidated and expressed either by infectious helper viruses or by plasmid-encoded proteins. The latter approach is based on co-expression of both genome analogs with predetermined termini and viral proteins from transfected plasmids using the transient vaccinia virus T7 RNA polymerase expression system, or expression vectors based on pol II or pol I promoters. This approach allows for the analysis of *cis*-and *trans*-acting factors required for virus replication and transcription, and moreover, it has recently allowed the generation and rescue of infectious viruses from several different families entirely from cloned cDNAs (recently reviewed in (Conzelmann 1998; Roberts and Rose 1998). These include viruses with nonsegmented genomes, such as rabies (Schnell et al. 1994), respiratory syncytial (Collins et al. 1995) and measles (Radecke et al. 1995) viruses, and also those with a segmented genome, bunyavirus (Bridgen and Elliott 1996) and influenza virus (Neumann et al. 1999). Similar procedures are potentially applicable to LCMV and should facilitate the investigation of the arenavirus molecular genetics, virus-host interactions, and pathogenesis.

4 Reverse Genetics of LCMV

4.1 *Cis*-Acting Sequences Required for Transcription and Replication of an LCMV Minigenome

Evidence obtained with other NS RNA viruses has shown that all *cis*-acting signals required for encapsidation and viral polymerase entry are located within the terminal noncoding sequences (UTR) of the viral genomes. Arenavirus genomes exhibit sequence conservation at their 3′-ends and 3′-5′ termini complementarity. These findings led us to hypothesize that also for the arenaviruses, the UTR contain *cis*-acting signals required for transcription and replication of the viral genome RNA. This hypothesis predicts that a reporter gene placed under the control of these *cis*-acting signals will be replicated and transcribed by the LCMV polymerase, as has been shown with other NS RNA viruses. To test this hypothesis, we constructed an LCMV minigenome (MG), or minireplicon, designated LCMVSCAT1 (LEE et al. 2000). The LCMVSCAT1 plasmid contains the coding region of the CAT gene, in antisense orientation with respect to the T7 promoter, placed between the 5′ and 3′-UTR of the LCMV genome S RNA. The LCMV 3′-UTR contains nt 3316–3376 (genome polarity), including the initiation codon (ATG) of the NP, whereas the LCMV 5′-UTR contains nt 1–78, followed by nt 1484–1694 (genome polarity) containing the intergenic region (IGR) present in the LCMV S RNA (LEE et al. 2000). Based on results with other NS RNA viruses, we expected that the precise termini of the LCMVSCAT1 RNA would be required for transcription and replication by the LCMV polymerase. The precise 5′-end of LCMVSCAT1 RNA was determined by the position of the T7 promoter relative to the viral cDNA. To generate the precise 3′-end sequence found in the LCMV genome RNA, we introduced a *Mvn*I restriction site at the end of the 3′-UTR of LCMV SCAT1. Plasmid digestion with *Mvn*I and transcription by T7 RNA polymerase generates an LCMV RNA analog, containing three extra Gs at its 5′-end, and the precise 3′-end sequence (5′-GCG-3′) found in the LCMV genome RNA.

We predicted that if LCMVSCAT1 RNA contained all the *cis*-acting signals required, it should then be encapsidated by the LCMV NP and subsequently, once in a RNP stage, transcribed and replicated by the LCMV polymerase. To test this hypothesis, we used a helper virus-dependent system to rescue LCMV model genome expression. In such a system, virus infection provides all the required *trans*-acting factors. Reproducible, although low, CAT activity was only detected in cells that were infected with LCMV and transfected with in vitro transcribed LCMVSCAT1 RNA. This finding indicated that the 5′- and 3′-UTR together with the IGR contain all the *cis*-acting signals required for LCMV RNA synthesis (LEE et al. 2000). However, there is evidence that viral genomes with short deletions in their 5'- and 3'-UTR are generated and accumulated during LCMV natural infection (MEYER and SOUTHERN 1997). It has been suggested that these truncated RNA genome molecules may play an important role in the outcome of the infection by modulating virus replication and transcription (MEYER and SOUTHERN 1997). Future studies using the LCMV minigenome system should allow experimental testing of this intriguing hypothesis.

Levels of NP have been proposed to be implicated in the regulation of LCMV RNA synthesis. Interestingly, we observed an apparent correlation between intracellular levels of NP and helper virus-dependent expression of CAT activity by the LCMV minigenome (LEE et al. 2000). Several possibilities could have accounted for low CAT activity. The use of in vitro transcribed and capped β-gal mRNA to transfect uninfected and LCMV-infected BHK-21 cells showed that the efficiency of RNA transfection in LCMV-infected cells was rather low and variable, which could help to explain the low levels of CAT activity obtained. Also, the LCMV system could be similar to the influenza virus and bunyavirus ones, which are also segmented, negative-strand RNA viruses. In these two viral systems, minireplicon-mediated reporter gene activity cannot be rescued by transfection of infected cells either with deproteinized RNA or with plasmid DNA that allows intracellular synthesis of the minigenome RNA (Ortin, personal communication; BRIDGEN and ELLIOTT 1996). Competition between authentic viral RNP and synthetic vRNA analog for polymerase factors has been proposed as one possible explanation. Therefore, we decided to explore the use of a helper virus-free, plasmid-mediated expression of the putative LCMV *trans*-acting factors (Fig. 2). The helper-free system would also allow us to assess the contribution of each individual LCMV gene product to virus replication, transcription, packaging, and maturation.

4.2 Viral *Trans*-Acting Factors Required for Efficient Replication and Transcription of LCMV Minigenome

4.2.1 Intracellular Co-Expression of LCMV Minigenome and Proteins

To avoid difficulties inherently associated with RNA transfection of cells, we followed the approach of transfecting a plasmid DNA, which allowed intracellular synthesis of LCMV minigenome with predetermined 5' and 3' termini through the use of a T7 promoter and ribozyme, respectively. The T7 RNA polymerase was provided using a recombinant vaccinia virus expressing T7 (vTF7-3). Initially, we designed a construct where the ribozyme sequence from the antigenomic strand of the hepatitis delta virus (HDV) was cloned downstream of the 3'-end of LCMV, followed by a T7 transcription termination sequence (T7 T). Therefore, the transcript generated by T7 polymerase will contain the genomic polarity of HDV ribozyme, which will provide autolytic cleavage at the 5'-end of the HDV ribozyme RNA (PATTNAIK et al. 1992), generating a 3'-end of the upstream RNA that will

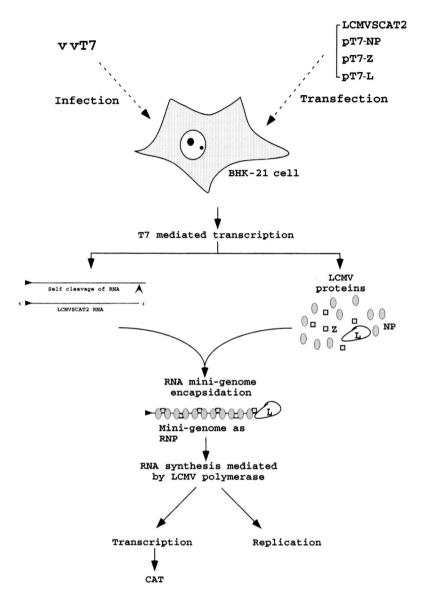

Fig. 2. Scheme of helper virus-independent rescue of LCMV minigenome

correspond to the authentic LCMV 3′ terminus. A similar approach has been successfully used with a variety of negative-strand RNA viruses (CONZELMANN 1998; ROBERTS and ROSE 1998). However, we found that this RNA, when intra-cellularly produced by T7, was very poorly processed. A possible explanation for this is that the last nucleotide at the 3′-end of the LCMV minigenome is guanosine (G), whereas the efficiency of autolytic cleavage by HDV ribozyme follows the pattern: C > U > A > G, with respect to the nucleotide located immediately 5′ to the site of cleavage (PERROTA and BEEN 1999). To solve this problem, we constructed plasmid pLCMVSCAT2, where an LCMV-specific hairpin ribozyme was substituted for the HDV ribozyme (PATTNAIK et al. 1992) (Fig. 3A). This ribozyme was designed to execute self-cleavage leaving in the upstream RNA the precise 3′ terminus of the LCMV S RNA (LEE et al. 2000). To examine the efficiency of pro-

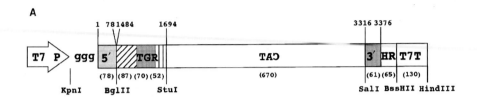

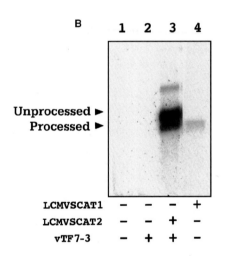

Fig. 3. A Schematic diagram of the LCMV minigenome LCMCSCAT2. Plasmid pLCMVSCAT2 was made by inserting an LCMV-specific 3′ hairpin ribozyme (*HR*) followed by a T7 RNA polymerase terminator (*T7 T*) into pLCMVSCAT1. Plasmid pLCMVSCAT1 was constructed by combining the following elements: the minimum T7 RNA polymerase promoter (*T7 P*) followed by three extra Gs, the 5′-UTR of the LCMV S RNA (nt 1–78), the IGR of the LCMV S RNA (nt 1484–1694), a DNA encoding the full-length CAT ORF in antisense orientation with respect to the T7 promoter, the 3′-UTR of the LCMV S RNA (nt 3316–3376). Viral sequences were derived from LCMV Arm 5. Nucleotide (nt) numbers correspond to those of the S RNA. *Numbers in parentheses* indicate the length of cDNA fragment. Restriction enzymes used for cloning were indicated at the *bottom* of the figure. *Hatched* and *striped boxes* represent the 3′-end of GP and NP, respectively. B Northern blot analysis of in vitro and intracellularly synthesized LCMV RNA minigenomes. BHK-21 cells were infected with vTF7-3 and subsequently transfected with pLCMVSCAT2. Total cellular RNA was prepared by using TRI reagent at 24h p.i. of vTF7-3. RNA (5μg) was analyzed by Northern blot using a CAT sense riboprobe. LCMV-SCAT1 RNA was prepared in vitro transcription with T7 RNA polymerase of *Mvn*I-digested template pLCMVSCAT1 DNA. Unprocessed and ribozyme-processed RNA species are indicated by *arrowheads* on the left side of the figure

cessing of intracellularly produced LCMVSCAT2 RNA, BHK-21 cells infected with vTF7-3 were transfected with plasmid pLCMVSCAT2. After 20h, total RNA was prepared and analyzed by Northern blot hybridization using a sense CAT riboprobe. Specific hybridization was detected only in RNA samples from cells that had been infected with vTF7-3 and transfected with plasmid pLCMVSCAT2 (Fig. 3B). We detected two main RNA species with approximate sizes of 1021 and 1216nt (Fig. 3B, lane 3). The smaller RNA species had the same electrophoretic mobility as the in vitro transcribed LCMVSCAT1 RNA (Fig. 3B, compare lanes 3 and 4), and corresponded to correctly processed LCMVSCAT2 RNA. The other RNA species had a predicted size compatible with RNA transcripts that were terminated at the T7 T site, but were not processed by the self-cleavage of the 3' hairpin ribozyme. Quantitation by densitometry indicated that approximately 22% of the intracellularly transcribed LCMVSCAT2 RNA was correctly processed by the LCMV-specific hairpin ribozyme.

We also used the vTF7-3 expression system (FUERST et al. 1986) to provide the LCMV *trans*-acting factors required to reconstitute intracellular replication and transcription of the LCMV minigenome. In this system, the cDNA encoding the gene of interest is placed under the control of a T7 RNA polymerase promoter, and followed downstream by a T7 transcription terminator element. These plasmids, when transfected into cells infected with vTF7-3, resulted in high levels of expression of the corresponding polypeptides. Levels of each individual LCMV protein required for optimal polymerase activity can be modulated by using different amounts of the corresponding plasmid in the transfection.

4.2.2 NP and L are the Minimal *Trans*-Acting Viral Factors Required for Efficient Replication and Transcription of an LCMV Minigenome

LCMV RNP isolated from infected cells can direct both replication and transcription of LCMV genome RNA in vitro (FULLER-PACE and SOUTHERN 1989). These viral RNP contain NP and L but not GP-1 and GP-2 polypeptides (FULLER-PACE and SOUTHERN 1989). Whether Z is associated with RNP during RNA synthesis remains to be determined. Nevertheless, Z has been implicated in both the replication and transcription of the genome RNA of the arenavirus Tacaribe (GARCIN et al. 1993). Therefore, we reasoned that coexpression of NP, L, and Z would be required to reconstitute intracellular replication and transcription of the LCMV minigenome. To examine this question, BHK-21 cells were infected with vTF7-3 and subsequently co-transfected with pLCMVSCAT2 and various combinations of plasmids encoding LCMV NP, Z, and L proteins. At 24h after vTF7-3 infection, cell extracts were prepared, and CAT activity was measured. It is expected that CAT could only be expressed after the formation of a functional LCMV RNP and subsequent transcription of the minigenome by the LCMV polymerase complex. Consistent with this hypothesis, high levels of CAT activity were obtained in cells co-transfected with the transcription plasmid pLCMV-SCAT2, together with plasmids expressing L, NP, and Z (Fig. 4, lane 9). Cells transfected only with NP or Z did not express detectable CAT activity (Fig. 4, lanes

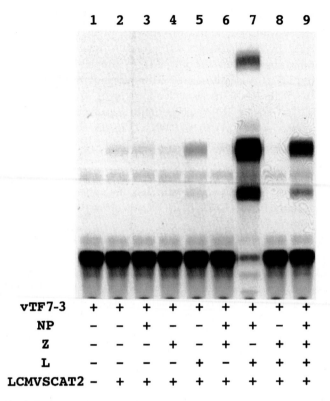

	1	2	3	4	5	6	7	8	9
vTF7-3	+	+	+	+	+	+	+	+	+
NP	–	–	+	–	–	+	+	–	+
Z	–	–	–	+	–	+	–	+	+
L	–	–	–	–	+	–	+	+	+
LCMVSCAT2	–	+	+	+	+	+	+	+	+

Fig. 4. Expression of LCMV minigenome in cells infected with vTF7-3 and transfected with pLCMV-SCAT2 and LCMV NP, Z, and L protein-encoding plasmids. BHK-21 cells were infected with vTF7-3 and then transfected with various combination of plasmids, pLCMVSCAT2, pCITE-NP, pUCIRES-Z, and pGEM-L. Cells were harvested at 24h p.i. and analyzed for CAT activity by thin layer chromatography (TLC). *Symbols* (+ and –) indicate the presence and the absence of both plasmid and vTF7-3

3 and 4). In contrast, and unexpectedly, cells transfected only with L showed detectable, although extremely low, levels of CAT activity (Fig. 4, lane 5). Intriguingly, inclusion of Z together with L and NP caused a significant reduction in the level of CAT activity (compare lanes 7 and 9, Fig. 4). These findings indicate that NP and L are the minimal *trans*-acting viral factors required for efficient CAT expression indicated by the LCMV minigenome.

Northern blot hybridization using an anti-sense CAT riboprobe showed two RNA species, ca. 700 and 1100nt (Fig. 5, lanes 4 and 5). The sizes of these two RNA species were compatible with being the nonpolyadenylated CAT mRNA and anti-minigenome RNA species, respectively, produced from the LCMVSCAT2 minigenome by the LCMV polymerase. Oligo (dT) fractionation confirmed that the two RNA species were nonpolyadenylated (Fig. 5, lanes 5 and 6). Thus, CAT activity correlated with synthesis of the CAT mRNA from the LCMV minigenome mediated by the LCMV polymerase.

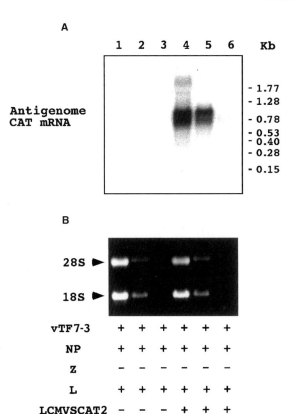

A

Antigenome CAT mRNA

Fig. 5A,B. Analysis of RNA synthesized intracellularly by LCMV polymerase components. BHK-21 cells were infected with vTF7-3 at a multiplicity of infection (MOI) of 3 then transfected with pLCMV-SCAT2 and LCMV NP, Z, and L protein-encoding plasmids. Total cellular RNA was isolated at 24h p.i. and fractionated by oligo (dT) chromatography. Total (*lanes 1* and *4*), poly A– (*lanes 2* and *5*) and poly A+ (*lanes 3* and *6*) RNA corresponding to equivalent amounts of cell numbers were analyzed by Northern blot hybridization using an antisense CAT riboprobe (*i*). *Symbols*, + and –, indicate the presence and the absence of both plasmid and vTF7-3. CAT mRNA and antigenome RNA are indicated by *arrowheads* on the *left*. **B** Bottom panel (*ii*) shows ethidium bromide staining of the formaldehyde agarose gel prior to transfer of the RNA samples to the membrane

4.3 Z Inhibits LCMV Minigenome Expression

To better understand the role played by Z in the control of LCMV RNA synthesis, we evaluated the effect of incrementally increasing the amount of the Z expression plasmid in the minigenome rescue assay. Z caused inhibition of CAT enzymatic activity in a dose-dependent manner (Fig. 6A). Co-expression of increasing amounts of Z plasmid resulted in a concomitant increase in the expression of Z protein (Fig. 6B). The amount of Z protein required to completely inhibit minigenome-derived CAT activity was slightly lower than that found in LCMV-infected cells (MOI of 3) at 24h p.i. Hence, this activity of Z could also operate during the natural course of LCMV infection consistent with the minigenome results, cells transiently expressing Z exhibited decreased susceptibility to infection with LCMV (CORNU and DE LA TORRE 2001). This inhibitory effect associated with the Z plasmid was lost when two stop codons were introduced at the N-terminus of the Z ORF, indicating that inhibition of the LCMV minigenome expression by Z is a function of the protein rather than due to hybrid arrest of the minigenome by the Z mRNA. In addition, co-expression of Z protein did not affect NP and L plasmid-

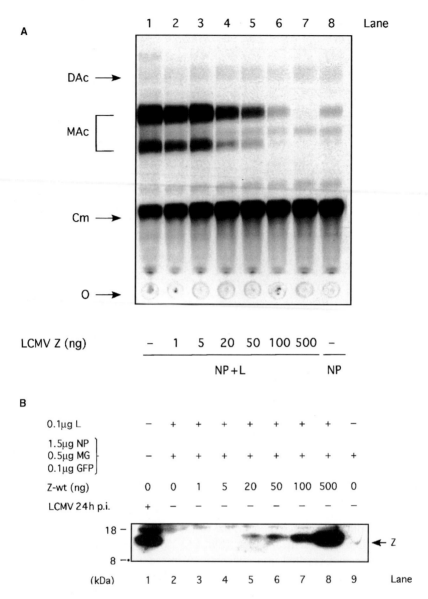

(Cornu and de la Torre 2001).

mediated expression, suggesting that Z-mediated inhibition of LCMV minigenome expression was not due to Z-mediated downregulation of NP and/or L expression (Cornu and de la Torre 2001).

The role of Z in the life cycle of arenaviruses is poorly understood at present. Based on results from in vitro transcription combined with immunodepletion experiments of the Z protein from Tacaribe virus, it was proposed that Z is required for both genome replication and mRNA synthesis (Garcin et al. 1993). The apparent discrepancies between these findings and our results could be related to

Fig. 6A,B. LCMV Z inhibits CAT expression by the LCMVSCAT2 minigenome in a dose-dependent manner. BHK-21 cells were infected with vTF7-3 and subsequently co-transfected with: pLCMVSCAT2 (0.5µg), pCITE-NP (1.5µg), pGEM-L (0.1µg), pTMI-GFP (0.1µg), and increasing amounts of pUCIRES-Z as indicated. In all the samples, the total amount of DNA was kept constant (2.7µg) by adding the appropriate amount of plasmid pTMI. The use of pTMI-GFP allowed us to determine the efficiency of transfection, based on the number of GFP-positive cells, prior to harvesting the cells. **A** Expression of LCMV minigenome. Cells were harvested at 24h p.i. and analyzed for CAT activity by thin layer chromatography. CAT activity in *lane 8* corresponds to extracts from cells that did not receive plasmid pGEM-L. *O*, origin; *Cm*, chloramphenicol; *Mac*, monoacetylated Cm; *DAc*, diacetylated Cm. **B** Expression of Z protein. Cell lysates from vTF7-3 infected and transfected cells (*lanes 2–9*) or from LCMV-infected cells (*lane 1*) were analyzed for levels of Z protein expression by Western blot using a rabbit serum to Z

possible differences between Tacaribe virus and LCMV with respect to Z functions. It is also possible that the antibody to Tacaribe Z protein used in the immunodepletion studies affected cellular factors required for virus RNA synthesis. For several negative-strand RNA viruses, the role of cellular components, especially proteins associated with the cytoskeleton, in virus replication and transcription has been documented (CIAMPOR 1988; LAI 1998).

Moreover, biochemical and immunological studies have shown that Z is a structural component of the virion, where it is apparently closely associated with NP (SALVATO et al. 1992). Therefore, immunodepletion of Z might have caused depletion of NP, too. However, treatment of LCMV with nonionic detergents showed that Z partitions into the hydrophobic phase rather than remaining associated with the viral nucleocapsid. These findings have led to the proposal that Z might be the arenavirus counterpart of the matrix (M) proteins found in other negative-strand RNA viruses. For several negative-strand RNA viruses, the association of the M protein with the RNP core appears to shut down virus transcription (CONZELMANN 1998). Whether Z plays an equivalent role remains to be determined.

Z has also been shown to interact with several host cell proteins. The association of Z with the eukaryotic initiation factor 4 E (eIF-4 E) has been implicated in the repression of protein synthesis in an eIF-4 E-dependent manner (DWYER 2000). This could explain the reduced expression of cyclin D1 in LCMV-infected cells, as it is known to be eIF-4 E sensitive. This Z/eIF-4 E interaction has been proposed as a mechanism for the slower growth of LCMV-infected cells, which could provide a viral strategy for establishing persistence. In addition, Z interacts also with the promyelocytic leukemia (PML) protein (BORDEN et al. 1998), leading to the relocation of PML nuclear bodies to the cytoplasm, which has been proposed to be responsible for the noncytolytic nature of LCMV (BORDEN et al. 1998). Together, these observations raise intriguing questions about a spectrum of potential functions played by the Z protein in the biology of arenavirus. The investigation of some of these questions will benefit from the use of the system described here. Precedents for proteins with roles as negative regulatory factors can be found in other negative-strand viruses. The RSV NS1 protein has been shown to be a potent inhibitor of transcription and replication of the RSV minigenome (ATREYA et al. 1998). In addition, the RSV M2 mRNA encodes a negative regulatory factor from its downstream ORF (COLLINS et al. 1996). The Sendai virus V protein was shown to inhibit the replication of a defective interfering (DI) genome (HORIKAMI et al. 1996); whereas the Sendai virus C protein strongly inhibited the amplification of an internal deletion type of DI genome, as well as of a complete infectious genome (CADD et al. 1996).

4.4 Formation and Budding of Infectious LCMV-Like Particles Requires GP and Z

Production of LCMV occurs by budding at the surface of infected cells. For most negative-strand RNA viruses, this process is assumed to depend on the interaction between the ribonucleoprotein core and the virus-encoded transmembrane glyco-proteins (GP) (GAROFF et al. 1998). The matrix (M) protein is thought to play an essential role in this interaction. Moreover, budding of rabies virus and vesicular stomatitis virus (VSV) does not require the presence of GP, suggesting an intrinsic budding activity of the M protein (MEBATSION et al. 1996; ROBISON and WHITT 2000). Nevertheless, GP enhances budding dramatically. The LCMV spike glyco-protein complex, composed of noncovalently linked tetramers of GP-1 and GP-2, is responsible for both viral attachment and fusion with cell membranes (CAO et al. 1998). Therefore, expression of LCMV GP is expected to be required for the formation of infectious LCMV-like particles. Arenaviruses do not encode an obvious counterpart of the M protein, but evidence suggests that one of the roles of Z might be related to virion morphogenesis. We therefore examined the role of Z and G in the generation of LCMV-like infectious particles using the minigenome system. The prediction would be that the supernatant of cells co-transfected with the minigenome-encoding plasmid, together with plasmids encoding NP and L, as well as Z and GP will contain infectious LCMV-like particles. This possibility was tested by examining the ability of the supernatant from transfected cells to drive CAT expression in fresh cells. In this case, the *trans*-acting factors (NP and L) required for minigenome expression were provided by co-infection with helper LCMV. Unexpectedly, we observed that although the GPC precursor was effi-ciently expressed using the vTF7-3 system, its processing was severely impaired. To overcome this interference of vaccinia virus infection with the processing of LCMV GP, we expressed the viral *trans*-acting factors as well as Z and GP under the control of a pol II promoter. We also included an additional plasmid expressing T7 RNA pol also under the control of a pol II promoter. Absence of Z and/or GP in the transfection mix did not affect the levels of CAT activity in cell lysates (Fig. 7A, lane 1), but prevented CAT expression in fresh cells co-infected with the super-natant of transfected cells and helper LCMV (Fig. 7B, lanes 1 and 2). These findings suggest that efficient packaging and budding of infectious LCMV-like particles require both Z and GP. As predicted, incubation of the supernatant of transfected cells with an anti-LCMV neutralizing antibody, but not with an unre-lated serum, prevented the transfer of CAT activity to fresh monolayers.

Could Z play a role in budding similar to that assigned to the M proteins of other negative-strand viruses? It is worth noting that the *N*-terminus of the M of

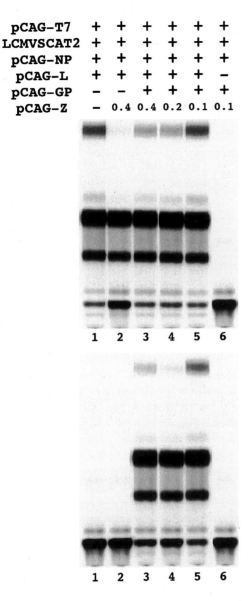

pCAG–T7	+	+	+	+	+	+
LCMVSCAT2	+	+	+	+	+	+
pCAG–NP	+	+	+	+	+	+
pCAG–L	+	+	+	+	+	–
pCAG–GP	–	–	+	+	+	+
pCAG–Z	–	0.4	0.4	0.2	0.1	0.1

1 2 3 4 5 6

1 2 3 4 5 6

Fig. 7. Passage of LCMV minigenome detected by CAT activity. BHK-21 cells were transfected with the indicated combinations of plasmids. For this experiment, expression of NP, L, Z, and GP viral proteins, as well as T7 RNA polymerase, was driven by a pol II promoter. At 72h after transfection, the supernatants were collected and cell extracts prepared for CAT assay. Levels of CAT activity in the initially transfected cells were analyzed by TLC (*top panel*). Clarified medium supernatants were passaged onto fresh BHK-21 cell monolayers which were also coinfected with LCMV helper virus to provide the viral *trans*-acting factors required for LCMV minigenome replication and expression. Cell extracts were prepared and analyzed for CAT activity (*bottom panel*) 72h later

VSV and other rhabdoviruses contains a highly conserved PPPY sequence motif that closely resembles the PY motif in the late (L) domain in the Gag protein of Rous sarcoma virus (RSV) and some other retroviruses (WILLS et al. 1994; XIANG et al. 1996). Biochemical and genetic evidence indicates that as with the L domain present in retroviral Gag proteins, the PY motif is involved in promoting budding of VSV (CRAVEN et al. 1999; HARTY et al. 1999; JAYAKAR et al. 2000). Interestingly, the C-terminus of all sequenced arenavirus Z genes also contain a PY motif identical to that found in the M of VSV. The PPPY motif in the RSV L domain matches the consensus proline-rich motif required for interaction with the WW domain found in several regulatory and signal transduction proteins (SUDOL et al. 1995). This finding suggests that the PY motif present in the Z of arenaviruses could participate in the recruitment of WW-containing cellular proteins for the purpose of assembly and budding, as well as other possible processes involved in the virus lifecycle.

5 Perspectives

We are now in a position to conduct a detailed molecular characterization of the *cis*-acting sequences controlling LCMV RNA synthesis, as well as to probe the function of LCMV polypeptides in virus replication and transcription. This system has also provided us with the foundation to attempt the rescue of infectious LCMV entirely from plasmid DNAs and in the absence of helper virus.

The complex spectrum of different manifestations of LCMV infection illustrates the delicate balance in which the virus-host interaction hangs, and how minor differences in either the host or viral genetics can profoundly influence the outcome of infection. Important findings in this research area have been made based on the very laborious and limited approach of identification, isolation, and characterization of naturally and rarely occurring LCMV mutants with phenotypes of interest. The ability to generate predetermined specific mutations within the LCMV genome and analyze their phenotypic expression will significantly contribute to the elucidation of the molecular mechanisms underlying LCMV-host interactions, including the bases of LCMV persistence and associated disease. Evidence indicates that LCMV remains present in the USA and Europe and capable of causing significant morbidity in infected individuals, likely being a neglected human pathogen (JAHRLING and PETERS 1992; BUCHMEIER and ZAJAC 1999). Moreover, new arenaviruses are being discovered in the Americas on the average of one every 3 years, with some of them causing severe hemorrhagic fever (PETERS et al. 1996). Therefore, it is important to develop effective vaccine strategies and antiviral therapies for the control and treatment of these emerging human pathogens, a task that will be facilitated by the ability to apply a reverse genetic approach to study the arenaviruses.

References

Atreya PL, Peeples ME, Collins PL (1998) The NS1 protein of human respiratory syncytial virus is a potent inhibitor of minigenome transcription and RNA replication. J Virol 72:1452–1461

Auperin DD, Romanowski V, Galinski M, Bishop DHL (1984) Sequencing studies of Pichinde arenavirus S RNA indicate a novel coding strategy, an ambisense viral S RNA. J Virol 52:897–904

Borden KL, Campbell Dwyer ES, Salvato MS (1998) An arenavirus RING (zinc-binding) protein binds the oncoprotein promyelocyte leukemia protein (PML) and relocates PML nuclear bodies to the cytoplasm. J Virol 72:758–766

Bridgen A, Elliott RM (1996) Rescue of segmented negative-strand RNA virus entirely from cloned complementary DNAs. Proc Natl Acad Sci USA 93:15400–15404

Buchmeier MJ, Zajac AJ (1999) Lymphocytic choriomeningitis virus. In: Ahmed R, Chen I (eds) Persistent viral infections. Wiley, New York

Buchmeier MJ, Southern PJ, Parekh BS, Wooddell MK, Oldstone MBA (1987) Site-specific antibodies define a cleavage site conserved among arenavirus GP-C glycoproteins. J Virol 61:982–985

Burns JW, Buchmeier MJ (1991) Protein-protein interactions in lymphocytic choriomeningitis virus. Virology 183:620–629

Burns JW, Buchmeier MJ (1993) Glycoproteins of the arenaviruses. In: Salvato MS (ed) The arenaviridae. Plenum Press, New York

Cadd T, Garcin D, Tapparel C, Itoh M, Homma M, Roux L, Curran J, Kolakofsky D (1996) The Sendai paramyxovirus accessory C proteins inhibit viral genome amplification in a promoter-specific fashion. J Virol 70:5067–5074

Cao W, Henry MD, Borrow P, Yamada H, Elder JH, Ravkov EV, Nichol ST, Compans RW, Campbell KP, Oldstone MBA (1998) Identification of alpha-dystroglycan as a receptor for lymphocytic choriomeningitis virus and Lassa fever virus. Science 282:2079–2081

Ciampor F (1988) The role of cytoskeleton and nuclear matrix in virus replication. Acta Virol 32:168–189

Cole GA, Nathanson N, Prendergast RA (1972) Requirement for theta-bearing cells in lymphocytic choriomeningitis virus-induced central nervous system disease. Nature 238:335–337

Collins PL, Hill MG, Camargo E, Grosfeld H, Chanock RM, Murphy BR (1995) Production of infectious human respiratory syncytial virus from cloned cDNA confirms an essential role for the transcription elongation factor from the 5′ proximal open reading frame of the M2 mRNA in gene expression and provides a capability for vaccine development. Proc Natl Acad Sci USA 92: 11563–11567

Collins PL, Hill MG, Cristina J, Grosfeld H (1996) Transcription elongation factor of respiratory syncytial virus, a nonsegmented negative-strand RNA virus. Proc Natl Acad Sci USA 93:81–85

Compans RW (1993) Arenavirus ultrastructure and morphogenesis. In: Salvato MS (ed) The arenaviridae. Plenum, New York

Conzelmann KK (1998) Nonsegmented negative-strand RNA viruses: genetics and manipulation of viral genomes. Annu Rev Genet 32:123–162

Cornu TI, de la Torre JC (2001) RING finger Z protein of lympocytic choriomeningitis virus (LCMV) inhibits transcription and RNA replication of an LCMV s-segment minigenome. J Virol 75:9415–9426

Craven RC, Harty RN, Paragas J, Palese P, Wills JW (1999) Late domain function identified in the vesicular stomatitis virus M protein by use of rhabdovirus-retrovirus chimeras. J Virol 73:3359–3365

Dwyer EA (2000) The lymphocytic choriomeningitis virus RING protein Z associates with eukaryotic initiation factor 4E and selectively represses translation in a RING-dependent manner. J Virol 74:3293–3300

Farber FE, Rawls WE (1975) Isolation of ribosome-like structures from Pichinde virus. J Gen Virol 26:21–31

Franze-Fernandez M-T, Zetina C, Iapalucci S, Lucero MA, Bouissou C, Lopez R, Rey O, Deheli M, Cohen GN, Zakin MM (1987) Molecular structure and early events in the replication of Tacaribe arenavirus S RNA. Virus Res 7:309–324

Franze-Fernandez M-T, Iapalucci S, Lopez N, Rossi C (1993) Subgenomic RNAs of Tacaribe virus. In: Salvato MS (ed) The arenaviridae. Plenum, New York

Fuerst TR, Niles EG, Studier FW, Moss B (1986) Eukaryotic transient expression system based on recombinant vaccinia virus that synthesizes bacteriophage T7 RNA polymerase. Proc Natl Acad Sci USA 83:8122–8126

Fuller-Pace FV, Southern PJ (1989) Detection of virus-specific RNA-dependent RNA polymerase activity in extracts from cells infected with lymphocytic choriomeningitis virus: in vitro synthesis of full-length viral RNA species. J Virol 63:1938

Garcia-Sastre A, Palese P (1993) Genetic manipulation of negative-strand RNA virus genomes. Annu Rev Microbiol 47:765–790

Garcin D, Kolakofsky D (1990) A novel mechanism for the initiation of Tacaribe arenavirus genome replication. J Virol 64:6196–6203

Garcin D, Kolakofsky D (1992) Tacaribe arenavirus RNA synthesis in vitro is primer dependent and suggests an unusual model for the initiation of genome replication. J Virol 66:1370–1376

Garcin D, Rochat S, Kolakofsky D (1993) The Tacaribe arenavirus small zinc finger protein is required for both mRNA synthesis and genome replication. J Virol 67:807–812

Garoff H, Hewson R, Opstelten DJE (1998) Virus maturation by budding. Microbiol Mol Biol Rev 62:1171–1190

Gliden DH, Cole GA, Monjan AA, Nathanson N (1972a) Immunopathogenesis of acute central nervous system disease produced by lymphocytic choriomeningitis virus. I. Cyclophosphamide-mediated induction by the virus-carrier state in adult mice. J Exp Med 135:860–873

Gliden DH, Cole GA, Nathanson N (1972b) Immunopathogenesis of acute central nervous system disease produced by lymphocytic choriomeningitis virus. II. Adoptive immunization of virus carriers. J Exp Med 135:874–889

Harty RN, Paragas J, Sudol M, Palese P (1999) A proline-rich motif within the matrix protein of vesicular stomatitis virus and rabies virus interacts with WW domains of cellular proteins: implications for viral budding. J Virol 73:2921–2929

Horikami SM, Smallwood S, Moyer SA (1996) The Sendai virus V protein interacts with the NP protein to regulate viral genome RNA replication. Virology 222:383–390

Iapalucci S, Lopez N, Rey O, Zakin MM, Cohen GN, Franze-Fernandez M-T (1989a) The 5' region of Tacaribe virus L RNA encodes a protein with a potential metal binding domain. Virology 173:357–361

Iapalucci S, Lopez R, Rey O, Lopez N, Franze-Fernandez M-T (1989b) Tacaribe virus L gene encodes a protein of 2210 amino acid residues. Virology 170:40–47

Jahrling PB, Peters CJ (1992) Lymphocytic choriomeningitis virus: a neglected pathogen of man. Arch Pathol Lab Med 116:486–488

Jayakar HR, Murti KG, Whitt MA (2000) Mutations in the PPPY motif of vesicular stomatitis virus matrix protein reduce virus budding by inhibiting a late step in virion release. J Virol 74:9818–9827

Lai MM (1998) Cellular factors in the transcription and replication of viral RNA genomes: a parallel to DNA-dependent RNA transcription. Virology 244:1–12

Lee KJ, Novella IS, Teng MN, Oldstone MBA, Torre JC de la (2000) NP and L proteins of lymphocytic choriomeningitis virus (LCMV) are sufficient for efficient transcription and replication of LCMV genomic RNA analogs. J Virol 74:3470–3477

Luytjes W, Krystal M, Enami M, Pavin JD, Palese P (1989) Amplification, expression, and packaging of foreign gene by influenza virus. Cell 59:1107–1113

Mannweiler K, Lehmann-Grube F (1973) Electron microscopy of LCM virus-infected L cells. In: Lehmann-Grube F (ed) Lymphocytic choriomeningitis virus and other arenaviruses. Springer Verlag, Berlin Heidelberg New York

Mebatsion T, Konig M, Conzelmann KK (1996) Budding of rabies virus particles in the absence of the spike glycoprotein. Cell 84:941–951

Meyer BJ, Southern PJ (1993) Concurrent sequence of analysis of 5' and 3' RNA termini by intramolecular circularization reveals 5' nontemplated bases and 3' terminal heterogeneity for lymphocytic choriomeningitis virus mRNAs. J Virol 67:2621–2627

Meyer BJ, Southern PJ (1994) Sequence heterogeneity in the termini of lymphocytic choriomeningitis virus genomic and antigenomic RNAs. J Virol 68:7659–7664

Meyer BJ, Southern PJ (1997) A novel type of defective viral genome suggests a unique strategy to establish and maintain persistent lymphocytic choriomeningitis virus infections. J Virol 71:6757–6764

Neumann G, Watanabe T, Ito H, Watanabe S, Goto H, Gao P, Hughes M, Perez DR, Donis R, Hoffmann E, Hobom G, Kawaoka Y (1999) Generation of influenza A viruses entirely from cloned cDNAs. Proc Natl Acad Sci USA 96:9345–9350

Oldstone MBA (1975) Virus neutralization and virus-induced immune complex disease. Virus-antibody union resulting in immunoprotection or immunologic injury – two sides of the same coin. Prog Med Virol 19:84–119

Oldstone MBA (1998) Viral persistence: mechanisms and consequences. Curr Opin Microbiol 1:436–441

Oldstone MBA, Dixon FJ (1967) Lymphocytic choriomeningitis: production of antibody by 'tolerant' infected mice. Science 158:1193–1195

Oldstone MBA, Dixon FJ (1969) Pathogenesis of chronic disease associated with persistent lymphocytic choriomeningitis viral infection. I. Relationship of antibody production to disease in neonatally-infected mice. J Exp Med 129:483–505

Oldstone MBA, Sinha YN, Blout P, Tishon A, Rodriguez M, Wedel R von, Lampert PW (1982) Virus-induced alterations in homeostasis: alterations in differentiated functions of infected cells in vivo. Science 218:1125–1127

Pattnaik AK, Ball LA, LeGrone AW, Wertz GW (1992) Infectious defective interfering particles of VSV from transcripts of a cDNA clone. Cell 69:1011–1020

Pedersen IR (1979) Structural components and replication of arenaviruses. Adv Virus Res 24:277–330

Perrota AT, Been MD (1999) The self-cleaving domain from the genomic RNA of hepatitis delta virus: sequence requirements and the effects of denaturant. Nucleic Acid Res 18:6821

Peters CJ, Buchmeier MB, Rollin PE, Ksiazek TG (1996) Arenaviruses. In: Fields BW, Knipe DM, Howley DM, et al. (eds) Fields virology, 3rd edn.

Radecke F, Spielhofer P, Schneider H, Kaelin K, Huber M, Dotsch C, Christiansen G, Billeter MA (1995) Rescue of measles viruses from cloned DNA. EMBO J 14:5773–5784

Raju R, Raju L, Hacker D, Garcin D, Compans RW, Kolakofsky D (1990) Nontemplated bases at the 5′ ends of Tacaribe virus mRNAs. Virology 174:53–59

Roberts A, Rose JK (1998) Recovery of negative-strand RNA viruses from plasmid DNAs: a positive approach revitalizes a negative field. Virology 247:1–6

Robison CS, Whitt MA (2000) The membrane-proximal stem region of vesicular stomatitis virus G protein confers efficient virus assembly. J Virol 74:2239–2246

Romanowski V, Matsuura Y, Bishop DHL (1985) Complete sequence of the S RNA of lymphocytic choriomeningitis virus (WE strain) compared to that of Pichinde arenavirus. Virus Res. 3:101–114

Rowe WP (1954) Naval Medical Research Institute Report, Vol 12. National Naval Medical Center, Bethesda, pp 167–220

Salvato M, Shimomaye EM, Oldstone MBA (1989) The primary structure of the lymphocytic chorio-meningitis virus L gene encodes a putative RNA polymerase. Virology 169:377–384

Salvato MS (1993) Molecular biology of the prototype arenavirus, lymphocytic choriomeningitis virus. In: Salvato MS (ed) The arenaviridae. Plenum, New York

Salvato MS, Shimomaye EM (1989) The completed sequence of lymphocytic choriomeningitis virus reveals a unique RNA structure and a gene for a zinc finger protein. Virology 173:1–10

Salvato MS, Schweighofer KJ, Burns J, Shimomaye EM (1992) Biochemical and immunological evidence that the 11-kDa zinc-binding protein of lymphocytic choriomeningitis virus is a structural component of the virus. Virus Res 22:185–198

Schnell M, Mebatsion T, Conzelmann KK (1994) Infectious rabies viruses from cloned cDNA. EMBO J 13:4195–4203

Singh MK, Fuller-Pace FV, Buchmeier MJ, Southern PJ (1987) Analysis of genomic L RNA segment of lymphocytic choriomeningitis virus. Virology 161:448–456

Southern PJ, Singh MK, Riviere Y, Jacoby DR, Buchmeier MJ, Oldstone MBA (1987) Molecular characterization of the genomic S RNA segment from lymphocytic choriomeningitis virus. Virology 157:145–155

Sudol M, Bork P, Einbond A, Kastury K, Druck T, Negrini M, Huebner K, Lehman D (1995) Char-acterization of the mammalian YAP (Yes-associated protein) gene and its role in defining a novel protein module, the WW domain. J Biol Chem 270:14733–14741

Tordo N, DeHaan P, Goldbach R, Poch O (1992) Evolution of negative-stranded RNA genomes. Semin Virol 3:341–357

Torre JC de la, Oldstone MBA (1996) The anatomy of viral persistence: mechanisms of persistence and associated disease. Adv Virus Res 46:311–343

Wills JW, Cameron CE, Wilson CB, Xiang Y, Bennett RP, Leis J (1994) An assembly domain of the Rous sarcoma virus Gag protein required late in budding. J Virol 68:6605–6618

Wright KE, Spiro RC, Burns JW, Buchmeier MJ (1990) Post-translational processing of the glycopro-teins of lymphocytic choriomeningitis virus. Virology 177:175–183

Xiang Y, Cameron CE, Wills JW, Leis J (1996) Fine mapping and characterization of the Rous sarcoma virus Pr76gag late assembly domain. J Virol 70:5695–5700

Young PR, Howard CR (1983) Fine structure of Pichinde virus nucleocapsids. J Gen Virol 64:833–842

Zinkernagel RM, Doherty PC (1974a) Immunologic surveillance against altered self components by sensitized T lymphocytes in lymphocytic choriomeningitis. Nature 251:547–548

Zinkernagel RM, Doherty PC (1974b) Restriction of in vitro T cell-mediated cytotoxicity in lymphocytic choriomeningitis within a syngeneic or semiallogeneic system. Nature 248:701–702

Zinkernagel RM, Doherty PC (1979) MHC-restricted cytotoxic T cells: studies on the biological role of polymorphic major transplantation antigens determining T-cell restriction specificity, function, and responsiveness. Adv Immunol 27:51–177

Subject Index

Current Topics in Microbiology and Immunology

Volumes published since 1989 (and still available)

Vol. 239: **Vogt, Peter K.; Jackson, Andrew O. (Eds.):** Satellites and Defective Viral RNAs. 1999. 39 figs. XVI, 179 pp. ISBN 3-540-65049-0

Vol. 240: **Hammond, John; McGarvey, Peter; Yusibov, Vidadi (Eds.):** Plant Biotechnology. 1999. 12 figs. XII, 196 pp. ISBN 3-540-65104-7

Vol. 241: **Westblom, Tore U.; Czinn, Steven J.; Nedrud, John G. (Eds.):** Gastroduodenal Disease and Helicobacter pylori. 1999. 35 figs. XI, 313 pp. ISBN 3-540-65084-9

Vol. 242: **Hagedorn, Curt H.; Rice, Charles M. (Eds.):** The Hepatitis C Viruses. 2000. 47 figs. IX, 379 pp. ISBN 3-540-65358-9

Vol. 243: **Famulok, Michael; Winnacker, Ernst-L.; Wong, Chi-Huey (Eds.):** Combinatorial Chemistry in Biology. 1999. 48 figs. IX, 189 pp. ISBN 3-540-65704-5

Vol. 244: **Daëron, Marc; Vivier, Eric (Eds.):** Immunoreceptor Tyrosine-Based Inhibition Motifs. 1999. 20 figs. VIII, 179 pp. ISBN 3-540-65789-4

Vol. 245/I: **Justement, Louis B.; Siminovitch, Katherine A. (Eds.):** Signal Transduction and the Coordination of B Lymphocyte Development and Function I. 2000. 22 figs. XVI, 274 pp. ISBN 3-540-66002-X

Vol. 245/II: **Justement, Louis B.; Siminovitch, Katherine A. (Eds.):** Signal Transduction on the Coordination of B Lymphocyte Development and Function II. 2000. 13 figs. XV, 172 pp. ISBN 3-540-66003-8

Vol. 246: **Melchers, Fritz; Potter, Michael (Eds.):** Mechanisms of B Cell Neoplasia 1998. 1999. 111 figs. XXIX, 415 pp. ISBN 3-540-65759-2

Vol. 247: **Wagner, Hermann (Ed.):** Immunobiology of Bacterial CpG-DNA. 2000. 34 figs. IX, 246 pp. ISBN 3-540-66400-9

Vol. 248: **du Pasquier, Louis; Litman, Gary W. (Eds.):** Origin and Evolution of the Vertebrate Immune System. 2000. 81 figs. IX, 324 pp. ISBN 3-540-66414-9

Vol. 249: **Jones, Peter A.; Vogt, Peter K. (Eds.):** DNA Methylation and Cancer. 2000. 16 figs. IX, 169 pp. ISBN 3-540-66608-7

Vol. 250: **Aktories, Klaus; Wilkins, Tracy, D. (Eds.):** Clostridium difficile. 2000. 20 figs. IX, 143 pp. ISBN 3-540-67291-5

Vol. 251: **Melchers, Fritz (Ed.):** Lymphoid Organogenesis. 2000. 62 figs. XII, 215 pp. ISBN 3-540-67569-8

Vol. 252: **Potter, Michael; Melchers, Fritz (Eds.):** B1 Lymphocytes in B Cell Neoplasia. 2000. XIII, 326 pp. ISBN 3-540-67567-1

Vol. 253: **Gosztonyi, Georg (Ed.):** The Mechanisms of Neuronal Damage in Virus Infections of the Nervous System. 2001. approx. XVI, 270 pp. ISBN 3-540-67617-1

Vol. 254: **Privalsky, Martin L. (Ed.):** Transcriptional Corepressors. 2001. 25 figs. XIV, 190 pp. ISBN 3-540-67569-8

Vol. 255: **Hirai, Kanji (Ed.):** Marek's Disease. 2001. 22 figs. XII, 294 pp. ISBN 3-540-67798-4

Vol. 256: **Schmaljohn, Connie S.; Nichol, Stuart T. (Eds.):** Hantaviruses . 2001, 24 figs. XI, 196 pp. ISBN 3-540-41045-7

Vol. 257: **van der Goot, Gisou (Ed.):** Pore-Forming Toxins, 2001. 19 figs. IX, 166 pp. ISBN 3-540-41386-3

Vol. 258: **Takada, Kenzo (Ed.):** Epstein-Barr Virus and Human Cancer. 2001. 38 figs. IX, 233 pp. ISBN 3-540-41506-8

Vol. 259: **Hauber, Joachim, Vogt, Peter K. (Eds.):** Nuclear Export of Viral RNAs. 2001. 19 figs. IX, 131 pp. ISBN 3-540-41278-6

Vol. 260: **Burton, Didier R. (Ed.):** Antibodies in Viral Infection. 2001. 51 figs. IX, 309 pp. ISBN 3-540-41611-0

Vol. 261: **Trono, Didier (Ed.):** Lentiviral Vectors. 2002. 32 figs. X, 258 pp. ISBN 3-540-42190-4

Autumn Night Music

Summer is waning;
nights are gaining.
Evening trees have lost their song.
Katydids, the last to strum,
are packing up and moving on.

Music lovers, don't despair!
Autumn tunes are in the air.
Just tonight I heard a breeze
practicing inside the trees.

There *is* music after summer
with a different kind of strummer!

Fog Art

Fog art
is not what it draws
but how it erases.

Where there was a ship
just a mast remains
and the tip
of a bow.
The pier stretches
to nowhere now,
fades ghost-thin,
fades
and shows
and fades again.

Fog plays with shapes,
redesigns lines,
has a cool stroke.
Hang around it sometime
and be
part
of
the
art.

Color the Tiger

"Color the tiger on this sheet,"
my teacher said.
I carefully colored it
pink and red.
My teacher frowned
and shook her head,
"Tigers are orange and black."

She handed it back.

So I colored another one
orange and black,
and didn't bother to sign my name
because everyone's tiger
looked the same.

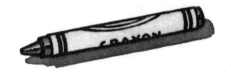

Candlelight

A sparrow of flame
on a twig of string

stretches
and puffs out its chest
to sing,
making its own kind of song,

melting the darkness around it
to pale honey-dawn.

Winter Morning at the Window

Crow wakes,
shrieks
"Awk! Awk!"

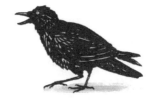

Sun peeks.
Ice on the roof
creaks.

I wake,
shiver and shake
wishing the frigid spell
would break.

A frost kiss
fogs the window glass.
I scribble on the mist,

meeting winter
touch to touch
with my fingertips.

Night Snow

This is ice
at its best,
bits of luminous white
overwhelming
the night sky
like a runaway
galaxy,
unstoppable stars
touching my face
with soft
cold fire!

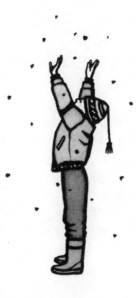

Spring to Summer

High
in this tree
I'm sitting under,
a bird makes music
bigger than itself.
Such ambition!
Is that why,
I wonder,
I hear spring
but I'm already
thinking "summer"?

House Painter

The painter cools the house
with fresh white paint.
I watch him in the summer's heat
and feel the soothing change.

And on the painter's face,
across his cheeks,
are flecks and streaks of splash,
like snowflake stains.

Spittle Bug

Please don't scold the spittle bug
whose splotch of frothy spittle

is hanging on a juicy stem;
remember, he's a little

green baby who will grow to be
a bigger, brown leaf-hopper,

but for now the foam's his home
and spitting's not

the least
improper.

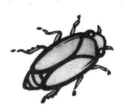

The Radish

Dear Grandma and Grandpa,

Here is
the second radish
from my garden.
It's bigger than
the one we ate.

It looks a little
strange
with that dent
down its middle
but I know you won't complain;
it *tastes* great.

Don't
put it in your salad;
eat it, right now,
plain.
       Love,
         You Know Who

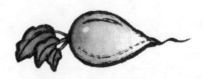

Acrobatics Recital

Like frogs, wheels,
bouncing balls
they roll,
leap,
jump,
fly,

spring
like snapped elastic,

bend and twist
like plastic.

I can't imagine how!

One is my regular
everyday sister,
but I hardly
know her
now.

An Old Nickelodeon Piano (circa 1920)

You put a nickel
in the slot
and hear it clatter
as it drops,

then piano keys
begin to play,
and drums will thump,
and horns will blow;
the mandolin will strum along
and with a bang
the cymbals clang.

All this goes on
without a strummer
or a drummer
or a hand.

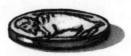

For a nickel,
just a nickel,
you have bought yourself
a band!

After the Rain

One bird
and scores of crickets
sing "all-clear!"

Puddles
all have smoothed
their rainy wrinkles.

Trees
are dripping
rain soup
from their chins,

and every spider's web
has caught some
twinkles.

An Ant on My Hand

Hi there,
little whisperwalker
ambling over Finger Ridge,
you tickle me!

There you go up Knuckle Hill,
to the peak,
around the bend,
down Thumb Gulch
and off again.

So long
and happy trails,
my friend!

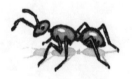

Wind

When I was very, very small
and hardly knew a thing at all,
the wind made me its toy,
shoved me playfully,
pushed me hard once
into a scratchy barberry bush.

Now when it bellows
and teases and slaps
I plant my feet
like two strong oaks;
my neck is a flagpole,
and only my hair flaps.

Bee Watch

I've been here
a while
by the lilies,
sunning,
watching a bumblebee
dive down deep

to disappear
in the world
of each flower
and stay long enough
to have fallen asleep.

Each time it's the same;
I watch and wait:
no bee, no hum
of its motor running,

then out it pops
like a jack-in-the-box!

The Lawn Sprinkler

We dash to the sprinkler
that sputters and spouts.
We scream from the cold stings,
run and shout.
Like bees to a flower,
we spend the day
buzzing around
in the waterspray.
Then, in the sun,
we lounge about
like a family of frogs
who are all croaked out!

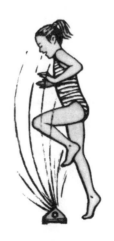

The Cook

With a twist
of hand and wrist
in one smooth stroke

he flips
two slippery eggs
in the pan
without breaking
a yolk!

Carolyn's Cat

She's a house cat
pampered like a child,
cuddled and petted
and very well fed,
a stranger
to the wild
outside.
(She's the kind of cat
you'd invite to tea.)

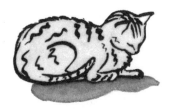

Her life, it seems,
is peaceful and good
with only her house
for a neighborhood:
the plump pillows,
the soft chairs,
the smooth wood.

But I saw her one night
posed perfectly still,
like a china cat,
on the windowsill,
meeting, with moonlike eyes,
the full moon's glow.

And I think
there are things
about Carolyn's cat
that even Carolyn
doesn't know.

On Rolling Down Grassy Hills

It's the "almost like flying"
feeling;
it's the speeding without really
trying;
it's the ground-hugging touch
from my head to my toes
and the strong, mysterious
smell of the earth
that I like
so much.

It's dandelions;
it's clover,
and bumps
I'm rolling over;
and the spinning mix
that tricks the eye
of trees and bushes,
grass and sky
and everything in between.

It's landing,
much too dizzy to walk,
too breathless to talk,
and buttered all over
with green.